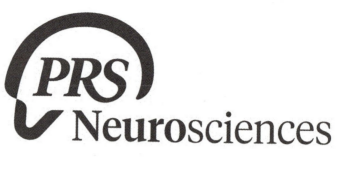

PRS Neurosciences

Presents

REBOOTING THE BRAIN®

Part 1 : The Journey Of 'HOPE'

by

Dr. Sharan Srinivasan
Dr. Prathiba Sharan

www.prsneurosciences.com

REBOOTING THE BRAIN®
Part I: The Journey Of 'HOPE'

Dr. Sharan Srinivasan and Dr. Prathiba Sharan

p. 307

cjn

m . 21.59 x 27.94

This book is dedicated to all our patients whose apparent 'hopelessness' in the face of neurological disabilities is the primary reason for us to do what we are currently doing! They have been our most significant and generous 'textbooks'; each patient has given us unique new learnings and validated our previous ones. And every small progress they make is like a 'victory' for us!

We also dedicate this book to all the caregivers who have 'unconditionally' trusted their loved ones under our care. This allowed our team to work fearlessly with them, and this 'championship team' delivered extraordinary results more often than not. Their resilience, unwavering determination, and relentless pursuit of helping their loved ones achieve functional independence inspire us to innovate and improve continuously. In your journey to re-integrate your loved ones back into the community, you illuminate the path for others and redefine what it means to succeed & thrive. Your courage and strength are a beacon of hope for a brighter tomorrow.

Finally, we would also like to dedicate this book to all our therapists (past, present, and future) who have worked tirelessly, day in and day out, trying their best to learn and try all the new techniques and technologies that we threw at them, without a murmur and with a smiling face, all with the sole commitment to help improve the quality of life of the patient and the caregivers. Thank you!

Category: HEA039110 - Health & Fitness: Diseases - Nervous System (incl. Brain)
ISBN: 978-1-957456-51-5

USPTO Trademark Registered - REBOOTING THE BRAIN

Dear Sir,

Greetings from Rights and Marks!

Congratulations!

Sub: U.S. Application Serial No. <u>79364480</u>

Mark: _REBOOTING THE BRAIN
Owner/Holder: PRS NEUROSCIENCES &
MECHATRONICS RESEARCH INSTITUTE
PVT LTD
Docket/Reference No.

Issue Date: April 23, 2024

We are pleased to inform you that your mark
has been registered with the United States
Patent and Trademark Office (USPTO). Your
United States trademark registration number is
7362312.

www.rebootingthebrain.com

DEDICATION

This book is dedicated to all our patients, whose apparent 'hopelessness' in the face of neurological disabilities is the primary reason for us to do what we are currently doing! They have been our most significant and generous 'textbooks'; each patient has given us unique new learnings and validated our previous ones. And every small progress they make is like a 'victory' for us!

We also dedicate this book to all the caregivers who have 'unconditionally' trusted their loved ones under our care. This allowed our team to work fearlessly with them, and this 'championship team' delivered extraordinary results more often than not. Their resilience, unwavering determination, and relentless pursuit of helping their loved ones achieve functional independence inspire us to innovate and improve continuously. In your journey to re-integrate your loved ones back into the community, you illuminate the path for others and redefine what it means to succeed & thrive. Your courage and strength are a beacon of hope for a brighter tomorrow.

Finally, we would also like to dedicate this book to all our therapists (past, present, and future) who have worked tirelessly, day in and day out, trying their best to learn and try all the new techniques and technologies that we threw at them, without a murmur and with a smiling face, all with the sole commitment to help improve the quality of life of the patient and the caregivers. Thank you!

ENDORSEMENTS

Dr. Sharan is a world-class neurosurgeon who has always focused on the best possible outcome for the patient and family after the life-changing experience of surviving the operating table. Along with Dr Prathiba, their life's work can be summarized as advocating for neurologically disabled individuals (and their families) to fight their way back and achieve the best possible 'functional independence life' without breaking the bank!

As the former Senior Vice President of Handheld Software at BlackBerry, where I worked for more than fifteen years, and also an uncle who has watched this journey very closely, I must say that I am very proud of what Dr. Sharan has achieved!

In their quest to develop a cost-effective, scalable, and sustainable business model, Dr Sharan has embraced leading-edge technology and concepts to drive the best outcomes for his patients!

-Suresh Periyalwar
Technology Leader & Entrepreneur
Toronto, Canada

Neurosurgery, especially functional neurosurgery, is not a subject but a philosophy. This branch cannot be compared to any other stream of Medical Sciences because its victim is not an individual but the whole family. Its complexities and individualistic nature have deterred any attempt at brain transplantation so far, while practically every other organ of a human being has been successfully transplanted. The reader will find his passion in the coming chapters. The author starts with a narrative impregnated with real-life stories and takes you on a guided tour with thoughtful essays on some of the daily practical and ethical problems we caregivers encounter. In his approach to health for all, Dr. Sharan reveals the story of lesional procedures, their sabbatical in history, and their revival in recent years. His persistence and perseverance in helping the neediest are so astounding that his colleagues are encouraged and inspired. The book is a masterpiece for medical professionals, business tycoons, and general readers. It isn't easy to put it aside without going through it thoroughly.

Manjul Tripathi
MCh, MNAMS
Faculty, Neurosurgery & Radiosurgery
PGIMER, Chandigarh

Rebooting The Brain®

Dr. Sharan Srinivasan is a rare gem in the world of medicine. I have seen Dr. Sharan as an amazing communicator who captures one's attention when he gives a public talk or speaks to an individual. I see the same ability in this book, too. He is an awesome storyteller like Prof. V. S. Ramachandran of the fame of 'Phantom in the Brain' book. The result is an inspiring, stimulating, informative, and enjoyable book.

This book does yeoman's service in effortlessly educating people about the possibility of rehabilitation of patients with functional deficiencies due to brain or spinal cord injury, giving a whole new clarity and hope to their family members.

The prologue is a heart-to-heart talk by Dr. Sharan. "I strongly advocate compassionate capitalism in healthcare" is a profound statement that touched me.

The whole book is in an enjoyable conversational style. Throughout, one gets pleasantly shocked by the deep commitment of a physician to the ultimate functional independence of his patients & their social concerns.

It is at once highly readable and fully informative, devoid of the Greek and Latin usually used in the medical world that intimidates people. It is such an interesting narrative that you cannot keep the book down; it just grips you. With his inimitable style of comparing the brain and its functions to a hard disk and the software loaded on it, Dr. Sharan makes the usually inaccessible aspects of the brain's uniqueness and the disabilities arising due to its damage easily accessible to the reader.

Reading this book, anyone can get an exciting overview of how the human brain is organized and works. Sharan's examples are as simple, lucid, vivid, and illuminating as Ramakrishna Paramahamsa's stories that demystify profound philosophical truths. He makes us understand why neuro rehabilitation is a hard task that may take a long time. Comparing the brain to a smartphone and therapists to sports coaches is refreshingly original.

The book is a must-read for all physicians and researchers to know how better-than-state-of-the-art healthcare can be made affordable and for potential entrepreneurs to grasp what needs to drive them.

Prof. Ramakrishnan A. G., Ph.D.
Professor of Electrical Engineering & Neuroscience (Retd.), IISc, Bangalore
Adjunct faculty, IIT Hyderabad.

When one pours passion into one's profession and perseveres in the search for perfection, opportunities for showcasing excellence arise. Highlighting these truisms as it were, this semi-autobiographical, narrative-style book by my friend and colleague, Dr Sharan, gives us a ringside view of his life's mission so far, with all its ups and downs. This monumental effort, long in the making, should enthuse individuals and society at large to benefit from such rare-focused endeavors. I sense this journey has barely begun, and I eagerly await the sequel.

Prof. Dr Ravi C Nayar,
M.S (PGI), DNB, DLO (RCS London), DCCF (Paris), FRCS (Glasgow)
Bengaluru, India.
Formerly, HOD, ENT St Johns National Academy of Medical Sciences Bangalore.
Program Director, CCAMP Inter-institutional BioMedical Innovations Programme (CIBIP).

"Rebooting the Brain®" is not just a book; it's a handbook of neurological rehabilitation meticulously crafted by the dynamic duo Dr. Sharan and Dr. Prathiba. Within its pages, readers are not only treated to a captivating narrative of medical innovation but also guided through the intricate process of neurological recovery. Each chapter serves as a beacon of hope, illuminating the path forward for patients and caregivers alike. Through the lens of ground-breaking surgeries and personalized care, the book unveils the transformative potential of combining advanced technology with compassionate treatment. As a handbook, it offers practical insights and invaluable guidance, empowering readers to navigate the complexities of the brain and the need for rehab with confidence and optimism. "Rebooting the Brain®" is more than just a story; it's a roadmap to recovery and a testament to the resilience of the human spirit.

Prof. Stafford Michahial,
(P.hd) Medical Image Processing, VTU, Karnataka
M.Tech Digital Electronics & Communication: B.Tech Electronics & Communication, VTU,
Karnataka
IEEE(Member),IETE (Member), VRARA(President Bangalore chapter (2017- 2020)).
Group Chief Technology Officer (Group-CTO), PRS Neurosciences & Mechatronics Research
Institute (PNMRI)

"Rebooting the Brain®" is a brilliant, lucid, and compelling book. It is a pathbreaking book from a leading Neurosurgeon of today, Dr Sharan, and his wife, Dr. Prathiba, a neuro rehab expert, to others in the field. It is interesting to see both of them, with their team, have helped patients reboot their brains and are happy back in society. Amazing job done towards fellow beings. He may not be aware that his infectious smile does the initial job when he receives a patient with a smile. The patient feels that he/ she is in safe hands, and he/ she does what the team says. Once Faith is developed, rebooting becomes very easy. Love towards a suffering one is essential for the reorganization of the neural network. Their love for suffering has made them write the book. Love toward all living beings can do wonders. Love, compassion, concern for wellness. It will be a sight for the heavens to see.

Rebooting of the brain shows what happens when the neural substrate and its connections have gone wrong. Indirectly, the author, Dr Sharan, is saying how important neuroplasticity is, a fundamental property of the neural substrate in all living beings. Everyone can re-wire their brains with their life experiences, day in and day out, so that they evolve to be a better person in the future., in-turn a better society, a better community, at large, a better nation, and a better world. - God bless.

Prof. Dr. D. Narayana Rao
Neurophysiologist (retired)
1st MBBS neurosciences teacher of the authors. He taught us neurosciences in 1986-87!

This book is an eye-opener for everyone. We know that the human brain is a remarkable organ, but what we don't know is how complicated its composition and workings are. We are glad that Sharan and Prathiba have, with single-minded devotion, worked hard to find ways and means of putting the injured brain on the right track after various traumas so that the unfortunate patients have a good chance to recover and lead a life as normal as possible.

As a student of Neurosurgery, Sharan always talked about the great surgeries of his bosses, but also that many patients were not recovering fully due to lack of right rehabilitation. His mind was always towards developing such a useful program. It took Sharan and his wife Prathiba almost 11 years before they could start a workable rehabilitation center of their own. Their CAREPa-Re® concept has come out as an answer.

Neuro rehabilitation is in serious need of workable techniques to help a maximum number of patients, and that too at affordable costs. Hearty congratulations and hats off to Sharan and Prathiba for their mission of treating neurological and neurosurgical patients at a reasonable cost.

As proud parents, we wish them good luck. God Bless them.

Mrs. Amrutha Srinivasan & Mr. P.R. Srinivasan
(Parents of Dr. Sharan)

CONTENTS

ACKNOWLEDGMENTS

24/4/2024

To my readers,

Writing a book is never a solitary endeavor; it's a culmination of support, encouragement, and collaboration from many individuals along the way. As I reflect on the journey of bringing this book to fruition, I am filled with profound gratitude to all those who have contributed in different ways.

First and foremost, I extend my heartfelt appreciation to all my patients and their caregivers for their unwavering belief in me and for supporting me by providing an opportunity to treat them and gain experience and expertise as a clinician. They have also shared insightful feedback about their successes and failures with me and my team, making me a part of their journey.

I extend my heartfelt gratitude to the co-author of my life and this book, my wife, Dr. Prathiba Sharan, my family, and friends for their insightful feedback and encouragement throughout my career and life. Your belief in me has been a constant source of motivation. I want to thank them for their patience, understanding, and unwavering support during the entire process. Your encouragement sustained me through the highs and lows of this endeavor.

I am deeply thankful to the trustees and management of Bhagwan Mahaveer Jain Hospital for their belief in me and for allowing me to create a world-class center for movement disorders, neurosurgery, and neuro rehabilitation. Your generosity has made it possible to turn this vision into reality.

My pranaams go to all my Gurus - Dr. Takaomi Taira, Dr. A.S. Hegde, Dr. N.K. Venkataramana, Dr. Rajeshwari, Dr. Narayana Rao, and other Gurus, thank you for your invaluable guidance, expertise, and wisdom. Your insights have enriched me as a neurosurgeon, and the content of this book is immeasurably good.

Lastly, I extend my thanks to the leadership team at PRS Neurosciences for putting up with all my demands for the creation and execution of the myriad ideas I constantly have and to Stardom Books for their professionalism, dedication, and expertise in bringing this book to fruition.

I am profoundly grateful to all who have contributed, whether large or small, to the creation of this book. Your contributions have left an indelible mark on its pages, and I am honored to share this journey with you.

With deepest gratitude,
Dr. Sharan Srinivasan

FOREWORD

The Awakening Field of Functional Neurosciences

Laligam N. Sekhar, MD, FACS, FAANS,
Professor and Vice-Chairman
Varadaraya S. Shenoy, MD
Senior Research Fellow,
Department of Neurological Surgery
University of Washington, Seattle, USA

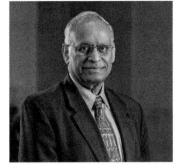

In this elegant book titled "**Rebooting the Brain®**," Drs. Sharan Srinivasan and Prathiba Sharan have presented a series of stories that lead to fascinating discussion topics on functional neurosciences. The entire neuro rehabilitation and neuromodulation field is awakening in the 21st century. Our successful treatment of many patients with neurological disorders, improved neurosurgical procedures on patients with neurological problems, and the proliferation of traumatic brain and spinal cord injuries have given rise to patients who have various disabilities. We are now thinking a lot about the quality of life of our surviving patients, which was not our concern some decades ago. Patients and their families also now demand more from their physicians and surgeons.

My first experience with chronic neurological deficits was with one of my relatives in the village of Laligam, near Dharmapuri, Tamil Nadu. He had progressive spastic paralysis due to a form of spinal degeneration and lived for many years in a mentally excellent condition, but required chronic care, which was only possible in his village home. The second bad experience occurred years later with my younger brother. He was studying at M.S. Ramaiah Medical College. He suffered a severe head injury in Bangalore when he was riding on the back of a motor scooter without a helmet. Fortunately, after his injury, he was eventually taken to NIMHANS in Bangalore, where he was provided exceptional care even though the physicians, surgeons, and nurses did not know who he was. I spent a month with him there, and over the years, I was distressed to see his prolonged recovery. He was able to finish his studies as a medical doctor with a delay of a year. However, he continued to have problems with seizures and mild mental disabilities, and he was never able to work as a specialist doctor, which was his goal in life. He also suffered an accelerated dementia, as is seen in some patients with severe head injuries. Since then, as a practicing neurosurgeon, I am constantly seeing patients who have disabilities either as a result of neurosurgical operations, stroke, or brain trauma. Many of these patients receive neuro-rehabilitative care, but after some time, they are forgotten and recede into the background.

Dr. Sharan and his colleagues have built a very elegant institute focused on rehabilitating such patients. In this book, they outline many patient stories and examples of such rehabilitation after stroke, trauma, and neuro-modulation surgeries for movement disorders. They emphasize the human touch and individualized patient care in all these rehabilitative efforts. This personalized and individualized care can only be delivered in specialist rehabilitation centers such as the one set up by Dr. Sharan and colleagues, and this center has become a model for other institutions in India and worldwide.

However, the kind of manpower needed to work one-on-one with many patients is very difficult. Here, I feel that using artificially intelligent (AI-enabled) robots that can perform both nursing care and patient education will be vital, not only in developed countries but also in countries such as India and China. Such AI-enabled rehabilitation robots can become essential to nursing and rehabilitative care and will play a significant role within the next ten years.

We are just starting many trials in the neuro-rehabilitative area, which may bear fruits. One of these that can be mentioned is Transcranial Magnetic Stimulation (TMS), which has been successfully used for conditions such as depression and post-traumatic stress disorder. Deep brain stimulation, as discussed by Dr. Sharan and his colleagues, may also be of use in this area. The kind of brain implants such as the one developed by the company **Neuralink** may find more usage for patients who have paralysis or other disorders. However, the use of these devices is still experimental and needs to be explored further. For patients who have spinal cord injury, researchers at the University of Washington, spearheaded by Dr. Chet Moritz and Dr. Christoph Hofstetter, have started using techniques of electrically bypassing an injured spinal cord and activating the muscles directly. The use of neural stem cells is also being tried for neuro-rehab; however, they are also in the experimental stages.

The question which may be asked is, who will pay for all these kinds of care? The answer may be to return the patients to a life that can be useful not only to them or to their families but also to society at large. We are living in an age of great turmoil caused by individuals. In Ukraine, we are seeing the effects of the aggression by Russians against the Ukrainians due to the evil nature of the Russian Leader. In Israel, we have witnessed massive destruction caused by terrorists coming over from the Gaza Strip, which has since then resulted in vast numbers of deaths and disability. In India, we have witnessed a great deal of corruption, violence, rapes, and murders, which have been mediated by some political interests, which in turn have resulted in a significant number of deaths and disability. We are also witnessing the effects of global warming caused by massive usage of carbon fuels, the destruction of trees, animals, and water bodies, and unmindful pollution with plastic and products. It is difficult for us as neurosurgeons to think about how to cure THIS human mental illness, which causes people to accumulate money in evil ways and to mediate attacks on other humans, animals, and plants. We are at the other end of the spectrum where we are trying to deal with the after-effects. I hope that neurosurgeons can lead a revolution wherein we can educate our fellow humans to stop these evil acts and create and elect the right leaders who can prevent these evil actions against humanity.

Why did we choose to write this book?

In the midst of the chaos...

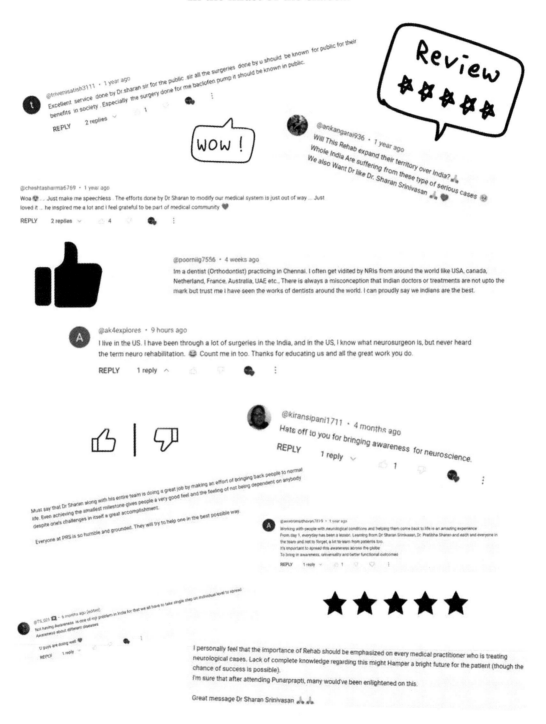

Find the method in the madness. Read on to find out more

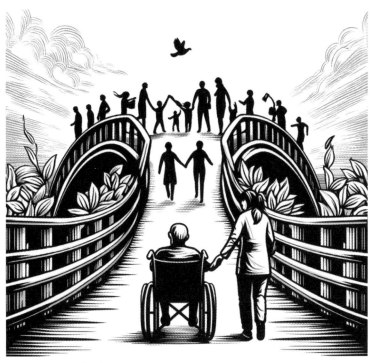

Part 1: The Journey Of 'HOPE'

One day, a friend of mine sent his branding consultant to learn more about our work and how to convey it to the world. As I spoke for over an hour, he transitioned from casual interest to rapt attention, his posture shifting from stooped to charged with positive energy. Inspiring those around me has always been essential to me, and that day was no different… it seemed to have had a profound effect on him as well. When he left, he excitedly called his boss, exclaiming, "Boss, they are selling 'HOPE' here!"

This journey of hope begins when patients and their families, once mired in feelings of helplessness and resignation, encounter the first glimmers of improvement through our multidisciplinary Functional Neurosciences approach. As such dependent patients realize that they're on the path to recovery and attain their functional independence, each step forward becomes a testament to resilience, turning despair into optimism and doubt into determination—a journey from hopelessness to hope, fueled by positive energy.

This journey is a testament to the human spirit's capacity for limitless adaptation and rejuvenation. As patients witness their own progress, hope blossoms, and the energy around them changes, igniting a flame of possibility and reigniting the belief in a brighter future. This journey of hope serves as a reminder of humanity's resilience, demonstrating that even in the worst of adversities, there's always light at the end of the tunnel. And as the saying goes – every dark cloud has a silver lining!

SECTION A: INTRODUCTION

PROLOGUE

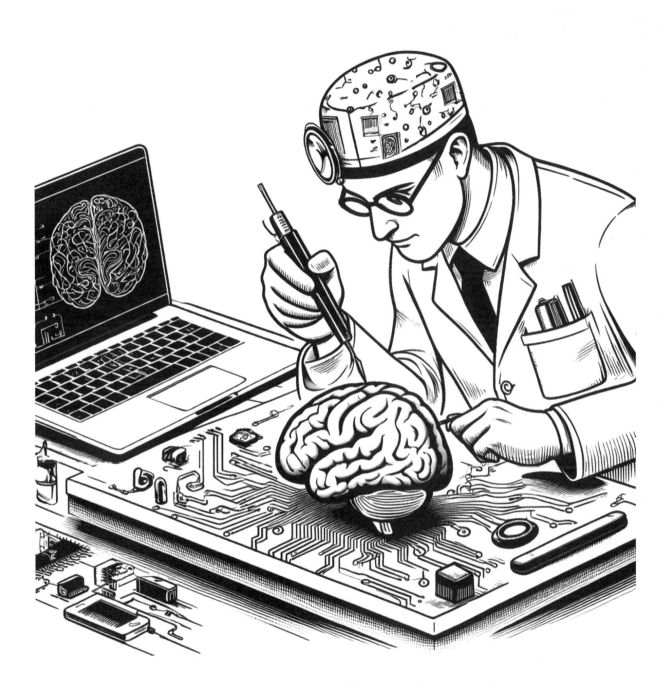

EXPLORING NEW FRONTIERS – THE PRS NEUROSCIENCES WAY!

Are you aware that a brain injury of any nature or cause is like the hard disk of your SMART device crashing?

You will have to reload all the software and then try and restore all saved files, folders, and apps so that your device is back to where it was before the crash! But here are the biggest challenges– who's got the spares for this software? Now, even if you have all these, how do we reload it? What sequence do we follow? How do we restore them?

What do we do if the original programs don't take on or run well?

What is our FATE?!?

There is no other organ in the human body that has its own software that is specific to each individual. Your heart and my heart do the same function of pumping blood, the same for our kidneys. Can you do neurosurgery or other things, like the way I do, or can I do what you are good at? Absolutely not!

Are you aware that all organs (like the heart, kidneys, lungs, liver, etc.) have their own specific 'Function Tests,' but there are no "Brain (or spinal cord) Function tests" available anywhere in the world??

I have always felt that medicine should not be overly commercial because this field uniquely involves handling human lives unconditionally, whether it's the CEO of a company or a beggar on the street. Both should be treated equally, as treatment should be based on the needs of the disease rather than the affordability – the COVID-19 pandemic is the best example for me to make all of you understand this.

Namaste, Pranaams; I am Sharan… Dr. Sharan Srinivasan, a Stereotactic & Functional neurosurgeon, to be more precise, just like the nature of my work. I was a neurosurgery aspirant since the 8th grade of my school. Do you remember what you wanted to be when you were a 14-year-old teenager? Are you living your dream? Me? For sure, I am!

Meet my wife, Dr. Prathiba, who has been my love since my first MBBS days. We became life partners, and we continue to be business partners. She is an empathetic physician and an excellent neuropsychologist, and she owns a fellowship in neuro rehabilitation. But more importantly, she is a great human being, like a "mother" to all those who come under her care. If I am the director of a movie called *"neuro rehabilitation – the newro way,"* she is the producer! Without her, the show stands still! I am the creator; she is the executor!

My wife Prathiba and I have always shared a deep connection. As she has supported me through my life's ups and downs and adopted my crazy dreams as her own, I felt she deserved a special trip for our 25th wedding anniversary. I decided on an Antarctic cruise (which was one of the items on my bucket list), and I began researching.

Initially considering a departure from New Zealand, I later discovered that the most popular routes start from Ushuaia, Argentina, the world's southernmost city, and crossing the world's most treacherous waters, the

Drake's Passage (which connects the Atlantic Ocean to the Pacific Ocean). The Drake's Passage is named after the English explorer Sir Francis Drake, who sailed through it during his circumnavigation of the globe in the late 16th century.

Despite its reputation as one of the world's most treacherous waters, with depths of up to four kilometers, our crossing was calm, taking just over 24 hours to reach the Antarctica continent. On the return, however, we faced over 8–10-meter waves, extending our journey to 36 hours. Initially, we considered taking friends with us but eventually decided to go alone, making new friends during the cruise.

The cruise itself was an expedition type, much like life, with just 150 guests, which allowed for a more personalized experience, including individual butlers and an attendant familiar with our Indian vegetarian preferences. He knew how Indians could not live without 'yogurt.' Throughout the cruise, we engaged with a diverse group of passengers, including several doctor couples from Canada, forming lasting friendships.

The strict environmental protocols on the ship ensured that we did not contaminate the pristine Antarctic environment. Our experiences in Antarctica were profoundly transformative, not just in witnessing the breath-taking landscapes but also in the connections we made, the adventures we had, and the stories we shared. This trip was more than just a celebration; it was a reaffirmation and an expression of our life's work and passions, particularly in 'Pushing the frontiers of Neuroscience,' which I spoke about in a lecture at the IISc, the Indian Institute of Science, Bengaluru, India.

This journey to the South Pole was symbolic of our explorative spirit, leading us to later rebrand our focus from being strictly a neuro rehabilitation company to a broader scope of 'Functional Neurosciences,' reflecting our continuous drive to innovate and expand our horizons, impacting the people who need these the most – those suffering from "Neurological Disabilities" due to brain, spinal cord or neuro-muscular issues.

You must be wondering why we even care to write this book. I could have spent this time making millions of dollars in the US or elsewhere and living a happy life with my family. Why did I stick around here in India and start working in a charitable hospital where the neurosciences department was non-existing when I joined? I could have joined one of the many corporate hospitals in Bengaluru, my hometown, or you may call it our *'karma Bhoomi.'*

Why are we willing to share our story of becoming one of the most successful entrepreneurs in the field of Functional Neurosciences (neuromodulation with advanced neuro rehabilitation) purely based on ethical practices and our entrepreneurial skills? Let me put it in an easy way. I have a utopian dream- the possibility for every neurologically disabled individual (and their families) to fight their way to achieve the best possible *functional independence level (FIL)'* – a dream of providing world-class yet affordable services, irrespective of their socio-economic status, race, region or religion, across the globe! It's too much for a doctor to dream, right? Well… I have found a way to do so! Will we succeed? Only time will tell. Do you want to know about it? Or, even better, do you want to join our team on this roller coaster journey? Do you need our help? Whatever the reason, you have found yourself in the right handbook!

Before we reveal our journey, one layer at a time, to you all, let me tell you something interesting about our medical education. Luckily for both of us, having 'earned' our merit seats to study medicine at the prestigious Bangalore Medical College and Research Institute (BMCRI), one of the top 5 medical schools in India, we obtained our MBBS degrees for a paltry INR 5000 or USD 60 as per the 2024 exchange rates!

Many of you must be thinking, "Man... that is just insane, unbelievable, impossible; this education must have been a fraud; how is that even possible??" But the truth is, it was possible, and we got our degrees, we did our postgraduate studies, we still have our licenses, and we have been in practice since 1994! You all know how expensive medical education is just because of the infrastructure itself. We may say that we are merit students, blah, blah, blah, that's all okay. But the truth is **that the public funds our education. This is the truth. If *we don't serve that public*, it just makes no sense to us.**

I pursued my 'neurosurgery' dream. I underwent my National Board-Certified training in neurosurgery at the prestigious Manipal Institute for Neurological Disorders (MIND), Manipal Hospital, Bangalore (MHB), one of the earliest premier quaternary care corporate hospitals in Bengaluru, India. I got this degree for INR seventy-five thousand (75,000) or USD 1000 dollars! Unheard of costs, right?

This is India for you– high-quality education at affordable costs. Finally, in August 2000, I officially qualified as a board-certified neurosurgeon in India, ready to take on the world and live my dreams. From 1982 till 2000, for 18 long years, I had kept this dream alive and made it happen! We have nothing to recover back from the system. God has been very nice to us. All we have to do is give back to the community that has funded our education!

Having been in the practice of neurosurgery since the year 2000, in the city that is called the 'Silicon Valley of India,' the 'Unicorn & start-up capital' of India as well, I strongly advocate that we need "Compassionate Capitalism" in the field of healthcare and 'making money' cannot be the sole yardstick to measure success, because for us, earning money is a key by-product of our activities, not the main objective, which is 'improving the QoL of our patients and their families.

I trained as an undergraduate in a government-run medical school with a free hospital service for the poor and later specialized in neurosurgery at one of India's leading corporate hospitals, offering a stark contrast in care experiences. Recognizing the need for quality yet affordable healthcare, I searched for the right hospital and found my fit at Bhagwan Mahaveer Jain Hospital (BMJH) in 2013. BMJH, a charitable institution under the Bhagwan Mahaveer Memorial Jain Trust, provides cutting-edge medical technology and advanced healthcare at affordable costs to all patients. When I joined, the Neurosciences Department was struggling, but I saw the potential for revitalization. Since then, the department has thrived, handling numerous consultations and surgeries monthly.

You see, our organization, PRS Neurosciences, is clinician-driven! Entrepreneurship runs in our family, and I was no exception. And like all entrepreneurs who want to solve the problems of the world, I also found my calling – 'patients with neurological disabilities' had nowhere to go to become 'able' again. After we initially dabbled with this idea with a small firm called 'Sharp Minds,' which we founded in 2009, we finally decided to 'bite the bullet' and formally start a company to help us take our mission forward. In 2011, we founded PRS Neurosciences & Mechatronics Research Institute (PNMRI) with support from our North American family.

When we started, my father, Puttur Rangaswamy Srinivasan, after whom the institute is named, gave me 'two golden pieces of advice'; the first one was - "You are starting a business, and 'business' means 'profits.' If you don't make a minimum of 25% profit, DO NOT call it a business. You do what you want (he already knew that both of us were doing charity in our practices and had founded our charity SAF in 2007 itself), but don't call it a business!" The second golden advice was "do not borrow money to start. Put in how much you have, but don't take a loan". His philosophy was firmly against borrowing to avoid the ethical compromises often forced by financial pressures.

This guidance has shaped and strengthened our philosophy and operations, emphasizing that medical services should always prioritize patient needs over business interests. Sounded idealistic, but was it practical? Feasible? Read on to find out.

My patients (and their families) were running out of money, selling their assets, family jewels like the 'mangalsutra,' etc, to meet the burgeoning expenses of the treatment to save their loved ones. This dichotomy was killing both of us mentally, but we didn't allow it to deter us. Both of us are 'champions,' and I asked myself a very interesting question - "how can I make money without my patient paying me more money?" I asked Dr. Prathiba the same, and both of us got thinking. This led us to what we are revealing to the world for the first time via this book – *The Philosophy of PRS Neurosciences, which is our personal philosophy.*

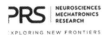

Philosophy of PRS Neurosciences

More for less – mass customization is the mantra

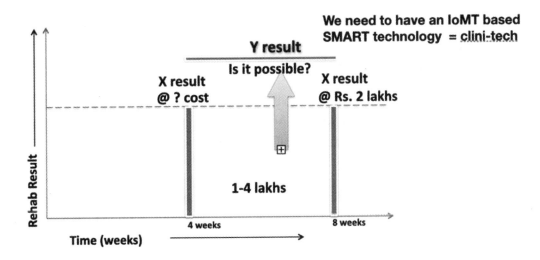

Let me explain - How can you achieve more for less?? - "if we take eight weeks to produce an 'X' result for a patient in neuro rehab, and we charge INR 400,000 for it, if we produce the same 'X' result in 4 weeks, how much can we charge?" After several possible 'right' answers, my answer was - "anywhere between INR 100,000 to 400,000, depending on the type of facility. Right?" The follow-up question to this was, "If 'X' is the best possible result today, and we want to create a result 'Y' that is better than 'X, then what do we need to do?" The answer was – affordable technology through research and data analysis.

If costs in the technology industry keep falling, why can the same thing not happen in healthcare? I felt that it could only happen with "Mass Customization." **This eventually led me to define our philosophy as the "8 weeks-4 weeks: X-Y" mantra.** I also thought about "mass customization in the space of Functional Neurosciences very early in my practice. I realized I was way ahead of my time, yet correct to the dot! I believed that with this 'thinking things through' process, I was confident that I could contribute positively to India's (and the global) GDP by not only saving patients money but also by making them 'productive citizens.'

This can be achieved by effectively managing recovery costs, ultimately reducing the overall financial burden borne by individuals. Is this idea generalizable? What technology of *'Internet of Medical Things (IoMT)'* do I need? How will I run it by decentralizing but without losing control of the quality of outcomes? Dr. Prathiba and I had a business to run without overloading the patients and their families – we built a Robin Hood model so that we, as an organization, could also sustain and grow profitably!

What is our concept of "Mass Customization?"

In the healthcare service industry, mass customization entails tailoring medical treatments, services, and experiences to meet the unique needs and preferences of individual patients. This precision and personalized approach acknowledges the diverse health conditions, requirements, preferences, and backgrounds of each patient. Through mass customization, healthcare providers aim to deliver tailored medical care while ensuring efficiency and effectiveness.

To achieve this, providers must leverage technologies such as standardized electronic health records and comprehensive data collection in a standardized format.

These technologies enable data analytics and telemedicine to gather and analyze patient information by identifying patterns and enabling the creation of customized treatment plans, medication regimens, and care delivery methods.

Mass customization in healthcare not only enhances patient outcomes but also facilitates the identification and application of preventive strategies, ultimately reducing the average length of hospital stays and medical expenses. This is what our customized, proprietary software 'newro LOGICS' does.

This approach enhances patient and caregiver satisfaction while improving the overall quality of care by ensuring that treatments closely align with each patient's specific needs and circumstances. And if we as an organization do this well and smartly, we can still make decent money!

Our philosophy meant that patient care is paramount, the patient (and their families) needs to be at the center of whatever we do, we focus primarily on their outcomes, and treating each patient with dignity is non-negotiable. This core philosophy of PRS Neurosciences, encapsulated in ***our "8 weeks-4 weeks: X-Y"*** mantra, focuses on delivering high-quality, profitable, yet cost-effective neuromodulation and neuro-rehabilitation services.

Our commitment extends beyond mere treatment; we also focus on preventative care to reduce long-term costs and ensure sustainable treatment pathways for our patients, emphasizing that they should not exhaust their financial resources before their rehabilitation journey is complete. Our research wing is constantly focused on innovation as we continue with the integration of machine learning and artificial intelligence into our newro LOGICS platform to refine our clinical and clini-tech algorithms and improve service delivery, ensuring that our operations remain aligned with our core mantra. This is essential, as any deviation from this mantra is not considered within our strategic objectives.

We did not want to remain as a mom-and-pop enterprise. So, I was very clear that we will always be 'process-based' and not person-based, and scaling up involves Internet of Medical Things (IoMT) based technology, both hardware and software, along with extensive data analytics, Artificial Intelligence (AI), and Machine Learning (ML). Serving disabled patients across the country globally, and across different payment segments requires active public participation. That's where our NGO Swaasthya Aarogya Foundation (SAF), an 80G charitable trust formed in 2007, comes into play to help raise funds. The Ministry of Social Justice and Empowerment, Government of India, which manages disability welfare, has an annual budget of 800-900 crores but often spends only 200-300 crores. There's a disconnect; millions of people with disabilities are not receiving adequate support due to a lack of effective intermediaries to utilize these funds. We aim to address this by making rehabilitation services affordable and accessible.

Affordability and accessibility are crucial, meaning we must penetrate into smaller towns. I looked at leveraging technology to standardize processes and adapt them to multiple languages. When seeking hospital software, many providers did not understand our needs and suggested expensive, generic solutions. After several failed attempts with other developers who could not tailor the software to our needs, we, on our third attempt, have successfully built a world-class rehab operating system platform for both patient and business management called **"newro LOGICS."**

This pursuit of affordable technology led me to avoid expensive international equipment and focus on building homegrown *'Atmanirbhar Bharat'* technologies with AR and VR, which seemed promising for 'immersive' rehabilitation experiences to re-wire the damaged 'functional' brain circuits. Our strategy involves using cutting-edge technology not only to facilitate rehabilitation but also to teach essential life skills through the "tell, show, try, do" method, optimized by AR and VR for both onsite and remote tele-rehab.

Though I have a clear vision and mission for my enterprise, it was and continues to be extremely hard to explain to many doctors the practicality and importance of Functional Neurosciences in patient recovery. In this field, there are peaks of appreciation to valleys of hopelessness and depression! This journey is inevitable for the patients (and their families). We all play our roles in this journey, along with the patient and family, but we can never replace them as the drivers in this process!

We are on a BIG global mission – to build a 'profitable unicorn' that delivers compassionate care at affordable costs and delivers to their homes and to all those who need it. We are looking for strategic business partners and investors who are 'Compassionate Capitalists' and are willing to join our Functional Neurosciences bandwagon. Are you one of them? If so, please reach out to us.

Being an avid reader of the 'Reader's Digest books in my childhood, I came across a quote in one of their editions that profoundly impacted me: "I was crying that I had no shoes on my feet until I met a man with no feet." This taught me to appreciate what I have.

Another story from another Reader's Digest edition, about the race to the South Pole by daredevil explorers Robert Scott and another named Roald Amundsen, way back in 1911, captivated and inspired me, planting the seed of visiting Antarctica one day. Basically, I am an explorer and love exploring the unknown. This child-like enthusiasm has remained to this day and fuels all my research desires.

We call ourselves and our team members – "Brain Rebooters!"

Overall, PRS Neurosciences provides top-tier, cost-effective neuromodulation and neuro rehabilitation to those in need, employing innovative yet appropriate and affordable technologies and practices to deliver superior care. We maintain a focus on preventive care to manage costs effectively, ensuring patients do not exhaust their financial resources before completing their rehabilitation.

Our approach is encapsulated in our core mantra: ***"8 weeks-4 weeks: X-Y,"*** *guiding all our endeavors.*

Through this book, we invite you to join us as we take you on a unique journey into the realms of neuromodulation and neuro rehabilitation, collectively named by us "Functional Neurosciences." You will be able to visualize what I, Dr. Prathiba, and my team of rehabilitation experts go through to achieve 'restoration of function.' We are great storytellers. We have shared tales of our journey through the Drake-passage of Functional Neurosciences, with neurological and emotional tides much higher than the 8-10 meter waves we encountered!

Some of you will find hope, and others will find inspiration through stories of those who walked down the path with neurological disorders and disabilities and reclaimed their life. You can step into our shoes as healthcare professionals and experience what we do in our daily lives while treating those who seek us! You will learn about some fascinating but 'misbehaving' functional neurological circuits and how we deal with their dysfunctions!

So, ladies and gentlemen, if you want to join us to become "Brain Rebooters", fasten your seat belts as we take off and enjoy this journey filled with facts from neurosciences mixed with some limbic system stimulants! Enjoy the journey because the destinations are totally unpredictable! Hope to meet you at the very end.

Pilot:
Dr. Sharan Srinivasan
Stereotactic & Functional neurosurgeon
Chairman & Managing Director
PRS Neurosciences & Mechatronics Research Institute (PNMRI)
Head of Neurosciences
Bhagwan Mahaveer Jain Hospital, Bengaluru, India

Co-pilot:
Dr. Prathiba Sharan
CEO, Director - Rehab Services, Head of Cognitive Rehab Services
PRS Neurosciences & Mechatronics Research Institute (PNMRI)
Bengaluru, India.

1

THE WORLD (AND INDIA) CANNOT AFFORD DISABILITY!

Functional Neurosciences is the art & science of reloading software, files, folders, and apps into a crashed hard disk (the human brain) without any backed-up data, USB port, or Wi-Fi enablement.

No BACKUP…PACKUP!!!

–Dr. Sharan Srinivasan
Stereotactic & Functional Neurosurgeon

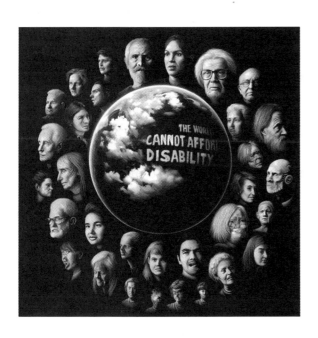

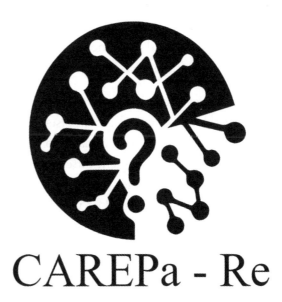

CAREPa - Re

December 2019...Dr. Prathiba receives a WhatsApp message from an unknown number at 3 am. She opens the message... It is from a US phone, a person named Sajiv Gulati, reaching out desperately needing help to rehabilitate his wife, Nina Gulati, who had suffered a major brain stroke a few months earlier in Chicago and is currently bedridden and basically in bad shape.

Dr. Prathiba - "Talking about Nina's experience, I think this is one patient who gave me the confidence that our rehab results are not inferior to any Western countries, which I had thought were much, much superior before having this experience with Nina. So, though she was a US citizen, and the stroke happened in the US, they were well to do, with a huge medical insurance cover, and they tried a lot with the insurance and stuff like that to get into the best of the rehab facilities there.

Unfortunately, Nina wasn't able to get any relief from there for various reasons. So, Sanjiv was frustrated; he decided to bring her to India for rehab as he also had family support (which had lots of doctors in India and abroad) and began googling 'best neuro rehab centers in India,' and we appeared! So, he basically found us online, and we had long chats on WhatsApp, WhatsApp calls, and so on. That's when I realized that there is this one man who really loves his wife and is willing to do anything to get his wife back to normalcy. So, he was willing to bring her to Bangalore and take the therapy as long as she needed. I think that it takes a lot from a husband, especially somebody from out of the country. He had to sort out his work and his business and come over to India with a caregiver. He initially decided to stay here for almost a month.

When Nina came, she really was like a baby. She just did not understand what people spoke. She kept calling him Guddu. That's all she knew. And he kept calling her Guddu. And they were a cute little couple. But then there's nothing more beyond that. She had a lot of behavioral problems, all the choiciest English 'swear' words, but could not do anything by herself. A lot of challenges. Even a small kid would do much beyond that, I guess.

Nina had to be dealt with in a different way for some time because there were times that she would get very abusive and very difficult with the therapists. She wouldn't cooperate with the therapists. So, the therapists found it very difficult to deal with Nina at some point of time during the long hours of therapy. So, I had to counsel the therapists and give them different ways and modes of dealing with Nina so that they could make friends with her. There were times that therapists sat with her, sang songs, watched movies, played puzzles with her, read stories for her, just chatted up with her, and had fun with her. Different tactics eventually helped all of them become friends with her, and she started cooperating with the therapists.

With almost five hours of therapy per day, lasting for almost eight months, Nina came to a level where she was able to identify alphabets and numbers, talk coherently in a few sentences, and identify a lot of her relatives, children, brothers, sisters, family members, and friends. She was able to, with support, walk to the bathroom and indicate her toilet needs. All these things were achieved in eight months with intense therapy. Unfortunately, because of the COVID, they had to go back to the US. So, Sanjiv decided to take her back to the US, and he said he would try and continue the rehab in the US, considering that the first wave of COVID had its own impact globally... Nobody had an idea how it would take a turn and what would happen after that.

But I guess it was after a month that I again received a call from Sanjiv saying that he was really finding it difficult to find therapists who would come and do the therapies. What we were doing five hours a day, and real intense and multi-disciplinary therapy, he was hardly getting five hours a week of basic therapy, I guess. And Nina started deteriorating. So, it was disheartening, I guess, more for him than her. Seeing his wife deteriorating, he, I think, had to take a tough call this time to bring her back to India.

Nina was very reluctant to come back to India because she stayed at the hospital for the first time. So obviously, he was finding it very, very difficult to convince her to come back to India for therapy. She had come to a level where she would understand what therapies were, what therapists did, and how difficult it was. So, it was not easy for Sanjiv to convince her to come back. But somehow, he managed to convince her, saying that he was taking Nina to India to stay in a resort, and that's how she got convinced.

Luckily, we had a resort where we had our services, and that's where Nina started taking her therapy. During the middle of the raging COVID-19 pandemic, between the first and second lockdowns, when it opened again for international travel, he came down to India on the 15th of April 2021, to be precise. And we continued the therapy for close to a year, and Nina eventually walked back. I mean, that was something amazing. And now, after the whole rehab done here, and that continued over there at home, I think she has reached a level where she's very cohesive. She's happy living at home. She's singing karaoke songs. And I mean, I can't say 100 % back to normal, but then, yeah, 70 to 80% there, I think. It's a great achievement for a person like her. Though they belong to a very affordable category of people, it was a very long-term rehab that Sanjiv had to take Nina through. He really negotiated every bit and piece of it to make sure that, on one side, he did not spend too much money on Nina's therapies, and on the other side, he wanted to ensure she got all the comforts and facilities that Nina needed. He was making sure that he was available for calls at every beck, making sure all support was available. Though he was remotely monitoring Nina from the US, he made sure everything was taken care of over here.

Though he loved his wife a lot, he was not very easy to work with. He was a perfectionist. He wanted some things to be done in a particular way, and he wanted to achieve the results in a particular way. It was imperative to make him understand that healthcare cannot be like machines or software and that the results that we have been getting were not easy. Several hours of caregiver counseling went into making him understand. He also got some support from the attenders. They also had to be counseled because Nina had a lot of behavioral issues: how to manage her, how to put up with her, how to deal with her, how to motivate her, all the time keeping them on their toes, making sure she sleeps well, making sure she eats well, making sure she doesn't overindulge in anything. All these things were to be trained by the caregivers who were around with Nina for that long period of time. Life wasn't so easy for them either."

This story gave us the belief and confidence that we were running a 'world-class' service but at affordable rates. Especially when Sanjiv said that it would have cost him a fortune if it were to be done elsewhere in the world.

So, readers, buckle up your ISI-certified helmets, fasten your seatbelts, and get enough dose of caffeine and carbs because Dr. Sharan will be taking you through an amazing, cognitively stimulating, emotionally draining, rollercoaster journey of the world of 'Functional Neurosciences,' as he sees it. Have fun!

Trivia: India's first ever '100 % Made in India' helmet testing machine was built by my father, Mr. P.R. Srinivasan in 1980.

In the late 1970's, the Indian Air Force approached my father and asked him if he could make an indigenously built helmet testing machine with ISI standards as documented in the ISI Manual. My father studied the manual, looked at the design of the machine and built a 100 % Made in India Helmet Testing machine in Bengaluru. This machine was tested, approved and used by Indian Air Force for many years after that. Seeing the success of this machine, other companies manufacturing helmets for the public like STUDDS, FIBRO, ORIENT, etc. asked my father if he could make a similar machine for them to provide better protection to people driving 2 wheelers! This was probably the first ISI certified helmet testing machine in India!

INTRODUCTION

Have you ever wondered if there could be a third epidemic that has the power to devour the world? There are infectious diseases like HIV and Non-communicable diseases like heart disease, cancer, and diabetes. We have just emerged from a bruising pandemic! Now, what could possibly be the third epidemic?

In the quiet corners of hospitals and homes across the world, a silent epidemic rages on. It is a battle fought not with visible wounds or contagious pathogens but with the complicated workings of the human Brain (and spinal cord) mind. Our brain (and spinal cord) is a magical system. It controls our entire life, starting from birth until we breathe our last. It controls everything from walking to talking to eating to sleeping to breathing to interacting with the world around us. What if it gets damaged and misbehaves? Like the hard disk of our computer or other smart devices??? What will our fate be?? What happens to all the data, files, and folders that were saved inside that hard disk called the human brain?

I often face this question in my mind: What is worse to have? A brain injury or a spinal cord injury? Honestly speaking, it's a better life for a brain-injured person because they may forget what they went through because of the brain injury, but a person with a spinal cord injury never forgets what misfortunes he had to go through—such a hell for life long! You see, in Indian Vedic sciences, our spinal cord is considered an axis-mundi. It is seen as a bridge between heaven and earth, linking the individual soul (Jivatma) to the universal consciousness (Paramatma). In easier words, our spinal cord is the connection between our brain, representing our consciousness, and our body, representing the interaction with the environment! Such a delicate system of chords branching out from the brain makes it a critical element of the nervous system, an injury to which can be an unforgivable mistake!

The heart is important, but the brain is not.

What if your hands get stuck as you attempt to sip coffee out of your cup, and you can no longer think, feel, or sense anything and just drop the cup on the floor? Strange and scary, isn't it? People rush to the hospital, having slight heaviness in their chest. But how do they react when they get a severe headache? They take a Paracetamol/Saridon and suppress it for as long as they can.

Chest pain = ECG hasn't translated to headache = CT scan or MRI!

Little do people realize that once your brain stops functioning, your entire body could become a mere lifeless organ. Neurological disability is something that the world has not even bothered to understand and, hence, has been ignored for the longest time. We don't realize the consequences of our ignorance until and unless it knocks us down, keeps us tied to our beds, or even, at times, takes our lives. It devastates not only our lives but also all those loved ones around us. It can become a ruthless enemy, where survival seems much worse than dying.

As the sun sets on countless lives altered by this unseen foe, a desperate cry for hope keeps ringing like an alarm through the hearts of patients and their families. It is a cry for a return to normalcy, a plea to reclaim the independence that once felt so natural and taken for granted. In the face of this daunting challenge, we find the Family, the Individual, and the Lifeline - a trio united by a singular goal, a shared vision- to bring their beloved back to normal!

We have seen countless patients coming into our advanced rehabilitation centers with different ranges of neurological disabilities. Some couldn't move their hands and limbs on one side, some could only move their hands, and some could barely move their neck. We have seen people who have lost their ability to speak or have poor memory and cognition. Some were much worse – in a state of coma or unconsciousness. But do you think that's the worst part? Oh, you are mistaken! The worst of the worst part of the entire thing is what the caregivers/bystanders have to deal with. These patients hardly have any idea about what the hell is going on. It is the bystander who has to go through the entire struggle, from helping the patient sit straight to taking them for rehabilitation, changing diapers, and cleaning food that often drooped out of their mouths. Caregiver burden is a neglected topic. Do you think it is easy to go through that? It is an experience that transcends the boundaries of helplessness. It is really hard for us to console the bystanders.

Do you think neurological disorders or dysfunctions happen only after having a stroke, Cerebrovascular Accident (CVA), or a brain attack? Oh no, darling, not at all! Try riding your bike without a helmet, under the influence of alcohol, or at high speed, and I can assure you that you'll end up being my next patient.

People are so careless to the point where they're more concerned about their freshly straightened hair than their brains. They think of their brain as something as silly as cauliflower, it seems. If you are a person living in Karnataka, you will see riders wearing a helmet that resembles the bowl in which you serve curry at home without realizing that their brain could literally turn into splattered shattered curry on the road if there is an unfortunate road accident, *like a fried Bheja!*

We have dealt with a number of youngsters who have lost their senses and neurological functions due to road accidents, specifically worsened by not wearing a helmet. I realized that most of them have a screen guard to protect their mobile phones. They also consciously put on a nice strong silicon back cover for it. What about the brain? I mean, seriously! Their smartphones are more important than their brains. They are stupid, aren't they?

For the family, it's like trying to herd cats through a maze made of confusion and mental breakdowns when their loved one grapples with neurological disabilities. It's a rollercoaster ride of "Did we just make progress, or are we about to do a U-turn?". We call it a *'neurological chakravyuh,'* much worse than what Abhimanyu encountered in the Mahabharat war. The family is basically armed with a mix of superhero capes and endless pots of coffee, which eventually turn into the unofficial cheerleaders and chief strategists of this unfortunate adventure, which seems to be leading to nowhere. They're the emergency support system stashed in the backpack of the individual's hopes and dreams, ready to be whipped out at a moment's notice. Imagine waiting outside the ICU with a heart that beats one fifty times a minute, expecting the doctor to come out any moment and say, "Your loved has made it through," but instead, they come and say, "We're trying our best. Your loved one might not make it through, or even if he/she does, you will have to take care of him/her for the rest of your life." The bystanders' pain doesn't end after the lifesaving surgeries, but like I said, will go on and on until the loved one comes back to at least near normalcy.

Picture the disabled individual as a character in a quirky sci-fi movie, suddenly burdened with a new set of super-duper limitations they never ordered. Yet, in their eyes, there's a glimmer of "I-will-conquer-the-world" mixed with a pinch of "I-might-need-a-map-though." When families come to us with a loved one who has become disabled, bedridden, wheelchair-bound, with poor memory and speech, or in need of care, they are often grappling with a storm of questions and uncertainties:

- Will my loved one improve from their current state?
- Is it possible for them to fully recover and return to the person they were before?
- How much time will this journey of recovery require?
- What measures must we undertake to facilitate their improvement?
- Is there a realistic prospect of rehabilitation for them?

Addressing these concerns necessitates a comprehensive understanding of the patient's condition:

- The origin of the patient's medical condition, whether it's a result of a stroke, head injury, infection affecting the brain, spinal cord issues, or a progressive degenerative disease, is pivotal to charting the course of treatment.
- Evaluating the patient's present functional level is crucial to establishing a baseline.
- It is essential to identify the disabilities currently impeding the patient's functionality to tailor an effective rehabilitation program.
- Understanding the patient's and family's expectations is equally important. Are these expectations achievable? What milestones can they realistically hope to reach?
- Determining the necessary abilities the patient needs to regain is a crucial step in setting realistic goals.
- To ensure that the patient is on the path to recovery, we must have metrics in place to measure their progress effectively.
- Open lines of communication are vital to keep the patient and family informed, offering clarity and hope throughout the rehabilitation process.
- Providing regular reports to the patient and family can encapsulate progress, adapt rehabilitation strategies, and manage expectations.

Our approach involves a dialogue that balances professional assessments with compassionate communication, ensuring that the family and patient are integral to the recovery process and understand the possibilities and the realities of their unique situation. Meanwhile, as I said, the family turns into an amazing set of coaches, personal chefs, 24x7 private nurses, and motivational speakers. Together, they start the mission to rewrite the story of life, but it's more like trying to rewrite a manual in a foreign language with a broken keyboard.

The road ahead is filled with more twists and turns than a mystery novel, and we might even take a few wrong turns, thinking we've arrived at a conclusion but ending up at a different beginning. The story never ends until the caregiver and patient accept their fate.

HOPE, well, it's a vital ingredient that makes every ride worth the wait.

At PRS Neurosciences, we have been attempting to provide hope to people when they think they have lost everything. Here, tradition and innovation converge in an evidence-based setup, constructing a track forward that delivers a comprehensive and holistic nature of healing. It is a journey that recognizes the mind-body connection, weaving together the threads of ancient practices of Ayurveda and yoga with the cutting-edge techniques of modern neuro rehabilitation. In this 'Samanvaya' or synthesis, we discover a comprehensive approach that leaves no stone unturned, addressing not only the symptoms but the very core of neurological disabilities – which is functional independence.

In "Rebooting The Brain®," we are embarking on an exciting expedition of adventure and resilience, a testament to the ultimate power of the human spirit in the face of sudden unforgivable misadventures. Through the poignant stories of the patients, the unwavering determination of the loved ones, and the guiding light of HOPE, we have been bearing witness to several journeys that transcend the boundaries of disabilities. This book is a narrative of those triumphs, an epitome of strength, and a testament to the boundless potential of the human brain (and spinal cord).

We began the chapter by discussing the third epidemic. The moment you hear the word epidemic, you generally tend to relate it with the pandemic. We experienced it for ourselves and had to stay indoors for several months. We faced a shortage of food and groceries since the entire country went into lockdown, and we had no other way but to stay confined inside the four walls of our house. But much worse, during the second wave, we had serious shortages of ICU beds, ventilators, etc.

People died like flies, and nobody could do anything for those who got infected by the COVID-19 virus. Lives were lost, and even those who survived went through a harrowing experience. Ask anyone whose O2 saturation went down and who needed to be put on the ventilator. Many are still traumatized by those events. The hopelessness and helplessness experienced by both the public and the healthcare professionals were extreme.

Now, the challenge about the third epidemic is that it is really hard to come out of that vicious cycle. Your brain, being the most vital organ of your body, has a lot of work to do apart from just controlling your breath and body. You need to take care of it very well. According to my understanding, one-fifth of the accidents across the world happen in India. Why? We are blessed with countless careless youths who are inherently undisciplined. All right, let us not put the whole blame only on youths; it is all because we have numerous careless drivers on the roads, upgraded highways, and high-end cars, but drivers with outdated driving skills.

I feel that we humans are inherently INDISCIPLINED! And careless.

In the past, a stroke, heart attack, or cardiac arrest often meant a dire prognosis and high mortality, with few avenues for treatment. Today, the medical field has transformed, democratized, and brimming with advancements that frequently turn what were once fatal events into surmountable challenges. It's increasingly common to pull patients through such critical conditions, yet we are now faced with the subsequent challenges—survivors left bedridden and profoundly incapacitated. This raises crucial questions about the Quality of Life (QoL) for survivors and their families.

In an era of 'no-time,' living life at a breakneck speed and small family units, the prolonged care of a disabled loved one is seemingly an impossible and daunting prospect. Unlike those on kidney dialysis or living with cardiac blocks who can maintain daily routines with lifestyle adjustments, brain disorders present a uniquely complex hurdle. When the brain—the epicenter of our control and perception—begins to falter, the individual's world alters profoundly, often becoming a heavy burden for their caretakers.

Though humans can perform even with a weak heart, kidney failure (on dialysis), or weak liver, even with 100% of the brain working, it is many times difficult to navigate through this treacherous world!

In a society where delayed digital gratifications or a slow smartphone or Wi-Fi can trigger distress, the patience to care for someone with a neurological condition is scarce. We're all ensnared in virtual reality, often struggling with trivial tech issues, let alone the gravity of a neurological disease. In the rush of contemporary life, the time to care for those with strokes or dementia, *a real reality scenario,* is not a commodity everyone can afford. Thus, self-care and prevention become imperative—no one in the 21st century can afford the luxury of illness.

Like I tell many of my colleagues and associates – we CANNOT AFFORD to fall sick!

As neurological disabilities and disorders rise as the new epidemic, our lifestyle diseases act as gateways, allowing further deterioration of our neural health. The seduction of ignoring conditions like diabetes is strong until they culminate in a 'heart or brain attack.' This harsh reality underscores the importance of vigilance in our health and lifestyle choices.

The brain's misbehavior is akin to a smart device's software glitch, disrupting life in profound ways. A NIMHANS, India study from 2010 highlighted that over four (4) million people in India develop neurological disabilities annually due to traumatic brain injuries, strokes, and dementia. As these numbers grow yearly, so does the burden on our social systems. It paints a grim picture of lost potential, where individuals who could be driving the country's progress become silent statistics.

And these are 2010 stats. Imagine the stats of 2024! Our current demography is our biggest bane! Young, hot-headed, undisciplined drivers with fast vehicles, great highways, and fast food, with alcohol to roost– a fantastic recipe for disaster!

The conversation around these issues is not just about medical intervention but about a societal shift towards patience, understanding, and a proactive approach to health and wellness, and if prevention fails, a focus and investment on comprehensive rehabilitation, recognizing that the true strength of a nation lies not just in the health of its economy but also in the health & functionality of its people.

THE WORLD (AND INDIA) CANNOT AFFORD DISABILITY!

Parents (rich or poor, from developed or developing nations), especially those with children and young adults between the ages of fifteen and twenty-five who are neurologically disabled, often approach me with a heavy heart and one pressing concern: "Doc, once I'm gone, who will care for my child who can no longer tend to their own basic needs?" This question, laden with the fear of leaving their 'adult' child unattended, strikes at the core of a grim reality. In a world where even healthy individuals sometimes feel neglected and being 100% healthy doesn't guarantee success, the stark truth is that once a caregiver is gone, those with neurological impairments are often left 'abandoned' and with inadequate support.

The complexity of the human nervous system, with its central, peripheral, and autonomic components, dictates the level of dependency based on the severity and location of the damage. Neurological conditions like autism and cerebral palsy highlight how even the slightest deviation in neural development can lead to a lifetime of reliance on others. While society is bustling and time is a luxury we seldom have, the duty to care for our kin is inescapable.

All these diseases and disorders are very 'democratic.' They do not distinguish age, sex, region, race, religion, or socio-economic status.

In the realm of neurosurgery, where emergencies demand rapid assessment and 'lifesaving' actions, we strive to address the tangible, the 'hardware' of the brain. Yet, beyond the visible lies the intricate 'software'—the cognitive and functional essence of our being, invisible yet indispensable.

In my practice, we are not just surgeons but restorers of this neural 'software.' Our mission extends way beyond the operating table, and we must tirelessly work to rehabilitate and reintegrate individuals into life as fully as possible. I feel it is a combined social responsibility of the healthcare system, the government, WHO, NGOs, and the corporates – a unique kind of PPP – Public Private Partnerships.

I hail from a lineage steeped in innovation. My father, an industrialist in the 1970s, was a multiple patent holder and recipient of import substitution awards. My aunt holds a formidable portfolio of technology patents in North America, while my uncle headed a team of creative minds who built the Blackberry phone. Adding to this legacy is my sister, a speech-language pathologist in America, who has contributed her expertise to bridge communication gaps caused by foreign accents, authoring a guide to help individuals assimilate more smoothly into diverse linguistic environments. My BIL, a pharmacological researcher and c-suite and business advisor, has strived to improve efficiencies and impact lives.

Together, our experiences underscore a commitment to innovation and care, where nurturing the capacity to adapt through technology is paramount. In this journey, my role is to ensure that individuals facing neurological challenges receive the care and rehabilitation necessary to live dignified lives, even in the absence of their primary caregivers.

However, amidst this legacy of innovation and being a doctor, a grumbling concern emerged within me. I noticed the world has a lot of facilities, but then I could clearly see a critical lack of awareness and facilities to improve the quality of life (QoL) of people once they have survived a devastating health condition. While conventional treatments for stroke or head injuries were administered, patients continued to struggle. They'd express concerns like, "I'm not able to work," "I can't articulate as before," or "I am not normal," despite receiving medical clearance.

It struck me profoundly that while we carefully measure kidney, liver, heart, and thyroid functions, there's a huge absence—a lack of standardized brain (and spinal cord) function tests. We celebrate the successful removal of a clot or a seemingly clear scan, yet patients grapple with residual issues affecting their daily lives. Like a software glitch!

This realization led me to question - why can't we have a universal brain (and spinal cord) function test?

What distinguishes it from other physiological evaluations? It became quickly evident that the assessment of brain function is not universal—since each of us human beings is unique. It's a measure of something inherently essential, something that profoundly influences every aspect of our lives, yet somehow overlooked in the realm of standardized medical evaluations.

This awareness stirred within me a desire to bridge this gap. After all, how can we hope to correct or enhance something we CANNOT measure? Thus, my quest began—to initiate the inclusion of comprehensive brain function tests in our medical protocols, aiming to empower individuals from all walks of life to achieve a holistic state of health and well-being.

Consider fasting blood sugar or creatine levels or liver function tests—they remain consistent across individuals, making standardization effortless. But when it comes to assessing brain functions, it's an entirely different ball game. While an MRI or CT scan might reveal the structures, it doesn't discern between a neurosurgeon's brain, a scientist's brain, or even a construction worker's brain. It merely identifies structures and damages of a human brain but CANNOT delve into the intricate software, programs, and files within each brain – akin to our SMART devices. They all look the same from the outside- iPhone, Samsung, Dell, MacBook, etc; but there is no way to find out what files, folders, software, and apps are installed and saved on the hardware by just looking at the devices. We cannot find the hard disk space unless we go into the depths of each system.

Imagine your child in third grade being taught second-grade material or even advanced fifth-grade content. As a parent, you'd immediately question the discrepancy. You possess a clear understanding of what the third-grade curriculum includes, making you ask relevant questions. Similarly, understanding the nuances of brain function across different individuals is crucial. Just as you know the academic standards for your child, comprehending the intricacies of non-academic brain (and spinal cord) functions that are crucial for our day-to-day interactions with the world around us are not exactly scripted, though appearing standardized within families or small communities – a concept we call "Mass Customization."

Establishing a comprehensive method to assess brain (and spinal cord) functions across its diverse complexities is crucial in ensuring everyone's specific needs are met and addressed effectively.

Understanding the cognitive & mobility levels of a patient post-head injury or stroke is akin to determining which grade level they're functioning at. It's this crucial information that forms the baseline for appropriate cognitive, behavior, and memory therapies.

As a passionate clinical neuroscientist committed to evidence-based practices, I found myself at an impasse. The field lacked a definitive means to gauge a patient's brain (and spinal cord) functioning accurately post-injury. Without this foundational understanding, providing effective therapy becomes a shot in the dark. It's like sowing seeds across a field without knowing the quality of the soil—it's a tough battle, hoping something might take root. Like carpet bombing or mud on the wall, hoping some will stick.

The crucial question emerged: How can I determine where my patient's brain (and spinal cord) functions stand post-injury? Can I also predict their outcomes?? The families and patients want to hear that for sure! Without this knowledge, tailoring appropriate therapies becomes an elusive task, let alone standardization.

We can't afford to adopt a one-size-fits-all approach, especially when dealing with something as complex and individualized as the human brain. This is where I realized that we needed to put a "PPPP" plan in place – PPPP = Progress and Prognosis Prediction Process.

In the realm of neuro rehabilitation, the trio of SEFA, C2C, and RI stands as a pioneering paradigm, revolutionizing the way we assess, monitor, and predict outcomes for patients with neurological disabilities. SEFA, or Self Evaluation of Functional Abilities, empowers patients and caregivers alike with an accessible online tool for self-assessment, transcending linguistic and cultural barriers to provide personalized insights into functional limitations. Complementing SEFA, the C2C framework categorizes patients' functional abilities following brain or spinal cord injuries, offering clinicians a standardized, objective method for tracking progress and predicting outcomes. Anchored by C2C, the Rehabability Index (RI) emerges as a predictive powerhouse, estimating the dynamic relationship between neuro rehabilitation protocols and functional recovery, guiding decisions on the feasibility, duration, and cost-effectiveness of interventions. Together, SEFA, C2C, and RI form a comprehensive suite of tools, driving forward the frontier of neuro rehabilitation with innovation and precision.

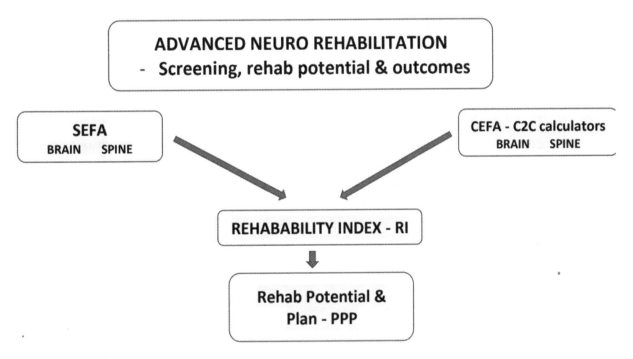

We at PRS Neurosciences have been helping people come out of such traumatic injuries and experiences. We have been communicating with patients from different parts of the country and globally who have reached out to us through word-of-mouth publicity and the World Wide Web. It's a recurring scenario my wife and I encounter—a common refrain from patients: "Why didn't my doctor inform us about your services earlier?" This lament often accompanies a realization that their valuable time was lost in seeking appropriate and targeted care. I vividly recall a lady who approached us three months ago. She lived just a kilometer away, yet it took her a painstaking six months to discover our services. Her husband had suffered a stroke, and they were under the impression that only medication or surgery held any hope, and after that, FATE. They were unaware of the possibilities in rehabilitation, assuming there was no other recourse.

This story is not an anomaly. Many individuals, like this woman, are navigating through a maze of misinformation, unaware that effective rehabilitation beyond medication or surgery exists. The prevailing belief that rehabilitation isn't a viable option prevails among numerous patients. As neurosurgery and neurorehab experts, Dr. Prathiba and I have seen firsthand the dire consequences of this lack of awareness. Patients get written off prematurely, not knowing that there are alternative pathways to recovery.

This is what I keep repeating ad nauseam – the human brain is still an 'old-fashioned' wired model and not

'Wi-Fi' enabled! Even if Google's Sundar Pichai's son is weak in mathematics, he needs mathematics tuition! No medicines will help, and neither can google! Even with all its tech and AI! If Sachin Tendulkar needs to refine his cover drive, he needs to practice for hours every day. He cannot just swallow some tablets, eat khichdi, watch TV endlessly, and hope for it to happen.

What I am trying to convey is simple – when our functional brain (and spinal cord) circuits are weak or malfunctioning, they need to be meticulously reconnected – what we call 'rewiring.'

Neurons that 'fire' together... 'wire' together. This is the simple principle of neuroplasticity.

Yet, we need to add precision and personalized medicine to this science to make it more meaningful for each patient.

Reflecting on all this, I realized the pressing need to bridge this gap in awareness and practice. It struck me deeply that despite being in a city like Bengaluru, the 'Silicon Valley of India,' a hub of medical excellence, most people, including healthcare professionals, remain oblivious to the possibilities of rehabilitation post-stroke or head injuries. Their lack of awareness leads them to medical facilities that might not offer the comprehensive care, precision, and personalized medicine that they truly need.

So, the question arises—how do we reach these individuals? How do we break through this wall of misinformation and ignorance, even amongst the educated and upwardly mobile, and bring hope and awareness to those who've been inadvertently excluded from knowing about available treatments? It's not just about promoting services; it's about ensuring that those who need it most are aware of the possibilities beyond conventional medical approaches. This realization has fueled my mission to not just treat patients but also to educate, to reach out beyond hospital walls, and to inform individuals that there's more to recovery than what meets the eye, that there's hope and possibility beyond what they might have been told.

Like the adage goes – it cannot always be "operation successful, but the patient died." From dependence to independence... it is a journey of 'hope' and 'possibility.'

Hardly anyone sees the patient as a whole and takes complete, end-to-end responsibility for the recovery – both physical and functional. The truth is, even if someone wants to do this, especially in neurosciences, ONE PERSON CANNOT handle all the complexities, and hence, a dedicated multi-disciplinary team was needed to do this. But this team has been trained on different curricula and different psyches, and hence, we need a common framework that helps all of them to think together and coherently with common goals in mind.

In the realm of Brain Analytics, navigating the intricate web of neural data is a complex and nuanced task. To tackle the intricacies, I champion a regimented approach, underscoring the importance of systematic, evidence-based methods in our analysis. In the absence of a disciplined methodology, the deluge of neural data risks becoming uncharted territory, obstructing our quest for actionable insights.

As we sail through this vast ocean of data, sharpening our focus on the desired outcomes is essential. With the rapid evolution of technology and the widespread adoption of advanced devices, the surge of raw, unstructured data becomes ever more imposing. This surge places a considerable burden on clinicians tasked with distilling copious amounts of information into practicable wisdom.

Take, for example, the process involving an MRI scan: the technician conducts the scan, and a radiologist interprets the images, but the ultimate judgment to proceed with surgery or medical line of treatment and the anticipation of the possible potential future complications rests with clinicians like me. The technician and radiologist provide crucial guidance, but the onus to make pivotal healthcare decisions returns to the treating doctors.

MRI reports, brimming with various findings, can often bewilder patients. I endeavor to clarify that not every recorded anomaly calls for immediate medical action. Many details in such reports are documented for comprehensive records, including medico-legal considerations. It's imperative to sift through this information to identify what is clinically significant versus what merely warrants monitoring. This refined judgment aligns with our commitment to a tailored, patient-centered approach, where interventions are thoughtfully considered and dictated not by mere data points but by the patient's overall & holistic well-being.

At PRS Neurosciences, we foster a 'person-centric approach.' This 'person-centric approach' underscores the importance of recognizing individual needs. I often emphasize to my team the necessity of having a method in the madness. To navigate this complex, arduous, and treacherous journey of attempting to restore abilities in the neurologically disabled, I came up with an evidence-based concept that eventually evolved over 5-7 years into a clinical decision-making framework.

Initially, this was called a 'model,' the CAREPa-Re® model *(pronounced KAIRPAIR, said together.)* Then, as the PRS Neurosciences team kept using, understanding, and distilling its various components, we converted it into a 'Principle' and finally, once the idea matured with constant use on the ground and the various processes and protocols were defined based on this 'Principle,' It was then adopted as a clinical 'Framework.'

The 'CAREPa' is predominantly used by the doctors and nurses involved in 'medical & surgical' care of the patients (hyper acute, acute, sub-acute, and even chronic), and the 'Re' is used predominantly by the rehab professionals (doctors, therapists, nurses, and others) involved predominantly in rehabilitation.

Even in the most advanced hospitals in the world, there has been very little conscious and organized attempt to bridge this gap, especially in neurosciences between **the CAREPa** (managed by the acute care neuro specialists) and the **Re** (Rehabilitation – managed predominantly by the neuro therapists).

During this exciting journey, I saw that it clearly broke into two distinct parts –

1. the CAREPa *(pronounced KAIRPA)* and
2. Re *(pronounced RAY).*

Said together, it is now called CAREPa-Re® (pronounced KAIRPA-RAY) Framework

@PRS Neurosciences

Model = Evidence Based Medicine/ Science
Principle = Evidence based Clinical Practice Guidelines (CPG)
Framework = Evidence Based Practice = newro LOGICS

Why? Because modern medicine has got so specialized, super-specialized, sub-specialized, and so complicated that everyone works in silos, and many times, they are running like parallel tracks which never meet!

This framework guides us in synthesizing complex data into a precise and impactful output akin to a laser beam. Let me break down the components of CAREPa-Re® for you:

- **C (Clinical):** This involves understanding the clinical symptoms exhibited by the patient.
- **A (Anatomical):** Examining and understanding the anatomical substrates involved, such as the frontal lobe, temporal lobe, parietal lobe, cortico-spinal tract, cerebellum, facial nerve, optic nerve, etc.
- **R (Radiological):** Utilizing radiological tools such as X-rays, CT scans, and MRIs to visualize, confirm, and understand the areas that are radiologically affected.
- **EPa (Etio-Pathology):** Considering the root cause or etiology of the condition, Ex: is there a cholesterol-induced narrowing in the blood vessel & the pathology – meaning whether this narrowing has eventually resulted in complete block or occlusion of that vessel and has resulted in a stroke – for Ex: Middle Cerebral Artery (MCA) stroke.
- **Re (Rehabilitation):** This represents the rehabilitation aspects of neurological disabilities.

Our standard phrase, "the CAREPa determines the Re," highlights the pivotal role of the CAREPa in shaping the rehabilitation approach. For instance, if the CAREPa indicates Alzheimer's, the Re (rehabilitation) would focus on palliative care. However, if the CAREPa suggests a non-progressive problem, the Re (rehabilitation) could aim for functional improvements, possibly even a cure.

The Re signifies subsequent CAREPa's that may emerge due to developments in the patient's condition, such as infections or other complications. These additional CAREPa's influence the ongoing rehabilitation efforts. If there is a lack of progress in Re (rehabilitation), we recognize that the issue likely lies within the CAREPa. In such cases, we revisit the CAREPa, conduct a thorough analysis using our CAREPa analyzer decision tree, engage in team discussions, and then re-enter the rehabilitation phase. This iterative, constant assessment and adjustment process between 'CAREPa' and 'Re' forms the foundation of our successful approach.

I'm counting on initiatives like videos or any means that can help me penetrate the market and spread awareness. The hope is that these efforts will educate people, directing them toward our approach—employing a unique combination of neuromodulation with new-age evidence-based neuro rehabilitation techniques alongside cutting-edge yet affordable 'Atmanirbhar Bharat' technologies designed <u>for precision and personalized medicine.</u>

The crux of our message lies in the seamless amalgamation of these methods. Together, they allow us to modulate neural function while simultaneously optimizing it. This dual approach aims not just to reduce disabilities but also to enhance overall functioning. Communicating this pivotal message is crucial: neurological recovery isn't a short-term fix. It's a long journey that demands a comprehensive, ongoing approach. It is not a 100-meter sprint but a marathon race with no clear finish line.

I want people to understand that a neurological disability following events like a stroke isn't a word without hope. Even if the initial outlook appears grim, it doesn't dictate the future entirely. Restoration is possible for many individuals, but it's a prolonged journey—one without a clearly defined finish line. If treated well, comprehensively, and completely, the number of such patients who have gone back to their lives is astounding! This concept, however, isn't widely understood. The complications of rebuilding brain circuits, the core aspect of our specialty, remain unknown to many.

Fixing a bone doesn't guarantee normal walking; it's about restoring function—a concept that's at the heart of our approach. Yet, this paradigm shift in understanding the complexities of brain function and rehabilitation remains a challenge to convey to the broader medical community and patients alike. Hence, I have embarked on this onerous task with this book – **Rebooting The Brain®.**

My team and I are not just practitioners; we're ambassadors of this new frontier in neurosciences called FUNCTIONAL NEUROSCIENCES. It's not merely about treating a disease or an injury; it's about guiding individuals end-to-end, from a coma to community or cot to community, on a path toward functional recovery, empowering them to regain control and independence in their lives. But breaking through the barriers of perception and educating people about this nuanced specialty is an ongoing endeavor—one that we are committed to, as it holds the promise of transforming lives beyond measure. When your phone's repaired but still not functioning properly, or your car struggles to run beyond 20 kilometers per hour, it's akin to the experience many individuals face post-stroke or head injury. The functionalities might be limited, and the hope for improvement wanes, leading many to give up on the idea of recovery.

This lack of demand for advanced neuro rehabilitation stems from a broader issue—people are unaware that hope exists beyond initial surgery and ICU treatments. There's a misconception that once conventional medical interventions have been exhausted, there's little else to be done. That's precisely the misinformation we aim to challenge and rectify. We have debunked the oft-said message – let the patient survive first, and then we worry about what comes next. This is not a sequential but a parallel activity. That is why we start our interventions very early. Right from the ICU, on-ventilator patients. We have a concept called keeping the body 'future-ready,' which we will be speaking about in upcoming chapters.

The essence of our approach lies in the combined power of Neuro Modulation with Advanced Neuro Rehabilitation—a method where we modulate and optimize neural function concurrently. Together, they constitute what we call 'Functional Neurosciences'. This tandem effort aims to diminish disabilities and elevate overall functioning. This is the message we're dedicated to conveying—a stroke, a head injury, or a spinal cord injury can't be resolved in a mere five or ten days of treatment. It's a misconception that we are keen on debunking.

We have made a web series titled **'Bheja Unfry,'** which is about the journey of our lives. It serves as a symbol of hope to people who are clueless about what to do after a severe injury. It's another medium through which we intend to communicate that there's a pathway to significant improvement, even when current conventional treatments seem to fall short. More importantly, we want to emphasize that this transformative approach isn't reserved for a select few—it's accessible and affordable. You can watch it on our YouTube channel (@prsneurosciences). We have created a few innovative assessment tests and have also signed up with a dedicated tech team who have been helping us construct a robust platform and also a few advanced neuro rehabilitation instruments that can track the progress of a patient from the comfort of their homes. The following chapters aren't just theoretical stuff, but each of them unfolds tons of surprises and knowledge that you might not have heard of before.

My journey towards becoming a neurosurgeon began in a way that I didn't initially recognize as a dream—it was much more profound than that. The seed was planted back in 1982, around my eighth standard. In those days, my mother used to subscribe to Readers Digest books, and I was an avid reader—something that hasn't changed even now.

This series of articles left a lasting impact on me. It was a section called "Drama in Real Life," where real events were vividly portrayed. I remember one story in particular—it was about a person skiing down the Alps who suddenly lost consciousness and tumbled down. When they found her, she was unconscious, and there were suspicions of a brain hemorrhage. In those days, such medical emergencies and even airlifting patients to specialized facilities were unheard of in India. This individual was airlifted to a sophisticated medical center where they diagnosed an aneurysm in her brain—a term that was new and intriguing to me at the time. She underwent surgery, was cared for in the ICU, and eventually recovered. The story ended on a positive note—' all is well that ends well,' as they say. It's fascinating how this article, depicting a real-life medical crisis and the subsequent successful intervention, struck a chord within me. It was like a window opening to a world of possibilities—a glimpse into a realm where medicine and the human brain intersected in such a profound and impactful manner.

That experience left an indelible mark on my young mind, igniting a curiosity and fascination with neurosurgery. It was then, at that tender age, that I made a decision—a seemingly premature one to others— that I wanted to become a neurosurgeon. The impact of that article, the drama in real life, and the sheer awe of witnessing the human brain's complexity and the possibility of healing within it— it was as if I had found my calling, even before fully understanding what it entailed. So, I was totally hooked on this story, which got my heart racing. I mean, I read it over and over just to relive that crazy adrenaline rush—it was addictively odd but totally thrilling.

Then, I stumbled onto this tale about a top-notch neurosurgeon from Canada. This guy was like a superhero, specializing in operating on kids with brain cancer. They painted this picture of his life, showing the rollercoaster of emotions, the stress of dealing with parents and grandparents, and the ups and downs of surgery. It made me realize, hey, even heroes have tough days, you know? But then, I dove into this article all about the brain itself. It turns out there's a ton we still don't know about. The mystery of it all fascinated me—I mean, we're talking uncharted territory here! That feeling of not having all the answers got me hyped up. I'm all about challenges and uncovering new stuff, so I thought, "Why not become a neurosurgeon and dig into this?"

I was dead set on it—neurosurgeon or nothing! I loved exploring, and the neurosciences bug had bitten me quite well. And the rest is history. In fact, even our company's tagline is – Exploring new frontiers!

By shedding light on this novel concept, we hope to ignite a spark of optimism in individuals who may have given up. It's about instilling the belief that beyond the perceived limits of recovery lies a realm where neural functions can be adapted, restored, and optimized, offering a renewed lease on life. Get ready for an adventurous trip where you will be introduced to some never-heard-before concepts and real-life incidents.

Every day, all around us, we see thousands of young, educated, intelligent people owning 4G or 5G smartphones, zipping around us in expensive two-wheelers but without helmets (the rider, the pillion, and even the children in between). We also see many professional car drivers and their passengers in the front and back seats, traveling in expensive cars but without wearing their seat belts. They are all part of the statistics that I will keep mentioning in this book!

So, wear your helmets, fasten your seatbelts, and drive safely cos you are getting into a neurosciences rollercoaster ride you CANNOT even IMAGINE!!

2

A CHILDHOOD DREAM THAT TRANSFORMED INTO A LIFELONG MISSION

"Take up one idea. Make that one idea your life - think of it, dream of it, live on that idea. Let the brain, muscles, nerves, every part of your body be full of that idea, and just leave every other idea alone. This is the way to success."

- Swami Vivekananda

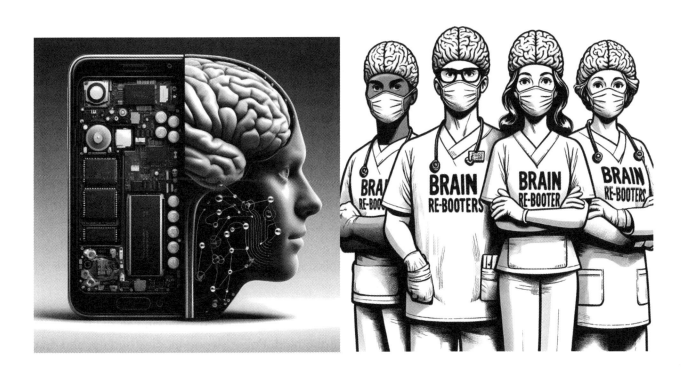

Let me share three patients' stories that impacted me profoundly.

So, let's start by rewinding the clock to 1995-'97, my second and third years as a budding neurosurgeon. There were THREE patients' stories (amongst countless others) that profoundly impacted my psyche and got me thinking.... neurosurgery doesn't just mean surgery, stitches removal, and done! I realized that it formed only a part of the larger picture in the patients' journey of recovery.

Picture this, dear reader- there's this IT pro's dad who faced a brain hemorrhage on the right side, causing paralysis on his left side. He is in this semi-conscious state, and we're trying to work some magic with meds' because the bleed wasn't the "big enough to operate" kind.

He was in the ICU at first, then strolled into the ward. Guess who's in charge of his case? Of course, yours truly, Dr.Sharan! When you're hanging with patients for weeks or months on end, you become good buddies with the caregivers—it's like having a squad. And there I was, the junior guy, making pals in the ward!

One day, the son of this patient asked me if we could repeat a brain scan to see what was happening to the clot. See, we'd learned from our wise seniors that if you don't go digging in to operate on a bleed, it usually dissolves in 8 to 12 weeks. So, when this guy asked me, "Hey doctor, how about a scan to check what's up?" I was thinking, "Okay, let's get that scan!"

Luck was on my side—the clot was making its disappearing act. And there I was, this tiny neurosurgeon in training, feeling like I just conquered Everest. All hyped up, I rush to him, waving my victory flag, like, "Guess what? The clot's gone!"

But then, he dropped a question that hit me like a truck: "So why's my dad still not talking, walking, eating?" Bam! Reality check. That moment, it hit me—physical healing isn't a straight ticket to getting back 'automatically' to normal function.

See, this dude thought that once the clot's gone, his dad's going to wake up, chat, stroll around, and everything's going to be great. I can't blame him because, hey, that's what we accidentally hinted at by not explaining things properly and clearly. He was all riled up, understandably. "Clot's gone. Why's my dad the same?" Ouch! That's when I realized— communication, folks, that's the key. We forgot to say, "Hey, sir, clot gone doesn't mean instant recovery." Lesson learned!

Here is the second event- buckle up for the pre-mobile phone era drama! It's my on-call night, and here comes this chap, a bit tipsy from the drink, who crashed on the road. Police swoop in, pick him up, and dump him at our hospital, no ID, no address... In our world, that's a big "Unknown Patient" label.

Now, our hospital's rulebook's crystal clear: if someone's in dire straits but unknown, we jump into action, no questions asked about family or cash. So, there I am, staring at this man's brain scan—a big clot waving hello. I'm the guy signing off on surgery, like, "Let's save a life, people!" So, into surgery we go, me leading the charge. Post-op, as we're wrapping things up, bam! The family is finally traced by the cops and the hospital squad from some other place.

Over the next month or so, this dude's on the mend—he wakes up, strolls about a bit, and says a few words. But here's the twist: memory problems, quirky behaviors—yeah, those stuck around! Eventually, I send him home, like, "Well, job done!" But talk about a twist?

So, this one day, the wife swings by for a checkup, and out of the blue, she drops a bombshell: "Why'd you save my husband? You should have let him DIE!!!!"." I'm standing there, feeling like this hero neurosurgeon, and then! Her words hit me like a ton of bricks. I'm like, "What's up, ma'am?" It turns out this guy's struggling big time. Alcoholic, wife abuse, the works. Can't handle life, let alone a job! It's a "can't even manage himself at home" kinda situation. She's like, "Doctor, I can't leave him alone to earn for the fam, and now my daughters, they're out of school 'cause we're broke!"

I'm sitting there, thinking I'm a hero for saving lives, but in reality, it's kicked the family into a tailspin. Hero to zero in a snap, who'd have thought? Talk about a plot twist! She dropped a truth bomb that hit harder than a ton of bricks!

She's like, "Look, Doc, if he had died, at least I could've got his job and saved my kids' lives. But nooo, this guy spent all his money on drinks, never cared for the family!" And there I am, thinking being a lifesaver's the top deal. Saving lives might make my day, but for the family, it's just not cutting it.

Here is the third one- this young businessman is newly married, and his wife is three months pregnant. Boom! A bad head injury hits him, and a clot sets up camp in the left side of his brain, the critical speech controls of Broca's and Wernicke's. Now, remember, the left brain's like the boss of the right side of your body and the talky bits, too. Clot is in both speech zones.

The senior surgeon rolls up his sleeves and does the magic surgery and boom, post-op looks like a win—no clot in the brain anymore! He's eventually out of the ICU, off the ventilator, and eventually walked out of the hospital. But hold up! He's walking around but with a glitch on the speech-o-meter. It's like he's in his own silent movie. The wife calls him by name, but there is no response. Kid, no recognition. It's like communication got lost on vacation and never returned. I'm standing there, scratching my head, thinking, "My goodness! What have we done? His entire speech circuits have gone for a toss. We have made him like an animal. Why? Cos, what differentiates we humans from animals is communication, and he was gone!"

These were the THREE patients' stories that really impacted me and got me thinking beyond neurosurgery into the realm of neuro rehabilitation.

The superpower of rehabilitation is not just to make your body move but to make communication and meaningful interactions with the surrounding environment possible. Everything in this world can be divided into two categories- living beings and nonliving beings. As living beings, we humans need to interact with the outside world; it can be with humans or with machines. The world is a beautiful place where humans and machines share a symbiotic relationship. Let me make it easier for you to understand using a real-life scenario. Think about your relationship with your phone. You won't disagree when I say your phone is a machine, would you? All possible outputs from your phone are given below:

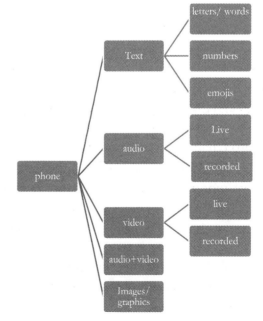

Why are we talking about phones when we're supposed to discuss neurosurgery and rehab? Think of it this way: everything you do on your phone falls into categories like text, audio, video, or notifications, like how your brain processes different stimuli.

When your phone beeps, you look at it immediately, right? It's a simple input (the beep) that prompts an output (you checking the phone). This is like how the brain responds to signals.

Your phone – whether Android or iOS – has hardware and software, and it works through connections, like the neural networks in our brains. Technology is often inspired by the human body.

So, what if your phone won't turn on? You'd try different chargers and sockets until you figure out the problem. It's all about troubleshooting to find the right diagnosis – whether it's the charger, software, or something else. Just like a broken phone disrupts your day, damage to your brain's 'machinery' can impact your life until it's repaired. And even if your phone turns on, if you can't use it because the touchscreen is broken, it's frustrating. Your phone's apps are controlled by its software. You need to know how your phone works to use it effectively, like deleting unused apps to free up space. Understanding the phone's capacity is key to using it well. This is like understanding your own abilities and limits.

Now let us try replacing "Machine" with "human brain."

Let's compare the human brain to a smartphone, which consists of hardware, software, and apps. Neuro rehabilitation experts, like tech experts troubleshooting a phone, need to fully understand the brain's capabilities to effectively assist their patients. When a phone stops charging, we might try different chargers or check the electrical socket—similar steps are taken by neuro specialists who must conduct detailed analyses to pinpoint issues within the brain.

When a phone becomes overloaded with apps and files, it can crash, much like how the brain can become overwhelmed under stress or anxiety, leading to a 'system overload' that manifests as cognitive or emotional difficulties. In such cases, the brain requires 'repairs' or therapeutic interventions, akin to how one might reset a phone or reduce its load by deleting apps.

Moreover, learning new skills, whether it's sports like tennis and swimming or mastering neuro rehabilitation techniques, involves a deep understanding of the fundamentals followed by dedicated practice. For instance, a beginner in tennis learns to hold a racket correctly and master basic shots under the guidance of a coach. Similarly, swimming training starts with overcoming the fear of water and progresses to learning proper stroke techniques and breathing methods. Consistent practice and guidance transform a novice into a proficient athlete.

In neuro rehabilitation, therapists apply a similar methodical and structured approach. They assess a patient's current cognitive and physical abilities, then implement a tailored therapy regimen that might include exercises to improve motor skills, tasks to enhance cognitive function, or strategies to manage emotional well-being. Therapists need to be as knowledgeable and dedicated as sports coaches, consistently applying their skills and learning new techniques to help patients overcome neurological challenges.

This detailed understanding and application of therapeutic methods enable neuro rehabilitation specialists to effectively guide patients through recovery, aiming to restore as much independence as possible and significantly enhance their quality of life.

Steps of becoming an expert in any skill

The human brain is estimated to have 100 billion neurons, and each of these can make 10,000 connections. So, the capacity of the human brain becomes 100 billion to the power of 10,000, literally limitless! Imagine **100 billion^{10000}** . **Wow!**

Let us try to understand the process of becoming an expert at 2 levels – external and internal.

First, let us look at the external aspect: As human beings, when we start learning any skill for the first time, we are all in a state called *'unconscious incompetence.'* This means we have absolutely no idea what the hell is going on and why! And, of course, we also have no clue how to perform that skill. Then, as we start observing and trying, we move to the next stage, called *'conscious incompetence .'* The only way one moves from the first to the second stage is by 'insights' or what we call the 'AHA' moments! Remember the idea bulb you see in comics or cartoons?? That's an idea or insight. Once we have the insights, we start moving to the third stage of becoming an expert, called *'conscious competence .'* This is where we have reasonable competence, but we need to remain constantly focused on the job at hand, lest we 'screw up .' And how do we move from the second to the third stage?? Practice. And finally, the ultimate stage of becoming an expert is *'unconscious competence.'.* And we can only reach this stage with more sustained practice. No wonder the oft-mentioned adage is that practice makes a man perfect! The task of learning to drive a car is a perfect example. In stage 4, you are driving as if in auto mode and talking simultaneously on the phone (with hands-free or car phone, of course!). These steps are what is physically visible from the outside.

Now, let me explain internally what changes occur inside our brains when the above process happens– the internal aspect. Initially, there will be a set of neurons (brain cells) that will make many random connections (synapses) as we progress from stage one to two of skilling. And then, once we get the hang of what's to be done and start practicing, unnecessary movements decrease, and our movements become smooth, aerodynamic, and elegant.

This is stage 3, and here, *'synaptic pruning'* begins to happen. Meaning, for example, from ten thousand random synaptic connections in stages one and two, pruning begins, and eventually, as we reach stage 4 of becoming an expert, most unnecessary and undesired synaptic connections would have withered away, and we may be left with say about three thousand connections to perform the skill!! Amazing, isn't it? No smart device in the world can ever do this as of today!

Now, when you come across patients who have lost all their known skills and come down to square one, the baby phase, where they are unconscious and incompetent, it is difficult to figure out which parts of the functional brain circuits are damaged. The entire discovery depends on the skill of the doctor and the therapists.

This is where our proprietary CAREPa-Re® Framework comes in handy. _Now, the therapist's goal is to bring the patient from unconscious incompetence to nonconscious competence._ You may have to literally walk through fire and back to bring that one beautiful aha moment to your patient. In my opinion, the easiest route that takes you from unconscious incompetence to nonconscious competence is nothing but practice, but in Functional Neurosciences dealing with damaged brain circuits. It is not such simple 1+1 =2 kinda stuff.

Patients tend to slow down due to lack of practice, and they are just as lazy as a four-year-old who doesn't like going to school. They say they will practice from home to skip hours, but they never do that. They become really slow and lazy. They won't do it as rigorously as we do it here in PRS Neurosciences with the guidance of our expert team. This is where we are adding AR & VR-assisted technologies to assist our rehab team in reskilling these patients.

Alright, so let's talk about reflexes. You know, those lightning-fast reactions our body pulls off without even asking for permission from our brain? For example, when you accidentally touch a hot stove, and your hand just decides to take a vacation without consulting your conscious mind, that's a reflex for you!

Now, there's this whole realm of automatic actions, too, but they're a tad different. We call them 'nonconscious,' not reflex. Picture this: you've been practicing a dance move or perfecting your pancake flip in the kitchen. The more you do it, the more automatic it becomes. It's like your body's own autopilot mode kicking in. But hey, don't confuse that with reflex; they're cousins but not the same!

Now, let's venture into the realm of consciousness. When someone takes an unexpected nap without signaling their brain, becoming unconscious, a bunch of conscious senses decide to clock out for a bit. You see when someone's "GCS" (that's our fancy medical scale for checking consciousness) hits eight or lower, things can get difficult. That's when even the rusty old cough reflex starts playing hide-and-seek. In worse situations, the fundamental drive to breathe is lost. And guess what? Asphyxiation (choking caused by lack of oxygen supply) due to aspiration, the not-so-fun game of "Can't Breathe," starts becoming a risk because of this disappearing act, and the oxygen saturation drops dangerously low.

At this point, let me share a trivia about how we manage someone who cannot breathe because of severe brain injury. So, what's the rescue plan? We use the tubes. We're talking about intubation and ventilation! That's our way of safeguarding the airway, making sure oxygen gets to where it's needed most. Because really, no one wants a cough reflex that decides to ghost on you when it's needed most, right?

Remember, it's all about keeping things clear and open in there. Alright, let's unravel the airway mystery! Picture this: the airway, that magical passage for our precious oxygen to reach our lungs and thence to the blood and farthest corners of our body, needs to be guarded like a treasure chest in a pirate movie. Why? To dodge the dreadful duo of asphyxiation and pneumonia.

Now, pneumonia gets its villainous spotlight when the cough reflex decides to take a toll on our patient, all because our buddy, the patient, is unwell. But fear not; this is temporary! Once they wake up from their unexpected nap, that cough reflex gets back in the game, and the threat level drops faster than a hot potato. Lesson learned- never rush to pull the tubes out early. Wait for the patient to regain consciousness and get the ability to swallow! And if things are very slow, then a tracheostomy is called for.

Ready for a fundamental lesson in neurosciences? So, how does our brain play CEO and give orders to the body? Think of it like a message relay race, with the brain as the lead player and the spinal cord as the messenger. Everything the brain wants to share gets couriered through the spinal code— I mean the spinal cord.

Let me share my story of how I decided to become the Brain Rebooter.

As mentioned in Chapter 1, I chased that dream of becoming a neurosurgeon through my schooling, from first Pre-University to second Pre-University. But here's the kicker: I didn't want to leave Bangalore. My sister's hostel life was a totally chaotic scene, with fights over food and insane bathroom lines. I mean, it was so crazy that once, my half-asleep sister started writing on our house walls, thinking she was in that hostel queue! No way was I signing up for that madness—I was all about staying home, soaking in my mom's delicious cooking – rasam rice and all!

So yeah, I chose to live the dream of becoming a neurosurgeon while keeping my taste buds happy. Hostel life and I? Not happening!

So, I did some serious digging and decided I wanted to do my MBBS at Bangalore Medical College—the best in Karnataka. But here's the catch: they only had 155 seats, and a mere 39 were up for grabs based on merit. That meant I had to snag one of those 39 spots, like trying to win a T20 match—you've got a target, and you're all in to chase it down.

My rank was 32 among those 39, and bam! That was my ticket to the world of neurosurgery. It felt like hitting the jackpot—I was on my way to chase that dream.

I spent a lot of time studying not just to get into a merit seat but with a deep and profound ambition to serve the community. I never thought of becoming a doctor because I could make more money. If that were the case, I would now be on the list of highest-paid doctors in the city. My purpose is truly different from what you probably know about the medical industry. Right now, I'm living my dream. I'm treating people with neurological disabilities, and I find a different sense of happiness in doing that.

You know when things just click, and people start thinking you're a wizard or something? It's like, "Whoa, slow down there, I'm no magician!" Seriously, anyone who thinks they're a god must be fooling themselves. We're just regular folks with skills. But here's the secret: if you use those skills for the greater good, something magical happens. Not every time, mind you, but enough times to make us believe in the power of those skills.

I'm knee-deep in helping my patients, and let me tell you, it's not just a job—it's living the dream. It's like finding that sweet spot where work doesn't feel like work anymore. It's like saying, "Hey, I'd do this even if I weren't getting paid for it!" Trust me, it's an unbelievable feeling. It's the kick I get when I succeed in what I love to do.

So, when those new docs stroll up to me, I hit them with the golden rule: "Don't become a doc just for the cash!" But I can see it in their eyes—thinking, "This guy's probably got cash raining down on him to talk like a saint!"

But hold up! I set the record straight: I am not anti-money. However, it's not all about the money. When that phone buzzes at 1 am on a Sunday, and it's not some late-night pizza delivery—but it's a kid needing an emergency, lifesaving brain surgery, I don't sprint to the hospital counting currency. It's about saving a life, plain and simple.

And let's get real: whether that child makes it or not, my paycheck's still cashing in. But if that little warrior pulls through? Man, what does their family get? Priceless! There's no stash of cash that can buy that kind of gratitude.

Money is just a bonus in this lifesaving gig. It's not like snagging the latest iPhone or a fancy kitchen gadget. This is about holding someone's life in your hands, and you can't slap a price tag on that!

You know, here's the thing people often miss: the stress we carry on our shoulders and the risks we take; it's a whole different ball game. Sure, there are some bad apples out there, but painting us all with the same brush? That's like saying all superheroes wear capes—totally unfair.

See, medical education's gone all commercial, just like any other gig. Who's running these schools? Not us docs, that's for sure! It's like someone else is calling the shots, and guess what? Money talks. You have to shell out big bucks for that medical degree, and when everything's about cash, well, how can medicine escape that cycle, right?

I always say healthcare shouldn't be all about money. Imagine if every time you sneezed, someone asked you for a buck. Crazy, right? We've gotta find that balance where saving lives isn't just another transaction. Otherwise, it's like turning a hospital into a vending machine, and trust me, nobody wants that! I have seen investors waiting eagerly in the queue to shake hands with me and seal a deal. But I did not really extend my hand for them to shake.

The quest for a 'compassionate capitalist' amidst this sea of ruthless money makers—I'm always on the lookout! When folks ask me about investing in medicine, I tell 'em straight up: I'm after someone with a heart, not just someone counting coins every three months like it's a game.

You see, I've got patients selling everything from their prized possessions to their livestock, their house, and land, and many married women sell their mangalsutra just to afford treatment. Now, I can't go handing that hard-earned cash to some fat cat swimming in money already. That's just not happening. But when I drop this truth bomb, some people get all gloomy, saying I'm too much of a dreamer, an idealist. I mean, come on, I'm not asking for the moon! It's just about making sure that money's got the right color—it's got to come from the right place, especially in this field.

For me, it's crystal clear—I know how I want to do things, and I'm loving every moment of it. I'm in my 24th year of practice, and I'm telling you, I've got enough fuel to go for another 22 years, fingers crossed! It's not just about me; it's about serving folks and being true to who I am.

But hey, don't get me wrong—I've got balance in my life. I'm not just all about work! There's a whole world outside these hospital walls, and I've got hobbies and downtime, too. You must keep your sanity intact while saving lives, right?

Two critical and unconnected events happened in 1999 when I was in my final year of training in neurosurgery. The first one was in January 1999... I developed a small, painless swelling on the right side of my upper neck/ lower jaw area. Since I didn't have any pain or fever, and I was running around like a mad guy, I would meet my ENT colleague in the corridor and show this to him, take some medications, and well... I just pushed the can down the road. By June of 1999, it had become quite big, and I could even see it in the mirror standing 10 feet afar! But still no pain or fever...but I got worried, met the ENT again, and initially got a FNAC (needle biopsy) done. And this was inconclusive. I didn't stop there and asked for an excision biopsy... and the result of the biopsy was?? Guess?? TB or Tuberculosis! Can you imagine?!?! I was stunned! I had no fever, no cough, no weight loss or tiredness, and all my tests were normal. Basically, there was nothing. Yet the biopsy showed that I had TB! I started my anti-TB treatment in June 1999, and not even three days had passed when two junior PGs who worked under me and were to take their interim exams and needed 'study leave' were denied it by the boss cos he thought that I might be going on sick leave. Both these PGs came to me and literally fell at my feet, and out of sympathy, I agreed to work! Can you imagine? On anti-TB treatment. Such was the intensity of the training and situations.

The second event was around September 1999. Just as I was recovering from my TB, I read an article in one of the leading medical journals on a non-medical topic... but the heading interested me – "divorce rates amongst doctors." And guess which specialty had the highest percentage??? NEUROSURGERY! Unbelievable? I was not surprised as I looked back at my own life and realized that I was heading towards such a grim statistic. Prathiba was already very upset with me, and she'd be like, "If I knew neurosurgery was this wild, I would never have agreed for you to become one!" And there I was, keeping my insane schedule under wraps. Picture this: Monday morning at seven to Tuesday night at 9 pm, Wednesday morning to Thursday night, Friday morning to Saturday night, Sunday morning to Monday night... and this 140-week cycle repeated for nearly five long years! It was like clockwork, but it was madness! But hey, I was diving into the most important part of the human body, right?

I had literally seen my 4-year-old daughter grow 'horizontally' (cos she would be asleep when I left home early in the morning and be asleep by the time I was back). That's when reality hit me—I needed to dial it down.

So, I hit pause, took a breather, and asked myself, "What's my dream future as a neurosurgeon?" The funny thing was, back then, counseling for young guys like me? No, didn't exist. Everyone was in their own zone; there was no playbook for this game. So, I looked around and spotted a few rockstar neurosurgeons—the Sachin Tendulkar of the neuro world. They were like my idols! I thought, "If I could scoop up their skills, catch the breaks they got—now that'd be the jackpot!" That's the real deal, my truth in the neurosurgery journey.

So there I was, standing at the crossroads of life, pondering the future ahead. I asked myself, "Do I like this future?" Well, not really. It seemed like everyone was becoming a slave to their jobs, with no time for themselves or their families. I could practically hear the collective family cribbing echoing in the background.

So, this is when I made a few life-altering decisions that I DO NOT regret to this day. ONE, I decided I needed to reclaim some precious time for myself. No more evening practices for me and no full-time corporate job where I'd be chained to my desk. I needed to keep my battery charged, you know? And TWO, I will develop a very good 'work-life' balance as I do not want to 'burn out.' I am happy to say that I have successfully achieved both, and I am proud of them.

It was the 2010-2011 India-Australia cricket match in Bangalore. Now, I'm a cricket fanatic, so I ditched all responsibilities and spent all five days at the Test match to watch my favorite cricket stars in action! I'm sitting at the gallery, witnessing Zaheer Khan impress everyone with his reverse swing, Tendulkar's double century, and all that jazz.

People were frantically calling me, asking, "Doc, Where are you?" My response? "I'm at the cricket match, living my best life!" They wanted to see me, and I'm like, "Sure, there are seventy other neurosurgeons in Bangalore. Take your pick, and I'll give you the address. But if you want to see me, it's either as an emergency – I'll rush there – or you wait for five days!"

I may not have mastered the art of time management every single time, but I've certainly tried. Life is too short to be stuck in a rut. So, in my quest for balance, I've become the self-proclaimed master of my time. It might not always be perfect, but hey, at least I've enjoyed the ride – and a five-day cricket match!

Alright, let's lay it out—there are five things in life that every soul craves- health, that's the boss. Then we've got happiness, peace of mind, love, and those precious relationships. But people think cash is the golden ticket to nabbing these goodies. Money's cool, no denying that, but these five gems? Not up for sale!

Once you get that, the magic happens. It's like hitting that jackpot—finding that sweet spot where life's all organized, where you're living the dream. And hey, I've hit that spot! My clan, from the family to the grandparents and beyond, are all on board with what I'm up to. We're talking about four generations of Tam-Brahms living under one roof and having a big, happy, joint family party. We recently bid adieu to my 93-year-old grandmother, whom I loved and shared a great relationship with.

I'm loving every bit of what I'm doing. Trust me, when you nail that balance, life's a whole lot brighter!

Now, I want you all to picture this- it's 1994, and I'm diving headfirst into neurosurgery. Now, let me tell you, neurosurgery isn't a piece of cake at all—it's a championship game, a solid six-year training after five and a half years of MBBS. I landed my spot at Manipal Hospital on Airport Road in Bangalore, spending time with great doctors like Dr. A.S. Hegde and Dr. Venkataramana—my first gurus in the neurosurgery realm. I soaked up knowledge like a sponge from those legends! While talking about gurus, I cannot forget Dr. Takaomi Taira. Being a famous Japanese neurosurgeon, he kind of adopted me under his wings, making me capable of performing complicated functional neurosurgeries on my own.

This person? Unreal. I mean, his teachings were priceless. Honestly, if I had nine lifetimes, I couldn't repay them. Their selfless mentorship paved my road, and now I'm all about passing on the knowledge to the juniors. Can't thank these gurus enough for shaping me into who I am today. So, here's this teeny-tiny seed of an idea called 'neuro rehabilitation' in my head, just hanging out, growing quietly. Years fly by, this seed's staring at me, going, "Hey, remember me?" Then, after a decade of staring contests with this idea, it's decision time! PRS Neurosciences—a bright idea that had to be mine to make a reality. It's like my superhero origin story but with more brainstorming and fewer capes!

Ah, the story behind PRS Neurosciences and Mechatronics Research Institute is a tale straight out of a family saga! You see, the "PRS" in our company name stands for a legend—my dad, the great entrepreneur Mr. Puttur Rangaswamy Srinivasan. His legacy inspired me to take the entrepreneurial plunge. And get this—our center's nestled in the same spot where my dad built his small-scale industry.

Neurosciences is like my forever flame. People say my wife's my first love, but nah, it's Neuroscience! Maybe both! I eat, sleep, and breathe it because it's a whole universe waiting to be explored. But Neuroscience can't roll solo. It needs its partner in crime—Mechatronics- robots, technology, and gizmos to help our patients get back on their feet. Neuroscience, Mechatronics, and Research—are like a trio that got lost in translation. They're not talking to each other! And that's the glitch. They need to cozy up, have their daily chats, share ideas, and play nice. Because, hey, teamwork makes the dream work, especially in the world of brain power and robots!

Imagine if I told you we could whip up a groundbreaking product that combines all three—Neuroscience, Mechatronics, and Research—isn't it one ultimate game-changer? Nope, that ain't happening. Why? Because the fancy international products out there are like luxury cars—unbelievably expensive! We're talking about "using an AK-47 to swat a fly" at a pricey level. It's way out of budget for most countries, mine included! So, here comes my typical Indian brainwave: "Gobi Manchurianising" the business was the only way forward!

Now, before you think I'm dishing out food recipes, here's the scoop: Gobi Manchurian, right? That desi-Chinese favorite? Turns out, it's not really Chinese—it's an Indian twist on a Chinese dish! That's what I'm getting at Jugaad, frugalizing and Indianizing. Making things affordable without compromising quality! Yep, you heard that right—cheap doesn't mean shoddy! Our mantra? Bringing top-notch neuro-modulation and advanced neuro-rehab services to every neurologically disabled patient in our country and beyond. Rich or not-so-rich, everyone deserves quality care!

Practically, we can't do such a huge thing all alone. We need brainy docs, fellow NGOs, corporate do-gooders flashing their CSR cards, the government squad, WHO champions, and even heavyweights like the Gates or the Obamas! It's like assembling the armies to fight the Mahabharat war of the 21st century. Against disability. Why? Because the World CANNOT AFFORD disability. Imagine this grand gathering where everyone's RSVPing and ready to pitch in. But here's the catch: What exactly are they bringing to the party? Money? Yeah, that's helpful. But what about the know-how? See, not everyone's got the skills for the main act. So, I realized I had to pave my own way, build my own toolkit, or should I say, "soft-ware," to get these services rolling.

The philosophy at PRS Neurosciences- top-notch neuro rehabilitation and neuromodulation services at prices that won't break the bank with world-class results. Now, I won't pretend we're magicians—100% success rates? No, that's just not happening. But even those who didn't hit the jackpot are doing miles better than before. We're always aiming higher. Tech's our best buddy, with AI, ML, and clinical skills. Well, let's just say we're flexing those to the max!

So, both of us are on a lifelong mission to build a dedicated, well-trained, empathic, and motivated team of "Brain Rebooters." Come, join the gang! The more... The merrier!

TWO (2) orbit shifts – the defining moments in my journey as a neurosurgeon

I had two proper orbit shifts in my life. The first shift happened when I decided to shift from being a 'structural neurosurgeon' to a 'functional neurosurgeon.' This even impacted the way I managed patients in acute care and ICU. The second one occurred when I chose to transition from just neuro rehab to the concept of Functional Neurosciences, which is a seamless symphony of neuro-modulation with advanced neuro rehabilitation. When both these things come together, we obtain the expected functional outcome. While undergoing these shifts, our team builds affordable goal standards that everyone can totally rely on.

SECTION B: NEUROMODULATION

3

THE WORLD OF MISBEHAVING BRAIN (AND SPINAL CORD) CIRCUITS

INTRODUCING, LESIONING v3.0

There is always a method in madness

~Shakespeare

Welcome to the world of misbehaving circuits in the brain and spinal cord…
and how to discipline them!

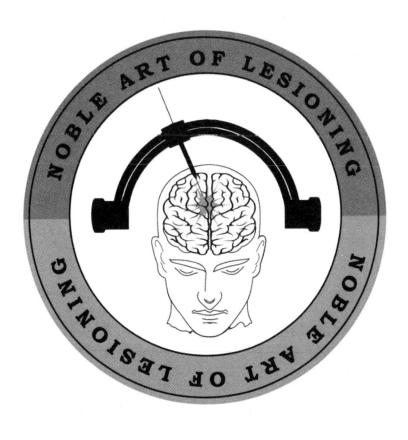

Lokesh – a police 'writer' whose hand just refused to write – a strange case called writer's cramp

Mr. Lokesh (name changed), who was in his early 40s, worked as a writer in the police department. As his work designation says – he was a "writer," meaning his job in the police station was to WRITE! Write reports, write FIRs, write evidence, etc. Fundamentally, all writing work was his responsibility. Around the 15th year of this, he ended up writing many times, over 100 pages per day, some of them in triplicate – meaning, he had to put extra pressure while writing.

About 2-3 years before he eventually met me, he began experiencing some difficulty in writing. He initially dismissed it as some possible discomfort due to overwork, etc., but gradually, it began bothering and troubling him. He felt that a 'strange force' that was preventing him from writing. And his once decent handwriting gradually became more and more illegible. He would have to take breaks while writing, and the task of writing a 5–6-page report became an ordeal. He was taking double time or even more, and it became both frustrating and desperate.

Why desperate? Because his seniors and other colleagues felt that he was bumming off. To overcome this problem and to save his job, he began bribing one of his juniors to write all the reports in his name, and he would only sign them. Eventually, this reached such a severe state that even signing his documents became impossible! By this time, he had met some doctors and a neurologist, and a diagnosis of "Writer's Cramp" had been made. Medications and even Botox were tried, but nothing helped.

He was frustrated and desperate, frequently praying to Lord Venkateshwara of Tirumala for a solution to this 'unsolvable' medical problem when he read about the 'guitar surgery' in the newspapers and saw it on TV (read about the guitar surgery in detail in the next chapter.) He saw some 'HOPE,' grabbed the next bus, and came to Jain Hospital to consult me.

When he approached me with his problem of being unable to sign a paper even though his colleagues were typing the documents for him, I realized the seriousness of his problem and understood his career and reputation were at stake! Dr. Sanjiv CC confirmed the diagnosis, and I offered him the same surgery as the guitarist – an MRI-guided Radio Frequency (RF) ablation of the Vo nucleus of the motor thalamus – what we call a 'Vo Thalamotomy.'

I decided to refer him for a pre-surgery occupational therapy evaluation as usual. Our occupational therapist conducted the initial evaluation for the writing activity and assessed the severity of the writer's cramp. We call it a task analysis. This evaluation includes understanding the task, breaking it down into segments, and correlating it to the performance components and performance context. Let me simplify it!

When the occupational therapist evaluated his handwriting, he realized that the involuntary muscle contraction was restricting him from holding the pen properly to write. Because of the fingers curling in, his alphabet formation and placement of the words on the reference line became as bad as a preschool kid!

His signatures did not match at all, which also became a problem when withdrawing money from the bank. Since this was a new experience for the occupational therapist as well, he was also not sure what should be communicated to the patient after the evaluation as to how the surgery would change the ability to write or what should be done after the surgery!

An interesting finding from the occupational therapy evaluation was that this guy had different levels of difficulty with different types of pens (ballpoint and gel pen), which he frequently used. It was also seen that writing while keeping the paper on the table versus writing with the paper on a clipboard held in hand, either sitting or standing, were two different tasks that required their own remediation! Amazing! The tricks that misbehaving brain circuits can play with us – physically, emotionally, and psychologically.

During the surgery, in the Operating Theatre, the occupational therapist had to periodically perform writing evaluations to see if there were any real-time improvements in his writing as the ablation was being done! To our surprise, his ability to prehend the pen and writing improved! The therapist and the neurologist were convinced that the patient's status improved! This was the start of his journey to recover from this debilitating disorder, which is blind to any radiological investigation and considered a 'supra-cortical problem' by many!

After the surgery, he underwent a meticulously designed therapy plan whereby a combination of a task-oriented approach along with a muscle retraining program targeting the pattern of muscles involved and isolation of each muscle from another, responsible for the generalization of the skill for writing, was conducted!

Over the rehab journey, there was a constant check on how the handwriting was improving. It took 3-4 months for him to start writing legibly, like before the cramps. Whenever he had 'performance anxiety, the previous muscle memory would crop up again, which demotivated him, but with constant practice, he overcame his anxiety and regained the ability to write at work!

He retrieved his functional ability to participate and regained his dignity in his department! His writing is back to 'normal,' and he is back to doing what he does best – work as a 'writer' in the police department.

Kudos to his determination and the success he achieved through a careful combination of neuromodulation and neuro rehabilitation, which I advocate to reduce the burden of neurological disability!

Let's now delve into the fascinating realm of managing misbehaving circuits within the brain and spinal cord. This section explores the intricate process of disciplining these neural pathways, offering insights into the art and science of neuromodulation.

So, welcome medical maestros and curious minds alike to the grand neurological circus. It's where movement disorders waltz through your nervous system. Step right up, and let's unravel the mystery in this not-so-serious but seriously informative chapter!

WHAT ARE MOVEMENT DISORDERS?

You see, movement disorders are like that one uncle at a family reunion who just can't stop dancing, even when the DJ has packed up and gone home. They're a bunch of neurological conditions that make your body do weird things, like the electric slide when you just want to stand still.

Movement disorders encompass a diverse array of neurological conditions that manifest through either abnormal involuntary movements or a lack of typical voluntary movements. These disorders can impact various facets of motor function, including speed, smoothness, quality, and ease of movement.

WHY DO THEY HAPPEN?

While some arise from specific brain damage, others stem from imbalances in neurotransmitters, the brain's chemical messengers. Clinically, pathologically, and genetically, movement disorders represent a heterogeneous group of diseases characterized by deficits in the planning, control, and execution of movements. They are broadly classified into two types:

- Hypokinetic disorders: These conditions are marked by a reduction in movement, presenting as akinesia (limited movement), bradykinesia (slow movement), rigidity (increased muscle tone), and sometimes cogwheel tremors. Examples include Parkinson's disease or parkinsonism.

- Hyperkinetic disorders: These disorders involve excessive movements, which may occur spontaneously, in response to voluntary actions, or triggered by external stimuli. They are often involuntary and encompass conditions such as essential tremors, dystonia, chorea, ballism, and athetosis.

That's some hardcore textbook science for you!

Parkinson's Disease: The Sneaky Bollywood Ninja Redux

Parkinson's disease is like a glitch in the dance routine of your brain's Bollywood blockbuster, causing tremors, stiffness, and trouble keeping up with the choreography, much like trying to follow the beat while the dance moves falter and stumble. Imagine watching an iconic Bollywood dance sequence, but instead of smooth moves, there are unexpected pauses and jerky motions, making it hard to follow the rhythm and flow.

Parkinson's disease emerges from changes in the brain's chemistry and structure, especially affecting the production of dopamine, a vital neurotransmitter. These changes disrupt the brain's ability to coordinate movements, leading to the signature symptoms of the condition.

While there's no magical cure for Parkinson's disease, treatments like medications, physiotherapy, and even dance therapy can help manage symptoms and enhance quality of life. If nothing else seems to work, then neuromodulation brain surgeries can help. Keep reading to know more about this.

Living with Parkinson's demands resilience, but with the support of neurologists and tailored treatments, many individuals find ways to navigate its challenges and continue to groove to life's Bollywood beats, finding rhythm amidst the vibrant chaos of the dance floor.

Dystonia: The Puppet Master's Prank

Dystonia is a disruption in the intricate dance between your brain and muscles, causing them to twist and contort involuntarily, akin to trying to follow a graceful rhythm while stumbling over unexpected obstacles. Picture yourself at a traditional Indian dance performance, but instead of moving with fluidity, your body is compelled to move in erratic and unpredictable ways, defying your intentions, as if some strange power has taken control over your body, akin to black magic!

Rooted in neurological intricacies, dystonia can arise from anomalies in brain function or genetic predispositions. Beyond its physical manifestations, it can erode confidence and impede daily activities.

While a definitive remedy for dystonia remains elusive, a multidisciplinary approach involving neurological expertise, medications, botulinum toxin injections, targeted therapies, or even neuromodulation surgeries to the brain can help mitigate symptoms and enhance the quality of life.

Living with dystonia requires resilience, but with the collaborative efforts of neurologists, functional neurosurgeons, and tailored interventions, many individuals find pathways to navigate its challenges and rediscover harmony amidst life's complexities, akin to finding rhythm amidst the diverse beats of Indian classical music. From head to toe, no muscle is spared.

Spasticity: The Tightrope Tango

Spasticity is like trying to drive a car with the hand brakes on! It is when certain muscles in your body become too tight, making it difficult to move smoothly. It's a bit like trying to dance gracefully, but your muscles feel stiff and jerky instead of flowing with the music.

Imagine doing a traditional Indian Bharatnatyam dance, but instead of your body moving fluidly, it feels like there's a tight rubber band holding you back, making your movements rigid and awkward. That's similar to what spasticity feels like. It can affect different parts of the body, such as the arms, legs, face, or even the muscles that control speech. This stiffness often happens after an injury to the brain or spinal cord, like a stroke, or conditions like cerebral palsy. While there's no quick fix for spasticity, there are treatments available to help manage it, such as therapy, medication, or even surgery.

Living with spasticity can be challenging, but like mastering a dance move, with the right help and practice, many people find ways to improve their mobility and enjoy life to the fullest.

Chronic Pain: The Uninvited Guest

Chronic pain is like carrying a heavy load on your shoulders every day, making it hard to enjoy life fully. It's a bit like the persistent ache you might feel after dancing for hours during a lively Garba or Dandiya night.

Imagine being at a vibrant Indian wedding celebration, but instead of joining in the festivities, you're held back by a constant, nagging pain that just won't go away. It's like having a stubborn knot in your muscles that just won't untangle. Chronic pain can come from various sources, like repetitive stress or injuries, arthritis, or conditions like fibromyalgia. It's not just a physical sensation; it can affect your mood, energy, and even your relationships.

While there may not be a cure for chronic pain, there are ways to manage it and improve your quality of life. This might include treatments like physiotherapy, medication, or even practices like yoga and meditation, which have been part of Indian culture for centuries. Living with chronic pain can be tough, but with the right support and strategies, many people find ways to ease their discomfort and rediscover joy in everyday life, just like finding solace in the soothing rhythms of classical Indian music.

Building a movement disorders practice:

Since 2016, I've had the privilege of collaborating with Dr. Sanjiv CC and his team, a seasoned neurologist and movement disorders specialist with over three decades of experience. Together with the specialized

Movement Disorders rehab team @PRS Neurosciences headed by V. Siddharth, we've delved into a spectrum of surgical interventions for Movement Disorders at PRS Neurosciences. Dr. Sanjiv's journey in specializing in movement disorders in Canada and the US back in 2001 laid the foundation for his commitment to Parkinson's disease and other movement disorders. His expertise spans dystonia, chorea, tremors, and injections, encompassing both medical and surgical management.

In our collaborative approach, Dr. Sanjiv and I kick off with medical management, utilizing a repertoire of drugs and sometimes injections like apomorphine. Should a case progress to a drug-resistant stage, we embark on detailed discussions with patients to explore surgical options.

Our Parkinson's management strategy involves a comprehensive blend of medical treatment coupled with multidisciplinary neuro rehabilitation. Before contemplating surgery, we emphasize sustaining patients with medicines and therapy. Neuro rehabilitation takes center stage in our holistic approach to managing Parkinson's and other movement disorders.

For dystonia cases, Dr. Sanjiv's keen eye identifies the type—focal or generalized—guiding our introduction of drugs. Focal dystonia finds relief in botulinum toxin injections administered once every three months. When dystonia persists despite drug intervention, surgery enters the picture. Procedures such as RF Ablation, aka Brain Lesioning, or DBS, become viable options, considering the patient's clinical diagnosis and financial considerations.

As a dynamic team, we actively engage in surgeries, contributing to the pre-operative, operative, and post-operative management. Our commitment extends beyond the operating room, with a shared passion for educational programs on movement disorders worldwide. Through national and international lectures, an active YouTube channel (@prsneurosciences), and conferences like the Noble Art of Lesioning (NoALCON), we strive to disseminate knowledge and contribute to the ever-evolving landscape of movement disorder care.

In our journey, we've performed 100s of surgeries, including staged bilateral stereotactic lesioning surgery for Parkinson's and dystonia patients, yielding significant benefits for the majority. Additionally, we've successfully conducted Deep Brain Stimulation (DBS) procedures, witnessing positive outcomes in several patients.

Patient selection is at the crux of our work. Rigorous evaluation and meticulous follow-up have revealed a noteworthy 72-80% improvement in specific cases. However, we recognize the reality that, despite our best efforts, some surgeries may face challenges. A remarkable instance involved a patient with task-specific dystonia related to professional guitar playing.

After finding relief through surgery at our center, he not only regained his ability to play but also resumed giving concerts. Another guitarist from Dhaka, Bangladesh, had multi-task dystonia, and he also recovered and is back to performing on stage.

Convincing and selecting the right patients for surgery present formidable challenges, and the choice of surgery must be made with precision. Our pre-surgical evaluations involve the application of various scales. In the operating room, we closely monitor signs, symptoms, and potential side effects. Post-surgery, brain imaging aids in detecting issues, and we tailor medication adjustments and rehabilitation programs accordingly.

Embarking on these procedures is no small feat; it demands mental preparedness to face the challenges ahead. Lesioning involves burning a small part of the 'misbehaving' brain circuits deep inside the brain (>8 cm usually) via a 14 mm hole in the skull.

While DBS entails a pacemaker attached to the chest, continuously stimulating the brain through battery-operated pacemakers and comes with a much higher cost, RF Ablation or Brain Lesioning proves to be a financially feasible alternative, especially for patients with predominantly one-sided symptoms and financial constraints.

Some patients make significant recoveries, attaining a reasonable state of normalcy, thanks to extensive and prolonged rehabilitation programming.

I am proud to say that we are one of the few centers in India and the developing world that is providing such a level of comprehensive care in this field.

HOW IS IT DIAGNOSED?

Diagnosing these disorders involves a neurologist's thorough detective work. Picture it: they're not merely inquiring about your chai intake but delving into the intricacies of your brain and nervous system. It's a medical masala mystery, and instead of the usual suspects, it's your dopamine levels playing tricks on you. It's like a medical whodunit, and it takes many months to even years to unearth the real culprits!

So, how does this neuro-mystery unravel?

1. **Medical History:** The neurologist becomes your medical detective, taking a detailed history of your symptoms and even investigating the family tree for any suspicious movement-related shenanigans.

2. **Physical Examination:** Think of it as your moment to shine – or wiggle and squirm. The neurologist assesses your motor skills, coordination, and muscle tone. It's like a dance-off but with medical precision.

3. **Neuroimaging:** This is where things get cinematic. MRIs or CT scans are the neurologist's way of peering inside your noggin, Sherlock Holmes-style. They're searching for any structural abnormalities, and no magnifying glass is spared. But interestingly, in most conditions, the MRI/CT scans are normal. Can you imagine? This is why, even in the 21st century, astute clinical acumen is mandatory for consistent good outcomes in the Movement Disorders practice.

4. **Blood Tests:** To rule out the possibility that your symptoms are just a result of too many tacos, they'll delve into your bloodstream. It's not a culinary critique; it's a way to eliminate other medical conditions and get to the root cause of the neuro-drama.

5. **Genetic Testing:** For those cases where it seems your genes are staging a rebellion, genetic testing steps in. It's like reading the genetic script to unveil any mutations that might be causing mischief.

6. **Electrophysiological Testing:** Cue the electric quizzes for your nerves and muscles – electromyography (EMG) and nerve conduction studies. It's the neurologist's version of testing your reflexes but with a spark of electricity thrown in for good measure.

7. **Dopaminergic Imaging:** Imagine James Bond entering the scene with a DAT scan. While it might sound like spy gear, it's a nuclear medicine test to check your dopamine levels. For disorders like Parkinson's, this high-tech scan is the secret agent in confirming the diagnosis.

In the world of neurology, solving the case of movement disorders involves a mix of Sherlockian deduction, medical flair, and a touch of James Bond sophistication. The neurologist becomes the detective, the brain the crime scene, and each test a clue leading to the elusive diagnosis. So, next time you're in the neurologist's office, remember – you're not just a patient; you're a character in the gripping tale of neuro-mysteries.

HOW IS IT TREATED?

Now, here is the fun part: the treatment. Medications and neurorehabilitation are the go-to remedy for many of these disorders. For Parkinson's, it's all about boosting that dopamine with meds. It's like giving your brain a double espresso.

Treating movement disorders is like orchestrating a blockbuster circus – a spectacle where neurologists, therapists, and your brain are all putting on their juggling hats. It's a multidisciplinary extravaganza, and each act is as crucial as the next. The treatment of movement disorders greatly varies depending on the specific disorder, its underlying cause, and the severity of symptoms. Some common approaches to treatment include:

1. **Medications:** It's the leading performer and the headliner in this pharmaceutical cabaret. For Parkinson's, imagine medications as the daring acrobats, gracefully flipping dopamine levels to keep your brain's equilibrium in check. Many movement disorders can be managed with medications.

2. **Physical Therapy:** Picture it as the tightrope act – physical therapy walks the fine line, improving mobility and easing muscle stiffness. Physical therapy also reduces pain in some movement disorders. It's the balancing act your body deserves.

3. **Occupational Therapy:** This is the daily-life choreography, helping you regain the smooth moves of functional independence. It's like a dance instructor for your everyday routines. This therapy assists individuals in regaining daily living skills and functional independence.

4. **Speech & Swallow Therapy:** Speech and swallow therapy for movement disorders focuses on improving communication and swallowing difficulties through exercises and techniques tailored to the individual's needs, enhancing quality of life and overall well-being.

5. **Cognitive therapy:** Cognitive therapy for movement disorders is like finely tuning the gears of your cognition, refining attention, memory, planning, and decision-making. It's the guiding hand that helps navigate the complexities of daily life with precision and clarity, enhancing not just your movements but also your overall quality of life.

6. **Botulinum Toxin Injections:** Enter the mysterious illusionist – Botox injections, magically easing symptoms like dystonia and essential tremor. These injections can help manage symptoms of conditions like dystonia and essential tremor. Abracadabra, muscle spasms are gone!

7. **Lifestyle Modifications:** Cue the dietary jugglers, the exercise acrobats, and the stress management clowns. They're the unsung heroes, balancing your routine and keeping your neuro-circus in top form.

Dietary changes, exercise, and stress management can all play a role in managing certain movement disorders.

8. **Supportive Care:** Last but not least, the emotional ringmasters – support groups and counseling. They're the heart of the circus, ensuring you never feel like you're doing the neuro-macarena alone. It's like having your personal cheerleading squad. Support groups and counseling can provide emotional and social support for individuals and families coping with movement disorders.

In this big medical field, managing movement disorders is all about the delicate art of juggling. Neurologists, therapists, and your brain are all key players, spinning plates to find the perfect balance. So, welcome to the neuro-circus – where the goal is not just to keep your moves smooth but to make your grooves unforgettable. Step right up!

The management of movement disorders is often a multidisciplinary effort involving neurologists, physical and occupational therapists, and other healthcare professionals to provide holistic care tailored to each patient's needs.

In a nutshell, managing these movement disorders is like throwing a grand, multi-act circus, with neurologists, therapists, and your brain all juggling for the spotlight – and it's all about finding the right balance to keep your moves smooth and your grooves in check.

Sorting Out Pills and Procedures: How We Tackle Movement Troubles

When addressing movement disorders, we typically start with medication and may consider surgery if necessary. It's like fine-tuning a dance routine: we begin slowly with medication as the primary strategy and switch to more invasive methods if the initial steps are not effective.

Initially, we assess the situation thoroughly. Medications are like the leading actors in our approach, carefully selected to manage and control the symptoms. They play a crucial role in the early stages, aiming to reduce the impact of the disorder and improve quality of life.

However, if symptoms persist and medications become less effective, we consider surgical options. Surgery is approached as a collaborative decision involving discussions with the patient and their support network to ensure everyone understands the potential outcomes and risks. Surgical interventions are seen as the final act in our treatment plan, employed when other methods fail to provide relief. They are meticulously planned and executed, akin to a well-rehearsed finale in a performance. In addition to medications and surgery, neurorehabilitation plays a critical role. This therapy works alongside other treatments to enhance movement control and daily functioning. It's an essential part of the overall management strategy, fine-tuning the body's responses and improving coordination.

Challenges in convincing patients to consider surgery include educating them about the benefits and risks and ensuring they are suitable candidates for the procedure. Surgical options vary: lesioning involves creating a precise burn in a specific brain area and is more cost-effective, while Deep Brain Stimulation (DBS) involves implanting a device that stimulates the brain, which is more expensive.

Overall, managing movement disorders requires a comprehensive approach that includes medication, possible surgery, and ongoing rehabilitation tailored to each patient's unique needs.

WHAT IS NEUROMODULATION?

Neuromodulation is a medical intervention that involves the targeted and controlled alteration of nervous system activity to treat various medical conditions. It encompasses a range of techniques that aim to modify neural signals, either electrically or chemically, to achieve therapeutic outcomes. Neuromodulation techniques are used to manage pain, improve neurological function, and treat certain psychiatric and movement disorders.

Neuromodulation and neurorehabilitation are relatively somewhat neglected specialties, especially in India. They are fields that haven't received enough attention. Take, for example, the United States, which has one-fifth of India's population. However, the U.S. boasts nearly 15,000 neurosurgeons, whereas in India, with five times the population of the U.S., we have only two and a half to three thousand neurosurgeons. The majority of us in India are primarily focused on saving lives, which is undoubtedly crucial. Still, a significant amount of our energy is dedicated to that aspect, and relatively few focus on enhancing the quality of life, especially in chronic situations.

This is where neuromodulation and neural rehabilitation come into play. At PRS Neurosciences, we focus on improving the quality of life of patients and their families. At the end of the day, we find ourselves striving to communicate this message to the public effectively. We aim to reach out to all those who are suffering from neurological diseases, experiencing disabilities, and seeking help.

Decoding Neuromodulation: Tailoring Treatment for Movement Disorders

Neuromodulation, the therapeutic alteration of nerve activity through targeted interventions, offers hope and relief for individuals grappling with movement disorders. In this exploration, we delve into the nuanced world of neuromodulation, particularly focusing on the distinctions between Deep Brain Stimulation (DBS) and Lesioning as treatments.

STEREOTACTIC NEUROSURGERY OR STEREOTAXY

It is a surgical intervention to precisely locate small targets deep inside the brain & to perform actions such as ablation (radio frequency or RF), biopsy, injections, stimulation implantation, radiosurgery, etc., Done by using an external 3D frame of reference, usually based on the Cartesian coordinate system.

FUNCTIONAL NEUROSURGERY

Functional neurosurgery is designed to improve the functioning of patients suffering from debilitating neurological disorders.

This specialized field encompasses surgeries in five key areas:

1. **Movement Disorders:** This includes conditions like dystonia, tremors, and Parkinson's Disease.

2. **Spasticity:** Conditions like focal or generalized spasticity arise from strokes, traumatic brain injuries, multiple sclerosis (MS), cerebral palsy (CP), and similar disorders.

3. **Chronic Pain:** Severe neuropathic pains resulting from brachial plexus injuries, Failed Back Surgery Syndromes (FBSS), or severe cancer pain are addressed in this category.

4. **Medically Refractory Epilepsy:** Targeting cases where epilepsy does not respond to conventional medical treatment.

5. **Psychiatry:** This includes treating severe and uncontrolled conditions such as OCD and depression.

While these disorders may not reduce life expectancy, they significantly impact the quality of life (QoL) and productivity of the affected individuals. Despite advances in medical science, research, and technology, no cure or preventative measures have been found for these diseases. Moreover, except for early-stage Parkinson's Disease, essential tremors, and mild spasticity, many of these conditions lack effective medical treatments for symptom management.

Functional neurosurgery plays a crucial role in providing relief and enhancing the lives of patients when other treatments fall short.

DBS VS. LESIONING v3.0:

Unraveling The Contrasts

Deep Brain Stimulation (DBS): DBS involves the insertion of an electrode into the brain, intricately connected to an Impulse Generator (IPG). This method selectively stimulates a targeted part of the nucleus, engendering the desired therapeutic effects. Notably, DBS allows for the simultaneous treatment of both sides of the brain. DBS, a more recent innovation since the mid-1990s, revolutionized movement disorder treatment.

This method entails implanting a pacemaker in the brain to modulate neural activity and alleviate symptoms. The inception of DBS was prompted by the limitations and complications associated with lesioning surgeries, primarily the destruction of specific brain circuits.

Lesioning v3.0: Lesioning has been a treatment option for movement disorders for a long time, over six decades in fact. It has undergone many a metamorphosis, as medical science and technologies evolved. I have broadly classified them into three versions.

Version v1.0: The pre-CT scan, ventriculography era.
Version v2.0: The early CT scan/ MRI era
Version v3.0: The post DBS era.

Proper patient selection and individualized treatment are crucial for successful lesioning outcomes. Some cases have shown better results with lesioning compared to DBS when performed correctly and in selected cases. Lesioning is proven to yield good results when properly executed.

Lesioning, in contrast, employs radiofrequency ablation or controlled burning of a specific brain area to achieve similar therapeutic results. Unlike DBS, lesioning is confined to treating one side of the brain. Crucially, lesioning stands out for not requiring a permanent implant, offering a distinctive advantage over DBS.

Evolutionary Insights: A Historical Perspective

The historical evolution of neuromodulation techniques reveals the dynamic interplay between lesioning and DBS. Lesioning surgeries, initially embracing small burning procedures, found renewed interest with the advent of DBS. The reversibility introduced by DBS not only transformed treatment approaches but also enhanced the understanding of brain anatomy, influencing and refining lesioning techniques positively, leading to the current avatar of Lesioning, what we call the Lesioning v3.0!

Comparison of DBS and Lesioning v3.0

Aspect	Deep Brain Stimulation (DBS)	Lesioning v3.0
Technological Advancements	DBS involves complex hardware, with rechargeable and non-rechargeable batteries, contributing to increased costs and procedural intricacies.	Lesioning surgeries have evolved from basic procedures to non-invasive options, adapting to technological progress.
Cost Considerations	DBS can be financially burdensome, with hardware costs ranging from 7 to 16 lakhs, depending on the type of battery used.	Lesioning surgeries are often perceived as more cost-effective, making them a potential alternative for those with budget constraints.
Indications and Uses	DBS is best indicated for bilateral symptoms in progressive diseases like Parkinson's or generalized dystonia, where continuous programming can adapt to disease progression. It is not the treatment of choice for FHD, one-side symptoms, etc.	Lesioning surgeries are considered for non-progressive diseases affecting one side of the body when medication fails. Also, bilateral surgeries are possible but better staged. Also, for FHD, it is the treatment of choice.
Mechanism	Involves placing an electrode in the brain connected to an impulse generator (IPG).	Involves radiofrequency ablation or burning of a targeted area or nucleus.
Stimulation Target	Stimulates a specific part of the nucleus to produce the desired effect.	Ablates or burns the targeted area or nucleus.
Treatment Area	Both sides of the brain can be treated	Limited to one side of the brain

	simultaneously.	usually but in skilled hands and in a staged manner, bilateral surgeries are possible and being done regularly globally.
Implant Requirement	Requires a permanent implant (IPG) throughout life.	Does not involve any permanent implants.
Reversibility	Reversible – adjustments can be made to the stimulation parameters.	Generally irreversible once the lesion is created.
Adjustability	Allows for adjustments in stimulation parameters to optimize treatment.	Treatment is typically fixed after lesion creation.
Management of Symptoms	Produces therapeutic effects by modulating neural activity. However, optimal results depend on the precision of electrode placement and abnormal responses of the adjacent brain to the stimulation.	Achieves similar results by eliminating or disrupting neural activity in the lesioned area.
Applicability	Widely used for various movement disorders like Parkinson's disease, essential tremor, etc.	Widely used for various movement disorders like Parkinson's disease, essential tremors, etc.
Safety and Risks	Both surgeries involve brain interventions but carry different risks. Safety considerations depend on the patient's specific condition and other factors.	

LESIONING v3.0

Lesioning Surgeries: A Historical Perspective

Lesioning surgeries have a venerable history, originating in the 1950s as a method to address movement disorders. The technique involves selectively destroying specific brain circuits associated with abnormal motor functions.

Over time, lesioning has evolved, with the latest iteration, version 3.0, representing the post-DBS era. Technological advancements have introduced non-invasive lesioning options like gamma knife and focused ultrasound, offering more flexibility in treating neurological issues.

Lesioning, a longstanding option in movement disorder treatment, has traversed decades as a reliable intervention. The key to its success lies in meticulous patient selection and the art of individualized treatment. As evidenced, certain cases have demonstrated superior outcomes with lesioning, outshining even the widely recognized Deep Brain Stimulation.

Lesioning's Financial Viability: Lesioning is considered financially viable, especially in developing economies and those living in remote geographies, presenting itself as a potentially cost-effective alternative. Its appeal lies in avoiding permanent implantation, a factor that can significantly reduce overall treatment expenses.

Advantages and Limitations: Lesioning is considered financially viable and avoids permanent implantation, making it a potentially cost-effective option. Lesioning surgeries can be planned in ways that the DBS stimulator can also be placed in the future. DBS, being reversible, allows for adjustments and removal, offering flexibility in treatment.

Choosing the Right Treatment: The choice between DBS and lesioning depends on factors such as the case, tailoring, surgical experience, precision, and the type of movement disorder. Both DBS and lesioning are viewed as valid treatment options, and one is not inherently better than the other. The decision on which treatment to use depends on individual cases and the specific requirements of the patient.

Choosing Wisely: Tailoring Treatment to the Individual: The crux of successful neuromodulation lies in the careful consideration of various factors. The choice between DBS and lesioning is a delicate decision, dependent on elements such as the specific case, tailoring requirements, surgical experience, precision, and the nature of the movement disorder at hand. It is crucial to understand that neither DBS nor lesioning is inherently superior; each has its unique advantages and limitations.

The landscape of neuromodulation for movement disorders is dynamic and multifaceted. By embracing individualized approaches and acknowledging the distinctive merits of both DBS and lesioning, healthcare professionals can navigate the complexities of treatment, offering tailored solutions that prioritize the unique needs and circumstances of each patient.

HOW DOES NEUROMODULATION HELP?

Neuromodulation helps by altering neural activity in a specific and controlled manner. The mechanisms behind its effectiveness can vary depending on the technique used, but the primary goals include:

1. **Pain Management:** Neuromodulation is often used to alleviate chronic pain, such as neuropathic pain, back pain, or migraine. By targeting and modifying pain pathways, it can provide relief when other treatments have been ineffective.

2. **Neurological Disorders:** In conditions like epilepsy, depression, or obsessive-compulsive disorder, neuromodulation techniques can help regulate abnormal neural activity, reducing symptoms and improving overall quality of life.

3. **Movement Disorders:** Neuromodulation can be employed to address movement disorders like Parkinson's disease or essential tremor. By stimulating or modulating specific brain regions, it can alleviate motor symptoms.

4. **Bladder and Bowel Dysfunction:** For individuals with urinary or fecal incontinence, neuromodulation can be used to modulate nerve signals to control bladder or bowel function.

There are several approaches to neuromodulation, which can broadly be categorized into pharmacological methods, bedside procedures (sometimes involving chemo denervation), and surgical techniques with or without device implantation.

Pharmacological Neuromodulation:

Pharmacological neuromodulation involves using medications to alter neural activity. This approach may include the use of medications that affect neurotransmitter levels, receptor activity, or ion channel function. For example:

1. **Antidepressants and Anxiolytics:** These drugs can modulate neural activity and are used to treat depression, anxiety, and other mood disorders.

2. **Antiepileptic Medications:** These drugs help control abnormal electrical activity in the brain, reducing the frequency and severity of seizures in epilepsy.

3. **Pain Medications:** Opioids and non-opioid pain medications can modulate pain pathways, providing relief in various pain conditions.

4. **Bedside Procedures with or without Chemodenervation:** Bedside procedures involve non-surgical interventions that can be performed in a clinical setting. They may include:

   a. **Nerve Blocks:** Injecting anesthetic agents near specific nerves to block pain signals and provide short-term pain relief.

   b. **Botox Injections:** Botulinum toxin (Botox) can be used to chemodenervate specific muscles, reducing muscle spasms in conditions like spasticity, dystonia, or even chronic migraines.

CLEARING MYTHS ABOUT STEREOTACTIC & FUNCTIONAL NEUROSURGERY

Myth 1: Stereotactic Surgery is a New and Unproven Technique

This myth is not true. Stereotactic surgery has a rich history dating back to the early 20th century. Over the years, it has evolved and gained greater precision, thanks to advancements in imaging technology, such as MRI and CT scans. Numerous clinical studies have shown the safety and efficacy of stereotactic surgeries for various neurological conditions, including brain tumors, movement disorders, and chronic pain.

Myth 2: Stereotactic Surgery is Only for Brain Tumors

Stereotactic surgery is not limited to brain tumor treatment. While it is widely used for tumor removal, it has a broader range of applications. It is employed for the treatment of epilepsy, Parkinson's disease, essential tremors, and even psychiatric conditions like obsessive-compulsive disorder. Stereotactic radiosurgery, a non-invasive variant, is also used for conditions like arteriovenous malformations and trigeminal neuralgia.

Myth 3: Stereotactic Surgery is Riskier Than Conventional Surgery

Stereotactic surgery is known for its precision and minimally invasive nature. The use of highly detailed imaging and computer guidance reduces the risk of damaging healthy tissue. This precision often leads to fewer complications and a quicker recovery compared to traditional open surgery. However, like any medical procedure, there are inherent risks, and the suitability of stereotactic surgery depends on the patient's specific condition and medical history.

Myth 4: Stereotactic Surgery is Extremely Expensive

Stereotactic surgeries can be expensive, but their cost varies widely depending on the specific procedure, location, and healthcare system. While the technology and expertise required may drive up the cost, it is essential to consider the long-term benefits. Stereotactic surgery often leads to shorter hospital stays, reduced rehabilitation needs, and improved outcomes, which can offset initial costs.

Myth 5: Stereotactic Surgery Replaces the Need for Traditional Open Surgery

Stereotactic surgery is not a one-size-fits-all solution and may not replace traditional open surgery in all cases. It is a valuable tool for specific conditions where precision and minimally invasive approaches are advantageous. However, open surgery may still be necessary for certain complex cases or when the target area cannot be adequately reached with stereotactic methods.

Stereotactic surgery is a well-established and effective approach in the field of neurology and neurosurgery. Many myths surrounding this technique are based on misconceptions, and healthcare professionals must stay informed about the latest advancements and clinical evidence to make informed decisions about its use. Stereotactic surgery is a valuable tool in the neurologist's and neurosurgeon's arsenal, offering precise and minimally invasive solutions for a wide range of neurological conditions.

Navigating the Complex Realities of Movement Disorders

Movement disorders present a complex challenge involving various treatments and the ongoing difficulties faced by patients. As part of the neuromodulation and neuro rehabilitation team, it's vital to recognize the diverse impacts of these conditions on individuals.

Occupational therapists see first-hand the physical struggles and emotional distress that patients and their families endure. Patients may deal with excessive movements or severe movement restrictions, leading to muscle atrophy and physical decline. Nutritional issues are common, with many patients experiencing difficulty swallowing and reduced appetite, which compromises their health. Symptoms often worsen at night, disrupting sleep and increasing psychological strain.

As movement disorders progress, the loss of independence in basic activities can diminish a person's quality of life, adding emotional and financial strain to families. This deep, personal struggle impacts not just the patient but their entire support network, highlighting the importance of comprehensive care in managing these conditions.

The Intersection of Culture, Economics, and Therapeutic Challenges in Movement Disorders

The complexities of managing movement disorders extend beyond the clinic into cultural and economic spheres. In India, cultural norms often encourage enduring pain quietly, leading individuals to avoid seeking medical help even when necessary. This cultural tendency contributes to delayed diagnoses and worsened health outcomes.

Economically, the cost of treatment poses a significant barrier. Most expenses for rehabilitation are out-of-pocket, with insurance companies frequently reluctant to provide coverage due to the unpredictable nature of movement disorders. This financial burden makes accessing necessary care challenging for many.

Despite these hurdles, the role of neurologists is crucial. They diagnose and collaborate with specialists like speech-language pathologists, physical therapists, and increasingly recognized occupational therapists to provide comprehensive care. Yet, there's a constant struggle between addressing symptoms and achieving functional recovery.

Communication between therapists and referring physicians is vital. Developing a common language—or a metaphorical API—helps bridge gaps in understanding and ensures a more cohesive treatment approach. This collaboration is essential for navigating the complex interplay of cultural, economic, and therapeutic factors in movement disorder care.

Harmonizing Expertise: A Holistic Model for Movement Disorder Management

In addressing movement disorders, a collaborative care model has been developed by a team including Dr. Sanjiv CC, a noted movement disorder specialist; Mr. V. Siddharth, an Advanced Neuro Rehabilitation Specialist; and myself, Dr. Sharan Srinivasan, a functional neurosurgeon. This model integrates neuromodulation and neuro rehabilitation, taking into account economic and cultural factors to ensure treatments are accessible and appropriate for each patient. For Parkinson's disease, we employ the Levodopa Challenge Test using the Unified Parkinson's Disability Rating Scale to assess the patient's response to medication, which helps determine suitability for surgical options. For dystonia, severity assessments are customized to the type of dystonia, providing a clear picture of each case.

This approach also involves a detailed analysis of daily activities to identify specific challenges faced by patients, which guides targeted neurorehabilitation strategies. By combining diverse expertise and understanding patient-specific contexts, this model exemplifies a comprehensive and evolving approach to movement disorder management, emphasizing personalized care and interdisciplinary collaboration.

Navigating Treatment Choices: A Patient-Centric Approach

The intricate dance between conservative management, neurorehabilitation, and functional stereotactic neurosurgery is steered by a meticulous decision-making algorithm. As part of the collaborative triad, consisting of a stereotactic neurosurgeon, a movement disorder specialist, and an ANRS, our focus is not merely on alleviating symptoms but on sculpting a personalized path to optimal functionality.

The initial hurdle lies in evaluating the severity of the patient's limitations. This involves scrutinizing various scores, each with its unique cutoff values. The amalgamation of neurologist, neurosurgeon, and occupational therapist experiences refine the understanding of the patient's condition.

Three pivotal questions guide our decision-making process:

1. **Severity Assessment:** Determining the seriousness of the patient's initial limitations sets the tone for subsequent interventions. Cutoff values, clinical experience, and nuanced understanding play crucial roles in this phase.

2. **Conservative vs. Surgical Management:** Assessing whether conservative management suffices or if surgical intervention is warranted demands a multifaceted approach. Patients naive to previous treatments or those who haven't explored conservative options undergo scrutiny to ascertain the most appropriate course.

3. **Expectations vs. Success Metrics: Setting Realistic Goals:** When managing movement disorders, it's crucial to have an open and realistic dialogue with patients to set achievable expectations. We aim for transparency, usually setting a success threshold of about a 40% improvement to maintain realistic expectations. However, our experience shows that over 75% of our patients see more than 80% improvement in their symptoms and a significant boost in their quality of life (QoL). *We operate on the principle of underpromising and overdelivering, which helps manage both patient and family expectations effectively in the complex realm of neurological disorders.*

For those opting for non-surgical management, we provide a tailored mix of multidisciplinary neuro rehabilitation interventions, medication adjustments, and task modifications.

Patients choosing functional stereotactic neurosurgery undergo thorough pre-operative and intra-operative evaluations, including video recordings and assessments by an Advanced Neuro Rehabilitation Specialist (ANRS). These evaluations serve as benchmarks for measuring postoperative improvements.

The use of video in evaluations is more than just for record-keeping; it's a powerful tool for demonstrating the transformative effects of our interventions. For example, a tailor suffering from debilitating Parkinson's Disease was filmed from a state of despair to a renewed sense of hope, showcasing the personalized impact of neuro rehabilitation and surgery.

Our patient-centric approach integrates expertise from various disciplines, forming a flexible framework that adapts to the unique needs, goals, and challenges of each patient, ensuring their priorities guide their treatment journey.

Deciphering the Decision-Making Algorithm: Balancing Severity, Conservative Management, and Surgical Prospects

The decision-making process within our collaborative triad is an intricate dance that balances the gravity of the patient's condition, the feasibility of conservative management, and the potential need for surgical intervention.

1. **Severity Assessment:**

   - Multifaceted Evaluation: The first step involves a comprehensive evaluation of the patient's initial limitations. Different scores, each with its cutoff values, become the bedrock of this assessment.

   - Diverse Experiences: The amalgamation of experiences from the neurologist, neurosurgeon, and ANRS refines the understanding of the patient's unique condition.

   - Outcome Expectations: The collaborative team endeavors to predict the kind of changes that can be anticipated based on the severity assessment.

2. **Conservative Management Feasibility:**

   - Bootstrapping Sessions: For patients who haven't undergone sufficient conservative treatments or medical management, a crucial question arises: can we still navigate with conservative approaches, or is the transition to more in-depth evaluations imperative?

   - Syndrome-Naive Patients: Those unfamiliar with standard medications like levodopa present a unique set of considerations requiring a nuanced evaluation. The decision-making algorithm contemplates the potential efficacy of these treatments.

3. **Surgical Management Considerations:**

   - Elective vs. Emergency: A pivotal question arises regarding the necessity of surgical intervention. It is clarified that this isn't about emergency surgeries; rather, elective surgery.

   - Functional Evaluation: The focus shifts to whether surgery is indispensable for restoring functionality. The decision-making process delves into the pros and cons of surgical intervention.

   - Post-Surgery Rehabilitation: Crucially, considerations extend beyond the surgical procedure itself. The team contemplates whether the patient can afford and commit to neuro rehabilitation post-surgery, recognizing its integral role in the holistic treatment plan.

In essence, the decision-making algorithm navigates through a labyrinth of factors, carefully considering the severity of the patient's condition, the viability of conservative approaches, and the potential implications of surgical interventions. This multifaceted approach, shaped by collaborative expertise, ensures that each patient's therapeutic journey is tailored to their unique needs and circumstances.

Navigating Success and Rehabilitation: A Patient's Journey through Dystonia and Surgery

In a compelling narrative, an occupational therapist recounts a poignant case of a software engineer grappling with focal hand dystonia. After undergoing surgery, the patient found himself adrift, attempting retraining with a therapist who lacked a comprehensive understanding of dystonia, the surgery's impact, and nil experience in handling a patient who has dystonia or operated for the same.

1. **The Challenge of Muscle Memories:**

- Unfulfilled Retraining: The software engineer's attempt at retraining post-surgery proved futile. The therapist, unaware of the nuances of dystonia, couldn't unlock the desired results.

- Persistent Muscle Memories: The therapist educates the patient on the persistence of muscle memories, emphasizing that even after surgery, neural pathways hold onto established patterns. This insight underscores the imperative need for neuro rehabilitation.

2. **Setting Realistic Expectations:**

- Managing Patient Expectations: The team adopts a cautious approach when discussing success rates, refraining from promising more than 40%. Patient participation becomes a pivotal factor, acknowledging the dynamic nature of individual commitment.

- Crucial Role of Rehabilitation: Emphasizing the criticality of rehabilitation, especially for younger patients, the team strives to ensure that those opting for surgery are willing to commit to the rehabilitation process post-surgery.

3. **Decision-Making Crossroads:**

- Conservative Management vs. Surgery: Let's delve into the considerations patients face when choosing between conservative management and functional stereotactic neurosurgery. This decision hinges on factors such as severity, potential for rehabilitation, and the feasibility of each option.

- Pre-Op Evaluation: The meticulous evaluation process involves a thorough pre-operative assessment, ensuring that all relevant aspects are considered before proceeding with surgery.

4. **Monitoring Functionality during Surgery:**

- ANRS Role: During surgeries, particularly stereotactic neurosurgery, the ANRS plays a crucial role. Their comprehensive evaluation aids in monitoring functionality, providing real-time feedback to the neurosurgeon and neurologist.

- End-to-End Understanding: The ANRS involvement grants an end-to-end understanding of the patient's progression, allowing them to detect any variations or worsening of functionality during the surgical procedure.

5. **Post-Surgery Rehabilitation:**

- Repeating Core Evaluations: Post-surgery, a series of evaluations and measurements help gauge the effectiveness of the intervention.

-Advanced Neurorehabilitaton Team's Role: The role shifts to targeted interventions, focusing on performance areas and contextualizing the benefits. Training regimens are customized based on the patient's specific needs, addressing both motor functions and skills.

A Tailor's Journey: (scan the QR code at the end of the book to see his videos and his journey)

Let me introduce to you the case study featuring a tailor, a poignant example of a young individual facing debilitating symptoms due to Parkinson's Disease.

The tailor's journey, from initial evaluation to surgical intervention and rehabilitation, exemplifies the intricate and impactful nature of the collaborative approach.

A 40-year-old tailor from Bengaluru named Shivanna grappled with the onset of Parkinson's disease at 38. His initial symptoms, starting with mild tremors in his left hand, gradually escalated to encompass his entire body over two years, significantly impacting his ability to work and perform daily tasks. As the disease progressed, Shivanna found himself unable to continue his livelihood as a tailor, which was the primary source of income for him and his family.

Seeking medical assistance, Shivanna consulted neurologists who prescribed conventional treatments, albeit with temporary relief and unpredictable effectiveness due to the on-and-off nature of Parkinson's medications. After years of struggling with the disease, which had significantly impacted his Quality of Life, Shivanna was recommended for Deep Brain Stimulation (DBS) surgery, a common procedure for Parkinson's patients. However, the exorbitant cost of the surgery, ranging from 15-20 lakh rupees, proved to be a significant barrier for Shivanna, who was financially disadvantaged.

Despite efforts to secure funding through government aid, Shivanna faced numerous obstacles and delays, exacerbating his condition and leading to a deterioration in his quality of life. Eventually, Shivanna was referred to me by the local MLA, and my medical team explored alternative surgical options, considering the feasibility and affordability of Shivanna's circumstances. They opted for a low-cost lesioning procedure targeting the right side of his brain, Pallidotomy, which showed promising results in alleviating his symptoms and restoring a significant degree of functionality to his left side and near total alleviation of his symptoms.

However, as time passed, Shivanna experienced a resurgence of symptoms on his left side, prompting further medical intervention. Amidst the challenges posed by the COVID-19 pandemic and associated lockdowns, Shivanna underwent a groundbreaking surgery known as Pallido-Thalamic tractotomy, also called PTT, a procedure previously unheard of in India but recognized internationally for its efficacy in treating Parkinson's symptoms.

Performed as a bilateral procedure, this surgery marked a significant milestone in Shivanna's treatment journey, offering hope for Parkinson's patients across the country. Not only did it provide relief from debilitating symptoms, but it also offered a more affordable alternative to traditional DBS surgery, making it accessible to a wider population, particularly those from economically disadvantaged backgrounds. He is probably the first ever patient in India to have undergone staged bilateral Lesioning v3.0 surgery to manage the motos symptoms of his PD.

Following the successful surgery, Shivanna experienced a remarkable improvement in his condition, with symptoms on both sides of his body significantly reduced, the on-off phenomena disappeared 100%, and he was back to his tailoring and other jobs. With renewed confidence and functionality, Shivanna embarked on a journey toward recovery, empowered by the innovative medical interventions that had transformed his life. As the first patient in India to undergo bilateral lesioning surgeries for Parkinson's disease symptoms and benefit from the Pallido-Thalamic tractotomy, also called the PTT procedure, Shivanna's story serves as a beacon of hope and inspiration for countless others grappling with similar challenges.

Empathy in Action: Farmer's Son and the Struggle for Functional Independence (scan the QR code at the end of the book to see his videos and his journey)

One of my ANRSs specialized in Movement disorders looked over the case of a 29-year-old farmer's son, a once-intelligent individual, who began experiencing involuntary movements. What initially seemed unusual in a village context escalated into severe retrocollis, progressing to generalized dystonia across his body. The depth of the clinician's empathy shines through as they recount the patient's profound challenges.

In the heart of a quaint town cradled by rolling hills, a young man battled a relentless foe—dystonia. What began as a slight tremor in his neck swiftly morphed into a merciless onslaught, with involuntary movements tightening their grip over his entire being.

Amidst the tumult of his worsening condition, a glimmer of hope emerged—a deep brain stimulator (DBS) implant. With cautious optimism, he underwent the procedure, clutching onto the promise of reprieve. Yet, fate dealt a harsh blow as the DBS battery faltered prematurely, leaving him with only a fraction of the relief he had hoped for.

However, hope often dims in the face of stark reality. For his family, burdened by economic hardship, the notion of replacing the depleted DBS battery loomed like an insurmountable obstacle. Their son's suffering served as a stark reminder of the gaping disparities that afflict society, where access to essential healthcare remains a privilege reserved for the fortunate few.

As days stretched into weeks and weeks into months, the young man found himself at a crossroads—his journey fraught with uncertainty. The removal of the dead DBS marked a pivotal moment, stripping away the false hope it had once provided. With its removal came a harsh reality—the loss of control over his movements, a stark reminder of the uphill battle ahead. And in place of that, he underwent simultaneous, bilateral pallidotomy. More details in chapter 7 on dystonia.

In the dimly lit corridors of the rehabilitation center, a new chapter unfolded—a testament to the resilience of the human spirit. Here, amidst the whirlwind of therapies—physical, occupational, speech, cognitive—the young man found sanctuary. Each session was a battle fought, a step closer to reclaiming what dystonia had stolen from him. And amidst it all, amidst the pain and the struggle, there echoed the young man's voice—a voice that spoke not of defeat but of resilience. His desire to regain control over his movements reverberated through the halls of the rehabilitation center, a rallying cry that resonated with all who knew his story.

In the end, his journey was not merely about physical rehabilitation but about reclaiming a sense of self—a journey guided by the beacon of functional independence. Through the haze of adversity, he aspired not only to regain movement but to achieve a compensated level of functional autonomy. Though the road ahead may be arduous, he marched forward with unwavering determination, his spirit unbroken, his resolve unyielding.

How Misbehaving Brain Circuit Impacts Rehabilitation Outcomes

Rehabilitation, especially in the context of neurological conditions, is a complex and multifaceted journey. It involves retraining the brain and body to regain lost functions and adapt to new circumstances. However, when a misbehaving brain circuit is involved, such as those seen in conditions like stroke, traumatic brain injury, or neurodegenerative disorders, the rehabilitation process can be particularly challenging.

The brain is an intricate network of interconnected circuits responsible for controlling various bodily functions. When one or more of these circuits is compromised, it can lead to significant disruptions in sensation and perception of the surrounding environment, motor skills, cognitive abilities, and even emotional well-being. For example, after a stroke, a disrupted circuit in the motor cortex can result in weakness or paralysis on one side of the body.

These misbehaving circuits can negatively impact rehabilitation outcomes in several ways:

1. **Limited Functional Recovery:** The damaged or dysfunctional circuit can impede the brain's ability to rewire and adapt, limiting the potential for functional recovery. This can lead to persistent motor deficits or cognitive impairments.

2. **Altered Motor Patterns:** Misbehaving circuits can cause abnormal muscle tone, coordination issues, or spasticity, making it more challenging to regain normal movement patterns during rehabilitation.

3. **Cognitive Challenges:** Cognitive functions, including memory, attention, and problem-solving, may be affected when brain circuits are disrupted. This can hinder a patient's ability to actively participate in rehabilitation and learn new skills.

4. **Emotional Impact:** Misbehaving circuits can contribute to mood disturbances, such as depression or anxiety, which can further complicate the rehabilitation process.

How Post-Operative Care Makes the Outcomes Multi-Fold

Post-operative care is a critical component of rehabilitation, and it plays a pivotal role in enhancing the overall outcomes. Post-operative care not only helps address the immediate aftermath of surgery but also creates an environment conducive to the brain's healing and adaptive processes. Here's how effective post-operative care can significantly improve rehabilitation outcomes:

1. **Early Mobilization:** Starting rehabilitation as early as possible after surgery can help prevent complications and promote faster recovery. Encouraging movement and exercises can stimulate the brain's adaptive capabilities.

2. **Pain Management:** Effective pain control is essential, as uncontrolled pain can hinder a patient's participation in rehabilitation activities. This is especially important in surgeries involving the brain, spine, or limbs.

3. **Supportive Environment:** Creating a supportive and positive environment can have a profound impact on a patient's emotional well-being. Emotional support can boost motivation and engagement in rehabilitation efforts.

4. **Customized, Measurable and comparable Rehabilitation Plans:** Tailoring rehabilitation plans to address the specific challenges posed by misbehaving brain circuits is crucial. Customization ensures that the rehabilitation targets the areas most affected by the neurological condition.

5. **Reinforcement of Neural Plasticity:** The brain's capacity for neural plasticity allows it to reorganize and adapt following injury or surgery. Post-operative care that focuses on repetitive and task-specific training can encourage these adaptive processes.

6. **Patient and Caregiver Education:** Informed patients and caregivers are more likely to participate actively in their rehabilitation. Providing patients with a clear understanding of their condition and the importance of rehabilitation can lead to better adherence and, ultimately, improved outcomes.

7. **Nutrition and adequate sleep** – Having adequate nutrition is akin to providing enough fuel to a vehicle to complete a journey. In neurologically impaired people, the nutritional needs are 1.5 times higher than those of a healthy individual. Similarly, getting a good night's sleep enables the brain to back up the data from what was taught and trained in the rehabilitation sessions.

The impact of misbehaving brain circuits on rehabilitation outcomes is significant but not insurmountable. Effective post-operative care is the bridge between surgery and successful rehabilitation. It creates an environment that promotes neural adaptation, encourages patient engagement, and addresses the unique challenges posed by neurological conditions, ultimately leading to more favorable rehabilitation outcomes.

4

THE "GUITAR SURGEON"

PRECISION BRAIN CIRCUIT BURNING AT ITS BEST!

'A fool with a tool is still a fool.'

-Prof. Dr. Takaomi Taira

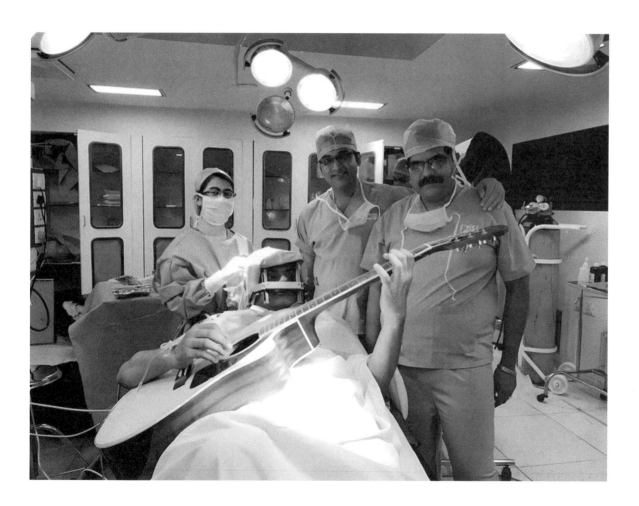

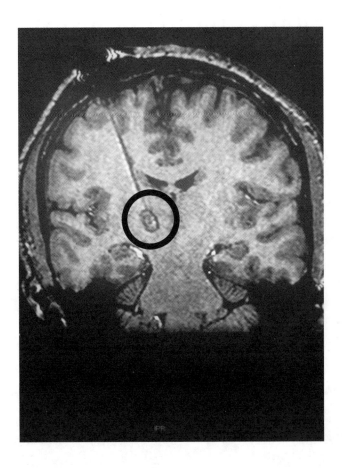

Hi, you see the above image, which is a scan of the brain and a circle marking a point where there is a lesion? Let me tell you the story of the owner of this brain!

Strumming Through Adversity: A Symphony Of Resilience

Meet Abhishek Prasad, a passionate guitarist whose fingers were staging a rebellion against his musical ambitions. As a functional neurosurgeon, I've encountered various fascinating cases, but Abhishek's story had a special melody to it.

Abhishek, hailing from the vibrant city of Bangalore, is an IT professional who decided to swap his laptop keypad for a guitar. Little did he know that his fingers were plotting a symphony of discomfort and cramps, particularly the rebellious trio of his left hand's 3rd, 4th, and 5th fingers.

Now, we've all experienced those nagging laptop-induced pains, right? The kind that makes you question your life choices but doesn't quite send you running to the doctor. Like most of you, Abhishek initially dismissed these musical rebellions, thinking they would magically strum away.

However, much like a poorly executed guitar solo, things went from bad to worse. The discomfort Abhishek felt escalated to the point where playing the guitar became an impossible feat. It was as if his fingers were on strike, demanding better working conditions. A diagnosis of Guitarist Dystonia, a type of Task -Specific Focal Hand Dystonia (TSFHD), was made by a neurologist & some medications were prescribed, but very little changed.

In his quest for relief, Abhishek was referred by a senior hand surgeon to PRS Neurosciences, the brainchild of yours truly. Now, you might be asking, "What's so special about this neurosurgeon and his neuroscience prowess?" Well, let me take you on a journey.

Picture this: a neurosurgeon fresh from special training in Tokyo, Japan- that is where I honed my skills in stereotactic & functional neurosurgery under the watchful eye of the esteemed Prof. Dr. Takaomi Taira. It was in those hallowed halls of Tokyo Women's Medical University (TWMU) that I learned the art of precision medicine, the dance of scalpels in harmony with neural pathways, which all culminated in the technique called Lesioning v3.0

Abhishek's case, a perplexing melody, even in the realm of neurological challenges, lacked the clarity offered by routine tests, leaving diagnostic markers elusive. This intricate composition, however, stirred my curiosity, setting the stage for an exploration into the depths of his symptoms. The spotlight shifted onto Abhishek's fingers, demanding a neurosurgical encore to decipher the enigma that silenced his musical pursuits.

As the discomfort intensified, Abhishek's once vibrant passion for music dimmed, replaced by a deep sense of frustration and desperation. His fingers, once nimble and precise, now betrayed him, echoing the notes slipping through his grasp. In this moment of despair, our paths crossed. A rare and unwelcome visitor named task-specific focal hand dystonia had settled into Abhishek's fingers, orchestrating involuntary muscle contractions that disrupted the graceful harmony he once had with his guitar. Confronted with a disheartening reality, Abhishek faced a dilemma that no musician would prefer to anticipate – the possibility of brain surgery OR QUIT playing the guitar!

I still remember that phone call very vividly. It was in December 2016, and when I answered his call, he told me that he was referred by this hand surgeon and that I had some treatment for his guitarist dystonia. I answered in the affirmative, and he asked me – "What is that treatment? What do you do?" And I casually told him that I needed to burn a small misbehaving circuit inside his brain! He was stunned, and his mom came online and asked the same question, following which they just hung up and never got back for the next nine months. The mere mention of such a drastic measure sent shockwaves through Abhishek and his family, triggering a wave of panic and uncertainty. The gravity of the decision to undergo brain surgery for a condition affecting his ability to play the guitar professionally felt surreal, like an unexpected crescendo in his life's composition.

When I tried calling him, he told me that his family thought that he was crazy to even contemplate brain surgery and that he should quit playing the guitar and just get back to his IT job. It was only when he started experiencing a similar cramp, even when he was typing on the keyboard, that he got back to me and agreed to the surgery, and the rest is history– a successful surgery. His wife, who was present in the OT, recorded the video of the entire surgery and posted it on social media. Immediately, the news went viral! More to that later.

In approaching Abhishek's case, my medical team recognized the seriousness of his condition. With a deep sense of responsibility, I proposed an unconventional solution – brain surgery that involved burning or 'lesioning' of the misbehaving brain circuits deep inside his motor thalamus, a Vo Thalamotomy– as a potential remedy for this perplexing neurological ailment. The recommendation acknowledged the profound impact it could have on Abhishek's life and his passion for the guitar, emphasizing the delicate balance between medical intervention and preserving the rhythm of his musical aspirations.

At PRS Neurosciences, an institution dedicated to pushing the boundaries of scientific understanding in the field of Functional Neurosciences, our journey with Abhishek became a testament to the convergence of medical expertise, patient resilience, and a shared commitment to explore new frontiers for overcoming challenges. Embracing the opportunity for exploration and discovery, we embarked on the unconventional path of stereotactic brain lesioning surgery, aiming to liberate Abhishek's fingers from the grip of the focal hand dystonia.

Abhishek, at a crossroads between the relentless severity of his symptoms and the pursuit of his passion, made the courageous decision to undergo the suggested brain surgery. In this intersection of cutting-edge science and personal choice, our collaboration unfolded as a symbol of hope for those facing similar neurological challenges. I had to hide my anxiety because I was doing this surgery for the first time! I had only assisted my professor in Japan. And I was all alone. Nobody in India did this kind of surgery, and hence, I had no one I could call in case something unforeseen happened. I had to replay the steps of the surgery in my mind so many times that I lost track. I read my notes multiple times to ensure that the neuronal network for such a highly skilled technique got hard-wired and etched in my brain! So much of self-training.

As the day of the surgery dawned, Abhishek, his guitar, and my surgical team stood prepared for this extraordinary performance. With the backdrop of a stereotactic procedure, Abhishek strummed his guitar, his fingers guided not only by the music in his soul but also by the skilled hands of the neurosurgical team. The fusion of neuroscience and art created a surreal ambiance, embodying the harmonious collaboration between music and medicine. The surgery itself happens in these FIVE steps.

Step 1: Fixing the stereotactic frame on the head. This must be fixed very precisely cos that is the base on which all my calculations start. I fixed it under local anesthesia with two screws into the forehead area and two crews in the back of the head, and all these four screws need to be screwed into his skull! As you see in the accompanying pic, he seems very happy despite all this cos he is sure that his fingers will recover and he will play the guitar again. We required four people to fix the frame, and I had practiced these moves multiple times with them in the days preceding the surgery.

Step 2: The patient is then sent for a stereotactic MRI, wherein we capture the 3D volumetric T1 images and the T2 axial and coronal images… with 1 mm thickness and no overlap. Before he is put into the console of the MRI machine, a localizer frame is mounted onto this frame, and this localizer has channels containing copper sulfate solution. My assistant had to ensure that there was not a SINGLE, even a small air bubble, in any of these channels cos, then the scan was of no use to me.

Step 3: These stereotactic MRI images are then imported onto the Surgiplan software dedicated to the planning of this surgery. I bought all the equipment used at the TWMU so that I could replicate my results. It normally takes 45-60 minutes to do the planning and to finally get the X, Y, and Z coordinates of the target and the entry point and the distance to the target from the entry point – this was 8.3 centimeters inside the brain in his case!

Step 4: Then we were ready to perform the actual surgery…. the patient is put on the operating table, and the head is anchored to the table securely so that it doesn't shake even ONE MILLIMETER! Then, all the key data needed is written on the whiteboard in the OT and double-checked by me and my assistant. Once the entry point is marked and the part prepped and draped, the actual surgery starts.

REMEMBER: These surgeries are done 100% under local anesthesia, and the patient is completely awake and talking to me and also hearing whatever is happening in the OT. Hence, keeping the atmosphere calm is critical for everyone's mental health. Once the 14 mm burr hole was drilled into the skull, the 'C' arc was fixed after verifying the X, Y, and Z coordinates of the target, and we were ready to start the key step of the surgery – the actual circuit burning or LESIONING! The lesion generator device also needs to be connected and in place, and the settings are made and verified – the 'high manual Hm' setting, a pulse width of 100 micro sec, a frequency of 133 MHz, and then the 1 x 4 monopolar electrode is carefully inserted into his brain and advanced till the pre-determined target. Just to let you readers know, this is totally blind surgery for me at this time, and I am only guided by the accuracy of the software and the feedback from the patient. I see nothing cos I am 8.3 centimeters inside the brain!

Step 5: The actual Lesioning procedure. The surgery starts with the AC in the Operation theatre at a temperature as low as 17 degrees Celsius. We neurosurgeons like low temperatures so that our brains are working most efficiently! Next, we focus on the actual lesioning procedures. This consists of a combination of macro stimulation with a graded increase in the current (given in milliamperes') and the voltage calculated using Ohm's law! Phew!…. We all do medicine to escape the complex mathematics, and here I am, attempting to do my first ever Vo thalamotomy for guitarist dystonia (I had done it for other types of FHDs), and I needed to check the impedance, calculate the voltage using the Ohm's law, etc etc, and parallelly check for any side-effects during the stimulation. We had planned seven lesions in total – each up to a temperature of 70 degrees centigrade and for a duration of 40 seconds: and along three parallel tracks – central (three lesions – zero, minus three, and minus five), posterior (2 lesions – zero and minus 3), and anterior (2 lesions – zero and minus 3).

Throughout the surgery, done at the Bhagwan Mahaveer Jain Hospital, Bengaluru, our expertise precision-targeted the specific areas in Abhishek's brain responsible for the guitarist dystonia, effectively reversing the condition.

The operation resonated with success, and as the circuit burning progressed (7 in total), his cramped fingers magically recovered 'on the operating table,' one finger at a time, to the delight of Abhishek and the entire surgical team and his wife inside the OT, watching with bated breath! Abhishek could once again embrace his guitar, creating melodies that had been silenced for far too long.

As the symphony of success reverberated through the surgical theatre, Abhishek's courage and the precision of the medical team intertwined into a harmonious crescendo. The intricate dance between the surgeon's scalpel and Abhishek's strumming fingers became a testament to the resilience of the human spirit. The rest, as I have said earlier in the chapter, is history. The news went viral, and I got the permanent tag – THE GUITAR SURGEON!

I still remember that day – it was two days after the surgery. I was at my high school reunion, doing the MC on stage, and the moment I finished and put on my phone, I had over 200 missed calls! And one of my journalist friends desperately called me and asked me, "Where the hell are you? Why aren't you answering the phone? The whole world is looking for you."

I was really perplexed and also concerned as to why the world was looking for me. After a 10-minute chat with him, I got the whole story.

The next three days were crazy for all of us – multiple TV channel interviews, regional, national, and international. BBC, CNN, Fox, ABC, Dubai Times, Singapore Times, NDTV, India Today, and an all-India front-page story in India's biggest newspaper, 'Times of India,' with the surgery pic shown below. Abhishek had his own interviews along with his guitar, wife, and all!

Dr. Prathiba says, "Abhishek's surgery was the first 'guitar' surgery Dr. Sharan did after he came back from Japan. It was a very stressful event for us because it was the first time he was doing it, and there were a lot of things that he had to put into place. As for getting viral, I had heard about it but really did not know what it meant. But then, I think Dr. Sharan mentioned he allowed Abhishek's wife to come into the last part of the surgical part. In the OT, she took a video and then put it up on Facebook, and it went viral. And really, when we traveled to Antarctica, when we saw Santiago, the capital of Chile, carrying his picture and news in Santiago, that is when we actually understood what going viral meant. I mean, it went all over; it was very exciting after that. And the results were amazing."

It all finally started sinking in. When I ventured to Tokyo for this fellowship (after a 4-year sadhana of chanting the 'Guru Sthotra' mantra written by Sri. Adi Shankaracharya every single day, and with the Sankalpa – God help me, to find my Guru), little did I realize that history was in the making!

Abhishek's story serves as a testament to the intersection of medical innovation and human resilience. The melody of his guitar, played amidst the intricate dance of this 'awake brain surgery,' resonates not only in the corridors of our institution but also in the hearts of those inspired by the potential for healing, discovery, and the harmonious blend of science and art.

Seeking my "Guru"

Amazing, isn't it? Did you guys get goosebumps? Did you google to see the video of the guitar surgery? All this sounds great, but I could never have done all this unless I was initiated into this by a "Guru." For about four years before I met my "Guru," I chanted Adi Shankaracharya's 'Guru Stotram' mantra every single day. And my Sankalpa was - "God, find me my teacher." And eventually, it happened!

Feb 2014, AIIMS New Delhi, in a conference, I saw 'Him' and immediately something inside me said - "He is your Guru." And then this amazing journey began. Do you guys want to know who he is? Prof. Takaomi Taira, from Tokyo, Japan, is the world's best functional neurosurgeon, especially for Lesioning v3.0!

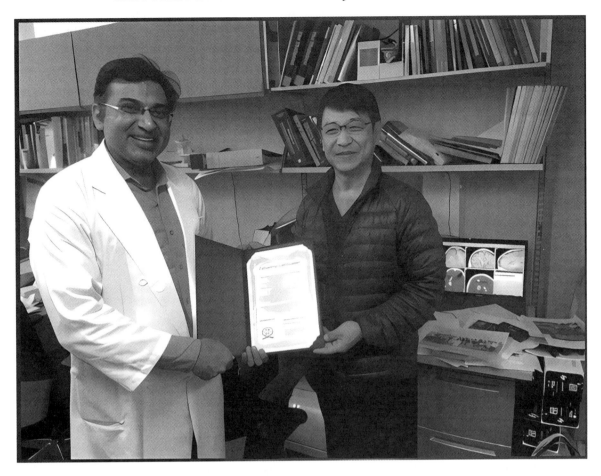

My Guru – Prof. Takaomi Taira, Tokyo Women's Medical University (TWMU)

Understanding Task-Specific Focal Hand Dystonia (TSFHD)

What is Task-Specific Focal Hand Dystonia (TSFHD)? Well, let's now explore what exactly this guitarist dystonia, or task-specific focal hand dystonia, really is and why it is important for a layperson to know about it because whatever has happened to Abhishek and thousands of others can also happen to any of us who do repetitive tasks every day – even like writing, typing, texting, etc.! None of us are immune from this, and there is no vaccine to prevent it.

To understand task-specific focal hand dystonia (TSFHD), let's first understand a little bit about dystonia. Dystonia is a neurological movement disorder characterized by involuntary muscle contractions that cause repetitive or twisting movements and can affect various parts of the body. It is like some strange magical power that moves parts of your body in weird ways and with writhing movements without your will. Sounds more like some voodoo or black magic stuff, doesn't it? And with all scans seemingly normal and many blood tests also so, it does validate this, and with no obvious medical solutions in sight, there have been umpteen cases where the family has sought the powers of the unknown in a desperate attempt to cure this.

Focal hand dystonia, which is usually 'task-specific,' is a specific type of dystonia that affects the hand and fingers, often making it difficult for individuals to perform fine motor tasks. It is as if your fingers are not listening to your brain'! The commonest type of TSFHD is known as the writer's cramp, while what Abhishek had is also called the guitarist cramp.

TSFHD is a specific subtype of focal hand dystonia that primarily manifests itself during highly specific or specialized, repetitive tasks like the musician's dystonia that Abhishek was cured of. This neurological disorder is characterized by abnormal muscle movements or spasms that affect the hand and fingers, typically when performing particular activities. The term 'task-specific' highlights the fact that the dystonia is triggered or worsened by specific actions.

Common examples of tasks that can trigger TSFHD include writing, playing a musical instrument, such as the piano, drums, violin, or guitar, typing on a keyboard, or other activities that require fine motor control of the hands and fingers or even those who blow the saxophone or trumpet, called Embouchures dystonia and this occurs around the muscles of the mouth. We have even seen TSFHD in those who do calligraphy!

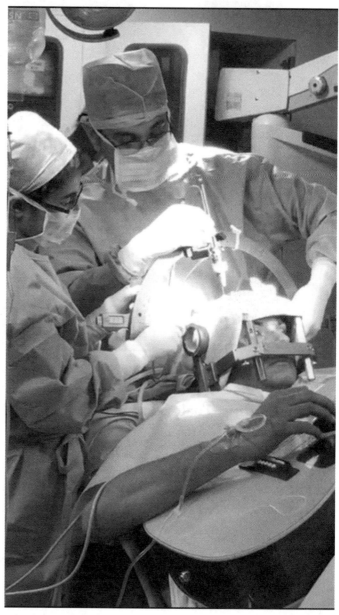

The exact cause of TSFHD is not fully understood, but it is believed to involve a combination of genetic, environmental, and neurobiological factors. Treatment options may include physical therapy, occupational therapy, medications, and, in some cases, botulinum toxin injections to alleviate the symptoms and help patients regain better control of their hands during these specific tasks. And if none of these work, then the final frontier is stereotactic lesioning surgery by a trained hand!

It's important to note that this condition can be challenging for individuals who rely on the affected hand for their livelihood or activities they are passionate about. Management often requires a multidisciplinary approach involving neurologists, physical therapists, and occupational therapists to improve function and quality of life for those affected.

Exploring the Nuances of Task-Specific Focal Hand Dystonia (TSFHD)

Within the domain of functional neurosurgery, a specialized discipline tackling disruptions in the brain's electrical activity, a peculiar anomaly emerges concerning guitars. The brain, a marvelously intricate organ, manifests these disruptions through symptoms like muscle spasticity or twitching. Dystonias, a unique subset, reveal abnormal muscle movements devoid of paralysis. An exceptional case unfolds where normalcy in hand function prevails until attempting to play the guitar. The patient articulates an indescribable force impeding his fingers, particularly in the left hand (but can happen in either hand), rendering them rigid and unresponsive.

Personalizing the Experience of TSFHD

In Abhishek's own words, the impact of TSFHD becomes vividly apparent. As the patient expressed, "These three fingers of the left hand, these two have become so stiff. I cannot bring them on the fretboard; I can't. God, it has become so stiff I cannot move at all. You can see that I'm trying, but I cannot move them at all." As the dystonia in his three fingers disappeared on the operating table, he said – "Doctor, this is MAGIC!"

MAGIC OR JADOO, as we call it in Hindi, is the name of the anthem of PRS Neurosciences – composed and sung by... guess who?? Abhishek Prasad, of course. Don't forget to tune into our YouTube channel (@prsneurosciences) to see the Jadoo song he performed in Punarpraapti 2023!

This firsthand account highlights the profound challenges posed by dystonia, specifically affecting the left hand's three fingers. The stiffness described impedes not only the patient's ability to bring the fingers onto the fretboard but also limits their overall smooth and coordinated movements.

The frustration and effort to overcome this stiffness are palpable in the patient's words, underscoring the intricate and disabling nature of task-specific focal hand dystonia in the context of playing the guitar.

Integrating such personal narratives enriches our understanding of the condition and its impact on individuals, emphasizing the urgency for comprehensive and effective intervention in functional neurosurgery.

Seeing his fantastic results on social media, Taskin Ali, a proficient professional guitarist from Dhaka with even more severe guitarist dystonia and other task-specific dystonia, came and got his surgery done.

Interestingly, both these guitarists performed recently in the first ever 'Noble Art of Lesioning' conference held in southeast Asia (NoALCON 2024, May 17th-19th) to a standing ovation!

Abhishek signed off with this message to everyone – even when you are in the depths of despair, never ever give up HOPE!

And like Lord Krishna told Arjuna in the Mahabharat war, you fight to WIN!

5

PARKINSON'S DISEASE - KAMPAVATA OR THE SHAKING PALSY

"I refer to having Parkinson's as a gift. People are dubious about this, but it's a gift that keeps taking because it's really opened me up to more compassion."

- Michael J Fox, Interview on CNN, 2010

"I float like a butterfly & sting like a bee..."

–Muhammed Ali – boxer

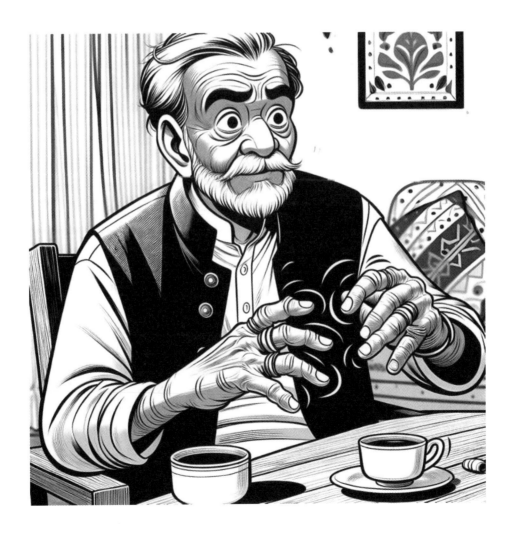

Navaraj Bhandari, a 48-year-old pharmacist from Nepal, presented a unique challenge when he walked into my OPD with his wife and brother at Bhagwan Mahaveer Jain Hospital, Vasanth Nagar. Renowned in his hometown as a well-respected man of knowledge, Navaraj found himself battling an enemy within—Idiopathic Parkinson's disease, which had escalated to severe resting tremors, severe motor fluctuations with frequent ON-OFF states, and disabling dyskinesias. His condition was so intense that during the OFF episodes at night, he would crawl on the floor and even pop in additional tablets... all this would keep his entire family awake at night, misinterpreted by some as a sign of supernatural forces at work. The family was helpless and clueless cos he was the smartest in the family.

Being a pharmacist has its own plusses and minuses. As the disease progressed, Navaraj quickly understood the phenomena of the ON-OFF phases, which most such patients describe as an experience akin to the roller coaster rides of drug addicts – from desperate withdrawal to pure ecstasy in la la land!

Navaraj's medical journey was marked by a struggle with 'medication dependency.' Initially prescribed Syndopa after his diagnosis, he became addicted, leading to severe dyskinetic episodes when he overdosed. These episodes transformed him dramatically—on medications, he resembled Mithun da, energetically performing to "I am a Disco Dancer," but without it, he became as immobile as a log, exemplifying the stark 'ON-OFF' motor fluctuations that are a hallmark of his disease.

His symptoms were profound and varied, complicating his daily life significantly. When off his medication, he faced not just physical immobility but also deep emotional turmoil, becoming a shell of his former self, filled with anxiety, despair, and frustration. For those who didn't know his suffering or the nature of this disease, he appeared schizophrenic! This stark contrast in his behavior underscored the complex nature of his treatment needs.

Determined to alleviate Navaraj's suffering, I referred him to our ANRS Siddharth for the Levodopa Challenge Test (LCT). Like ascending the steep and unpredictable slopes of Mount Everest, keeping Navaraj off his Syndopa medication overnight was a formidable challenge for him and his family. Yet, they managed to overcome this hurdle, and he arrived early the next morning for the LCT, feeling as agitated and restless as if caught in a storm high in the Himalayas.

Throughout the assessment, Navaraj's frustration was palpable, his emotions swirling like a tempest. He voiced his displeasure loudly, cursing and venting at Siddharth and the team for the delay and withholding his Syndopa, which he saw as essential to his well-being. However, as a pharmacist, Navaraj understood the necessity of the medical protocol, and his respect for the professionals in scrubs, despite his discomfort, remained intact, much like the enduring respect climbers hold for the majestic peaks.

The completion of the LCT yielded significant insights, revealing a path forward as clear as the view from a Himalayan summit. With an OFF-phase score of 132 and an ON-phase score of 60 on the Unified Parkinson's Disease Rating Scale (UPDRS), the results clearly demonstrated a positive reaction to levodopa. This affirmed that Navaraj was an excellent candidate for the proposed surgery and likely to experience considerable benefits from it, offering a chance to reclaim the peak of his health.

We opted for an MRI-guided stereotactic neurosurgery targeting the Globus Pallidus interna (GPi) nucleus of the basal ganglia. Why the GPi? Because of the myriad of motor symptoms he exhibited, this is the best target in the brain. The operation required meticulous planning and pinpoint precision to avoid the adjacent critical areas of the brain, with every feedback response from Navaraj being extremely crucial for the surgery's success. As he lay there, off medications, grumpy and deeply anxious, his pleas for Syndopa were heart-wrenching. There was a point that he didn't even care about the surgery. He just wanted the tablets!

During the surgery, as I ablated the targeted area, we encountered a tense moment when Navaraj's feedback reactions began to slow. Concerned, my finger immediately hit the STOP button on the lesion generator, thinking that we had hit the wrong area in the brain. Eventually, I discovered that he was simply cold in his feet —a reminder of how cold I keep the temperature in my OT and the simple human needs that persist even in high-tech medical scenarios. After ensuring his comfort, we proceeded, and the surgery concluded successfully with six lesions made. As the lesioning progressed from one to six, Siddharth and Dr. Sanjiv felt that his rigidity and bradykinesia were improving, and eventually, Navaraj himself told us that "he is feeling as if he has taken syndopa." This is the perfect and ultimate "on-table" feedback we expect from every PD patient of ours when we operate.

Postoperatively, the change in Navaraj was remarkable. His dyskinesias ceased, and the severe motor fluctuations he had suffered considerably reduced, but he said he was still not okay. He was not able to clearly articulate the challenge he was facing; he was stooping, falling, crying, and anxious. The same drama, and his wife was crying again, thinking the surgery had failed. She felt she had reached a dead-end now.

I immediately realized what the problem was – since it was a lesioning surgery, we only do one side at a time, and now we and Navaraj had the same problem faced by all such PD patients of mine – the operated side symptoms dramatically come down, but the non-operated side symptoms persist in the same manner. And the result? Optimizing the medications to achieve optimal dosing is a very delicate balancing act that our neurologist, Dr. Sanjiv, has perfected. Our multidisciplinary rehab team launched a comprehensive rehabilitation program addressing not just his physical symptoms but also his psychological and social needs.

When Navaraj returned to my clinic eight months later, he was a transformed man. The right side of his body showed minimal symptoms, but challenges persisted on the left, prompting plans for a second surgery to further improve his quality of life. His LCT was repeated, and the results revealed - that the OFF-phase score had reduced from 132 pre-surgery to 66 now, and the ON-phase score had reduced from 60 before the surgery to 11 now on the Unified Parkinson's Disease Rating Scale (UPDRS). The results clearly demonstrated a great result of the one-sided surgery, as well as the fact that his body had adapted well to the surgery. He is now a good candidate for the second-side surgery. Hopefully, by the time this book gets released, we should have done his surgery.

Navaraj's ongoing journey is a testament to the resilience of the human spirit and the transformative potential of targeted yet affordable medical interventions. Lesioning v3.0 is really a boon for millions of such patients who are suffering from Idiopathic Parkinson's Disease and cannot afford the DBS. Now, what do Navaraj Bhandari, the ordinary pharmacist, have in common with the world-famous Muhammad Ali and Michael J Fox? The same problem – Parkinson's Disease!

MICHAEL J. FOX AND MUHAMMAD ALI AND THEIR EXPERIENCE WITH PARKINSON'S DISEASE (PD)

Michael J. Fox and Muhammad Ali are both widely recognized figures who have faced the challenges of Parkinson's disease, albeit in different ways.

Michael J. Fox is a well-known Canadian-American actor, author, and advocate who gained fame for his roles in popular TV series like "Family Ties" and the "Back to the Future" film trilogy. In 1991, at the age of 29, Fox was diagnosed with Parkinson's disease, a progressive neurodegenerative disorder that affects movement control. This diagnosis came as a shock to him, as he was at the peak of his acting career.

Michael J. Fox's journey with Parkinson's disease has been marked by both personal challenges and remarkable advocacy efforts. Michael J. Fox's openness about his Parkinson's diagnosis and his commitment to advocating for research and treatment have made a significant impact on the Parkinson's community. He has become a symbol of hope for many individuals living with the disease and their families, and his foundation continues to raise funds and support scientific efforts to find a cure for Parkinson's.

Muhammad Ali:

Muhammad Ali, widely regarded as one of the greatest boxers in history, transcended the world of sports with his charisma, skill, and resilience. Born Cassius Marcellus Clay Jr. on January 17, 1942, in Louisville, Kentucky, Ali rose to fame with an Olympic gold medal in 1960 and went on to become the world heavyweight champion multiple times.

In 1984, Ali received the diagnosis that would reshape his life – Parkinson's disease. This progressive neurodegenerative disorder, which affects movement and can cause tremors and stiffness, was likely linked to the thousands of punches he took during his illustrious boxing career. Muhammad Ali's journey with Parkinson's unfolded against the backdrop of his iconic status and contributions to civil rights and humanitarian causes.

Both Michael J. Fox and Muhammad Ali's journeys with Parkinson's disease highlight the multidimensional approach to managing the condition. Medications, including those that address dopamine deficiency, play a crucial role.

Additionally, surgical interventions like DBS may be considered for individuals with specific needs or advanced symptoms. It's important to note that the management of Parkinson's is highly individualized, and treatment plans are tailored to each person's unique experience with the disease.

Both Michael J. Fox and Muhammad Ali, in their unique ways, have contributed significantly to the Parkinson's community. Fox's advocacy and the establishment of his foundation have advanced research efforts, while Ali's visibility has sparked discussions about the impact of sports-related head injuries on neurological health. Their experiences have brought attention to Parkinson's disease, fostering greater understanding and support for individuals affected by the condition.

Now, as soon as certain features are suspected in an individual for Parkinson's disease, such as tremors (especially resting tremors), rigidity (indicating stiffness and reduced mobility), or bradykinesia (slowness of movement, including a lack of arm swinging while walking), it becomes quite evident when you observe these patients. You'll never miss it. So, if any of these symptoms are happening, or if the voice is becoming slower, or if other features are manifesting, you need to start suspecting the presence of symptoms of Parkinson's.

In classical Parkinson's disease, there are motor and non-motor symptoms. Motor symptoms typically appear early. For instance, tremors, especially at rest, are quite common. These tremors occur when the person is at rest, and they resemble the motion of rolling a pill in their hand. Interestingly, these tremors often subside when the individual initiates an action or becomes aware of them. This is distinct from essential tremors, which are the most common type of tremor. Essential tremors do not occur when a person is at rest but only manifest when they are engaged in a specific activity. This distinction is essential because around one-third of Parkinson's patients experience hand tremors as one of their initial symptoms. Recognizing this difference is crucial because essential tremors can be mistaken for Parkinson's disease, causing unnecessary concern.

Furthermore, it's vital to understand that there's no rush for surgical procedures if you suspect Parkinson's. The differentiation between Parkinson's disease and Parkinsonism may take a few years. One of the early signs to watch for in patients is the presence of cognitive or memory issues. If they exhibit cognitive problems, memory lapses, or a decline in mental sharpness, there's a high likelihood of Parkinsonism or other Parkinson's variants rather than Parkinson's disease. Such patients typically do not benefit from surgical procedures.

How do we know if Parkinson's Disease has advanced enough to consider surgical management?

The 5-2-1 Rule for Parkinson's: Deciding the Path to Surgery

The 5-2-1 rule is a guideline devised by a panel of experts to help diagnose advanced Parkinson's disease (PD) and determine when to consider surgical interventions. This rule is applied to patients who are already on medication for PD and serves as a barometer for evaluating the progression of the disease and the efficacy of current treatments. Here's what the rule signifies:

- **5 Times Oral Levodopa Tablet Taken/Day:** This element of the rule indicates that if a patient needs to take oral levodopa medication five times a day to manage PD symptoms, their condition might be advancing.

- **2 Hours of OFF Time/Day:** "OFF" time refers to periods when the medication's effects are wearing off and PD symptoms become more pronounced. Two hours of "OFF" time per day suggests that the disease is progressing to a stage where medication alone isn't enough to manage symptoms effectively.

- **1 Hour/Day of Troublesome Dyskinesia:** Dyskinesia involves involuntary movements that can be distressing and disruptive. One hour of such symptoms per day signals a need for treatment reevaluation. Dyskinesia is often a side effect of long-term levodopa use, and its presence can complicate PD management.

When a patient with Parkinson's meets the 5-2-1 criteria, it implies that the disease has reached a stage where oral medications are not adequately controlling the symptoms. At this point, it is essential to consider advanced treatment options, such as surgery.

Surgeries like Lesioning v3.0 and Deep Brain Stimulation (DBS) can provide relief from symptoms and reduce both "OFF" time and dyskinetic episodes, improving the patient's quality of life. The decision to proceed with the surgery is made after careful consideration of the potential benefits and risks, patient preferences, and overall health status.

The 5-2-1 rule helps doctors and patients recognize when it's time to transition from a medical management focus to discussing surgical options as part of a comprehensive approach to treating Parkinson's disease.

Some individuals may also develop truncal ataxia (impaired coordination affecting the trunk) or balance problems early on, along with symptoms of autonomic dysfunction. These are often categorized as Parkinson's variants and do not respond well to surgical treatments.

LEVODOPA CHALLENGE TEST (LCT)
More Than Numbers!

It was a weekday at my office when I was sitting with Siddharth and discussing how we work on I2P for the upper limb (part of newro LOGICS) when Dr. Sanjiv came into my room and asked, "Sharan, I need someone to do the LCT for the patients and report! Who will do it?" I pointed to Siddharth and said – "he will do it!"

Siddharth is basically the guy who takes on things when thrown at without worrying about consequences! He said, "OKAY, I can do it, but I need to be trained as I have never done it before." We signed an 'LCT training pact,' and the journey started!

Since there was no fixed procedure already defined to conduct an LCT except for Siddharth, who cannot work without a process, he took on the task of creating a process that was 'future ready'! Let me first explain to you what this LCT is about!

The levodopa challenge test, also known as the levodopa/carbidopa test, is a diagnostic tool primarily used in the assessment of Parkinson's disease (PD) and related movement disorders.

Here's an outline of the procedure:

Purpose:

- **Diagnosis Confirmation:** The test helps to confirm a diagnosis of Parkinson's disease when the symptoms are ambiguous or when the diagnosis is uncertain.

- **Differential Diagnosis:** It aids in differentiating Parkinson's Disease from Parkinsonism and other similar conditions.

Procedure:
Preparation:

- The patient should not take any anti-Parkinson medications for at least 12 hours before the test.

- Baseline measurements of motor function and symptom severity are recorded.

Administration:

- The patient is given a single dose of levodopa (also known as L-dopa), usually in combination with carbidopa, to enhance its effectiveness and reduce side effects.

- The dosage typically used is 200 to 250 mg of levodopa combined with 50 to 100 mg of carbidopa.

Observation:

- The patient is closely monitored for a period of time after taking the medication, usually around 1 to 2 hours.

- During this time, clinicians observe for changes in motor function and symptom severity.

Assessment:

- Motor function and symptom severity are reassessed at regular intervals after the medication is administered.

- The Unified Parkinson's Disease Rating Scale (UPDRS) is often used to quantify changes in symptoms.

Interpretation:

- **Positive Response:** A significant improvement in motor function and symptom severity following levodopa administration, indicated by a wide difference between the On and OFF scores, suggests a diagnosis of Parkinson's disease.

- **Negative Response:** If there is little to no improvement in symptoms, it may indicate an alternative diagnosis or the presence of atypical Parkinsonism.

Considerations:

- **Duration of Observation:** The duration of observation may vary depending on the clinic's protocol but typically ranges from 1 to 2 hours.

- **Side Effects:** Levodopa can cause side effects such as nausea, vomiting, dizziness, and dyskinesias (involuntary movements), which should be monitored during the test.

- **Patient Safety:** Patients should be closely supervised during the test, especially if they experience significant changes in symptoms or side effects.

The levodopa challenge test provides valuable information to clinicians in confirming or ruling out a diagnosis of Parkinson's disease. However, it is just one part of the diagnostic process and should be interpreted in conjunction with other clinical findings and diagnostic tests.

In the context of the levodopa challenge test (LCT), clinical predictors in the Unified Parkinson's Disease Rating Scale (UPDRS) that may help determine a positive response typically involve motor function and symptom severity assessments. Here are some key clinical predictors in UPDRS that clinicians often consider:

Motor Examination (Part III of UPDRS):

Tremor: Assess the severity and frequency of resting tremor, postural tremor, and action tremor in different body parts.

Rigidity: Evaluate the resistance to passive movement in various joints, particularly in the neck, trunk, and limbs.

Bradykinesia: Look for slowness of movement, including reduced amplitude and speed of voluntary movements such as finger tapping, hand opening/closing, and leg agility.

Postural Stability and Gait: Assess the patient's ability to maintain balance, posture, and coordination during standing, walking, turning, and other activities.

Activities of Daily Living (Part II of UPDRS):

- Evaluate the impact of Parkinsonian symptoms on the patient's ability to perform daily activities such as dressing, eating, hygiene, and mobility.
- Assess functional independence and the need for assistance or adaptation in various tasks.

Motor Fluctuations and Dyskinesia:

- Monitor fluctuations in motor function throughout the levodopa challenge test, including "on" periods (when medication is effective) and "off" periods (when medication wears off).
- Note the presence and severity of dyskinesias, which are involuntary movements that may occur as a side effect of levodopa therapy.

Response to Levodopa:

- Document changes in motor function and symptom severity following levodopa administration during the test.
- Look for improvements in tremor, rigidity, bradykinesia, and overall motor performance compared to baseline assessments.

Time Course of Response:

- Observe the duration of the response to levodopa, including the onset of the ON-phase duration of the ON phase before the dyskinesias kick in.
- Note any fluctuations or variations in motor function over time during the observation period.

Subjective Patient Experience:

- Consider the patient's own perception of symptom relief and functional improvement following levodopa administration.
- Inquire about changes in symptom severity, mobility, and overall quality of life during the test.

By assessing these clinical predictors in UPDRS, clinicians can evaluate the response to levodopa during the challenge test and determine whether there is a positive response indicating a diagnosis of Parkinson's disease or related movement disorders.

The interpretation of UPDRS scores should be integrated with other clinical findings and diagnostic information to make informed decisions about diagnosis and management.

Knowing Siddharth and his compulsion to add flavor to whatever he does, I knew he would not be happy with what is standard procedure. He is an occupational therapist by profession and decided to combine his skill sets with the standard procedure of LCT!

Though I have never accompanied him physically in any LCT, I have heard that people love the way he speaks, interacts, and elicits the patient's complaints when he conducts the LCT. Some of the patients think that he is a neurologist, which he has to time and again clarify that he is not! He has gone beyond what we trained him to do!

He loves to write reports, but he likes to make things easier! Imagine what he did!

Having understood the process in depth and captured the communication during the evaluation, which answered the majority of the information, he split the process into three parts: pre-test (send out info brochures to the patient going to take up the test and ease them out by answering anything they want to know about the test, test (off phase -usually conducted early, test dose decision-based in the severity and other comorbidities), and post-test (which was usually quick and conclusive).

Then, he created an LCT calculator using a simple Excel spreadsheet and formulas. You will be amazed that this simple technique reduced the reporting time from 30 mins to 5 mins. All the data is captured at the source, and the final scores are automatically calculated and ready to report at the end of the phase test. The report is a simple ctrl+c and ctrl+v task with additional interpretation, providing a world-class output!

He trained more therapists to do the test effectively without a drop in the quality of the test! *Now, Siddharth wants to share one experience of LCT that changed his perspective towards LCT:*

The hummingbird sign

Here is what Siddharth has to say-

I am sharing the story of a 77-year-old man named Somnath (name changed), a devotee of the Ramakrishna Mission and an extremely social guy.

He used to walk to the mission ashram every day in the morning, clean the place with other volunteers, freshen up, go to his office, which was 30 mins from there, finish his job at 6:00 pm, go back to the ashram for the evening mediation and return home by 7:30 pm. He loved his family like any father would do and provided the best care in his capacity to this family.

He was brought to BMJH Girinagar by his son, who was very upset with his father because his father would constantly accuse him of having illicit relationships with his mother two years after he was diagnosed with Parkinson's Disease! You must be thinking that I'm speaking about someone who primarily has a psychiatric condition, right? But no. I am speaking about a patient who was diagnosed with Parkinson's disease in 2018 and continued to take his medications without fail. Imagine a father who was respected by his family like God starts shouting and accusing people around him!

When I met the son and his mother for the first time, I spoke to them objectively like I usually do. I started by preparing them for the LCT, as I would usually do when his son burst into tears. He held my hand and said, "Please believe me. I do not have any illicit relationships with my mother. I am married with a daughter. Please tell my dad that it is not true!"

I made him sit, offered him some water, and explained how some patients with Parkinson's disease hallucinate, may become delusional, and lose their sense of reality! Based on his history, I also told him that it might not be an idiopathic Parkinson's disease he is suffering from. It may be something else. The son was awestruck because he resonated with what I told him. He had done his end of the research and strongly believed it was not PD!

History elicited from the son was as follows:

2018- started with right-hand tremors (both action and resting), diagnosed with PD. Did not take Western medicine. Tried naturopathy and Ayurveda. The impact of management lasted for 15 days, and thereafter, I had to repeat the cycle.

2020- met a neurologist who put him on syndopa plus 125 mg TID, H&Y stage 2. MRI of the brain showed chronic lacunar infarcts.

2021- Visual hallucinations and night frights for which quetiapine was added

2021- Reduction in balance, no tremors, reduction in night frights

2022- Increase in delusional behavior, no significant tremors, but increased difficulty in balancing.

April 2023- Deterioration of balance with incidences of falls and delusions of persecution.

The day of LCT came- I reached around 8 am as usual. When I reached the hospital, Mr. Somnath wished me good morning! His son was smiling, but I was completely confused. What his son told me about his father and the man I saw looked completely different at that point. I went and asked him my usual question, "Your father is 12 hours off medication. How is he? Does he seem any different to you?". He said, "Siddharth, I think the medicine is causing the problem. This morning, when I came, he spoke to me like he used to do before we started Syndopa for him. He was asking me how my job was going and did not use any ill words for me or my mother! Can we stop his medication, please?"

I was still not able to grasp the situation, but I told him that we must not get carried away with the emotion. Let us objectively check what's happening.

We started the off-phase evaluation after 12 hours of medication. I took a detailed history to capture all the details. My clinician's suspicion was heightened. I believe this case is different from what I have seen earlier. I started the evaluation using the UPDRS scale. It took me 45 minutes to finish the off-phase eval, but the patient was so happy to move that he decided to show me all the possible movements he could do. I saw the happiness on his face and the hope that he was finally getting better. I identified that he had swallowing issues, but both the father and son brushed away the issue in the heat of the moment and said that it was not critical. His total off-phase score was 93.

Then, we administered the test dose of 250 mg of Syndopa Plus. We patiently waited for 1 hour. The patient did not appreciate any change in the medication. This was exactly what he informed me during the history verification. He was not aware when the medication worked and when it didn't. In the on-phase evaluation, he became more drowsier and inattentive. I was not able to connect the dots as the majority of the patients reported better attention and improved movement. I recall he never bent forward when he walked with or without the medication and was falling backward more often! It would not make sense if I continued to believe that this was Parkinson's Disease. His on-phase score was 94.

I completed the evaluation with him only to find out the difference between the on-phase and off-phase evaluation was 1! I thought I had wasted my time on this guy. I should have spoken to Sharan sir in the off phase and told him I don't think LCT will work in his case owing to his presentation!

We somehow managed to finish the test. I concluded two things. First thing, this is most probably not a case of PD and needs a re-assessment by a neurologist. Secondly, there is something fishy about this case that I am not able to put my finger on! I requested a swallow evaluation by our team, which got postponed due to a primary consultation with Dr. Sanjiv first. I reported my findings to Dr. Sharan and Dr. Sanjiv. We decided to shift him to the hospital where Dr. Sanjiv practices. Just before going to the hospital, after the on-phase evaluation finished, he became disoriented and restless and started abusing his son just like he did. I assumed there was a connection between the medication and the behavior changes, and I brought this to Dr. Sharan's and Dr. Sanjiv's attention.

While he was restless, the nursing staff fed him food so that he could be sent to Dr. Sanjiv at his clinic, which is roughly 30 minutes away from BMJH. Dr. Sanjiv evaluated him and asked him for an MRI. On the way back, our patient had a silent aspiration and became unconscious! I was at home when Sharan sir called and asked me if the patient had swallow issues! I agreed to that. He asked me – "why did you not get his swallow evaluated?" I informed him that it had been scheduled. He said that the patient had aspirated on the way back from the hospital and is in critical condition right now! His swallow evaluation was far more critical, and upon visiting Dr. Sanjiv, he was forced to ask me, "How could you compromise on that?"

For 5 minutes, I felt that the earth had stopped rotating. My heart rate would be approximately 100- 110, and I realized I had taken someone's life!

I told Sharan, sir, "I am ready to take the blame. What should I do to save him?"

Sharan sir said. "You cannot do anything, and we have to wait and watch!"

I was thinking to myself, "Did I learn anything at all from my work experience, or am I fooling myself into thinking that I am a thoroughbred healthcare professional?" In that 5 -10 minutes, I had thought through all possible ways this even can blacklist me!

After 10 minutes, I got a call from Sharan sir, which made me capable of breathing again. He said," Siddharth, that patient who aspirated is actually a case of Progressive Supranuclear Palsy, and he is in the advanced stages!

He is not a case of PD. The prognosis is poor. The blame is not on you, but be aware of these situations! You are an ANRS. I cannot accept this behavior from you". I also received a message from Sanjiv sir, "PSP, not PD!". It made me feel guilty instead of relaxed because I failed to correlate the symptoms I saw. The hallmark symptoms of PSP- are Parkinsonian symptoms, not flexed posture, frequent backward falls, breathing and swallowing issues, behavioral changes, hallucinations, and delusions! Usually, PSP does not respond to syndopa!

Do you know what the hallmark sign of PSP in a brain MRI is?- It is called a "Hummingbird Sign." I hated hummingbirds since then!

In the next ten days, we saw that his condition had drastically worsened. As an ANRS, I was constantly observing him in the ICU and his son outside the ICU. Mother was devastated. I would pray to God inside the ICU to please forgive me for my error and ask his son to forgive me outside. I honestly did not know how to cope with this!

Towards the 10th day, when they came, I became aware that Mr. Somnath would not survive seeing his son again and speaking with him as he did on the day we did the OFF-phase evaluation. I started detaching myself from him. I would see him objectively and try my best to forget what happened. That day, I realized how incapable I was of forgetting experiences!

I vaguely remember; it was mid-May 2023. I had gone to see another patient in the ICU, and I saw everyone gathered around Somnath. He was losing his vitals rapidly! I asked the nurse what happened. I got to know his son had withdrawn his ventilator support and decided to let him go following counseling from doctors. I could not hold myself anymore. I accepted I had killed a person! My LCT was an absolute failure. That damn hummingbird took his life!

I went out of the ICU. His son was there. I told him that it was me you believed, and you lost your father! My head was down in shame. He was smiling with tears in his eyes. He said, "Siddharth, because of you, I got to connect one last time with my dad. Because of your pressure, I got him down to the hospital. It was unfortunate we lost him. I am glad I met you. You explained to me my father's condition so well that I could counsel my entire family. I have gained a drastic change in my confidence to take care of my family. I wish my father could see me like this, but I guess he had to go on. I will be forever thankful to you!".

What did I learn? I learned LCT is not just a change in the score of UPDRS and the decision to operate or change the medicine or rehabilitate. The 3 hours of LCT is what every patient, therapist, and family member deserves to understand their movement disorder!

Since that day, I have added two more things to my LCT evaluation: prioritize the evaluations and look for the hummingbird!

In addition to Parkinson's disease, other variants include PSP (Progressive Supranuclear Palsy), MSA (Multi-System Atrophy), and vascular Parkinsonism. However, there's no need to be overly concerned or overwhelmed by these terms. Instead, it's recommended to consult your nearest movement disorder neurologist, who can provide a proper evaluation.

Parkinson's disease is the second most common degenerative neurological disease after Alzheimer's. Generally a concern for many in the middle-aged and elderly population, YOPD or Young Onset PD is also rapidly on the ascend. But what exactly is it, and how did it come about? Parkinson's, or Parkinsonism, goes way back to Dr. James Parkinson in the 1800s, who likely made his observations in a rather casual setting. Fast forward, and we've categorized Parkinson's into three types: tremor predominant, bradykinesia rigidity-based, and a mix of the two. There are also Parkinson's mimics, but we'll save that for another chat.

Now, let's cut to the chase—what's happening in Parkinson's? It's a movement disorder, a glitch in our body's software managing how we move. Picture it as a dopamine deficiency, and yes, dopamine agonists play a significant role in treating this.

"How do we diagnose it?" Clinical diagnosis is key. Typically, you notice a slowdown in movement or a hand tremor. Seeking medical help? Perfect. But remember, not any neurologist will do; you'll want one specializing in movement disorders, like our Dr. CC Sanjiv.

But wait, there's more! Dopamine scans, symptom progression, resting tremors—the journey continues. And then there's the "on-off" phase in motor symptoms, but let's not get ahead of ourselves.

Bottom line? There's a lot to unpack about Parkinson's—medicines, treatments, therapies—all designed to improve your quality of life.

So basically, Parkinson's disease is a progressive neurological condition that affects the movement of the body. It is characterized by tremors, stiffness, and slowness of movement.

This condition can be quite challenging to diagnose, as its symptoms can vary from person to person and take years to become apparent.

To make matters more complicated, there is no definitive test for diagnosing Parkinson's disease. This means that misdiagnosis is not uncommon, with rates ranging from 10% to 20% or even higher, depending on the expertise of the clinician.

Now, let's talk about Parkinsonism. Parkinsonism refers to a group of conditions that share similar symptoms with Parkinson's disease. These conditions may be caused by different underlying factors, such as medication side effects, brain damage, or even certain genetic disorders.

While Parkinsonism may present symptoms similar to those of Parkinson's disease, it is important to note that they are not the same. Parkinsonism is more of a broad term that encompasses a range of conditions, while Parkinson's disease is a specific and distinct condition.

Diving a bit deeper into the intricacies of what is commonly referred to as "parkinsonism," it's crucial to note that Parkinsonism itself is not a specific disease. When we mention Parkinsonism, we are talking about a cluster of clinical symptoms. These symptoms encompass slowness of movement, medically termed bradykinesia, tremors, which manifest as shaking of the hands or legs, and stiffness during movement, known as rigidity. Additionally, there's a notable postural instability, indicating an increased tendency to fall.

This set of disorders, characterized by these clinical presentations, falls under the umbrella term of Parkinsonism. Let's break it down into broad categories. The first and foremost is Parkinson's disease, also known as idiopathic Parkinsonism. The second category comprises degenerative disorders, but they affect areas of the brain beyond the substantia nigra.

This group is referred to as Parkinson's plus syndrome, encompassing disorders like multi-system atrophy (MSA), corticobasal degeneration (CBD), Progressive Supranuclear Palsy (PSP), and dementia with Lewy bodies. These symptoms may include cognitive impairments, muscle weakness, and problems with coordination. Parkinson's plus conditions are often more severe and progress more quickly than Parkinson's disease alone.

Moving, the third category involves Parkinsonism induced by external factors, such as toxins or certain medications. Notably, antipsychotic drugs, commonly used to treat psychiatric conditions like schizophrenia, and anti-epileptic drugs, employed in managing epilepsy or seizures, are common culprits. Drug-induced Parkinsonism can also be triggered by anti-emetics, medications used to alleviate vomiting or nausea, and certain other drugs like certain calcium channel blockers.

The final category within Parkinsonism arises due to various causes, including infections affecting the brain, such as bacterial or viral infections leading to encephalitis or meningitis. Moreover, changes in blood vessels, often stemming from conditions like prolonged diabetes or hypertension, contribute to Parkinsonism. Additionally, acute strokes near the basal ganglia area can produce symptoms resembling those of Parkinson's disease.

Understanding these nuances is critical for accurate diagnosis and tailored treatment approaches. If you find yourself grappling with these symptoms, seeking the expertise of a specialized neurologist is pivotal for a comprehensive evaluation and appropriate management.

While the terms Parkinson's disease, Parkinsonism, and Parkinson's plus may be confusing, they refer to different conditions with varying symptoms and underlying causes. It is important to consult a medical professional for an accurate diagnosis. Only through proper diagnosis can the appropriate treatment and care be provided.

While Parkinson's disease is commonly recognized as a movement disorder characterized by slowness and tremors, it extends beyond mere motor symptoms. Delving into the broader spectrum of challenges faced by individuals with Parkinson's, one realizes that slowness and tremors are merely the tip of the iceberg. Unfortunately, these additional problems often go unnoticed and unaddressed throughout the course of the disease.

It's crucial to comprehensively understand and identify the myriad of struggles that patients with Parkinson's disease encounter on a daily basis. Let's delve into the multifaceted aspects of Parkinson's, shedding light on the challenges faced by these individuals.

But before we talk about the challenges, it is pertinent to understand the diagnoses. Now, when we talk about diagnosing a disease, the first question that naturally arises is, 'How severe is it?'

Let's now jump into Parkinson's disease and its various stages.

Globally, Parkinson's is assessed using scales like the ***modified Hoehn and Yahr scale or modified H and Y scale.*** As we know, Parkinson's is a progressive disorder, commencing with minimal symptoms and potentially progressing to complete alleviation.

In the **initial stage 1**, about one-third of the body may be involved, typically starting with the Upper Limb. Gradually progressing to Stage 1.5, symptoms like tremors and tightness may extend to the axial body, forming a distinctive triangle change.

Stage 2 sees the emergence of symptoms on the other side, including tightness and rigidity, without any involvement of balance.

By **Stage 2.5**, balance impairments start to make an appearance, though not functionally disabling. Testing balance often involves a 'pull test,' showcasing good recovery.

Stage 3 witnesses a further development of balance impairments and symptoms affecting both upper and lower limbs, yet not severely hindering daily life.

As the disease progresses to **Stage 4,** significant balance impairments become apparent; necessitating walking aids like sticks or walkers. Despite this, individuals can often manage their daily activities, particularly in non-familiar environments.

Finally, **Stage 5, the last stage**, renders individuals wheelchair-bound or bed-bound. Even with assistance, they may manage a few steps, but manual aid becomes indispensable.

Now, onto some mind-blowing facts.

Fact one: the rate of Parkinson's progression varies widely, with some experiencing a slow progression over years or decades while others witness a much faster deterioration.

Fact two: if both right and left upper limbs exhibit similar symptoms, it's unlikely to be Parkinson's, prompting consideration of Parkinson's plus syndrome or drug-induced Parkinsonism.

Fact three: even before motor symptoms appear, non-motor symptoms such as olfactory loss (losing the sense of smell) may manifest. This may occur many months to years before the PD symptoms appear!

Fact four: in tremor-predominant PD, the symptoms remain unilateral for many years or even decades, unlike the mixed type or the bradykinesia-rigid types, which become bilateral very early.

In Parkinson's Disease tremors often take center stage, presenting in three distinct forms. The most common is the resting tremor, making its grand entrance when you take a break and graciously bowing out when activity resumes. Picture the thumb's delicate forward and backward dance, known as the pill-rolling tremor. Sometimes, it extends its performance to the head or limbs, turning a simple nod into a "no" or shaking up the legs.

Next in our trio is the postural tremor, a tremor with a flair for drama that surfaces when you strike a pose. Trying to maintain a specific position, like extending your hand, can trigger this particular tremor.

Last but not least, the action tremor takes the stage when you engage in action, whether it's savoring a meal or scratching an itch. It adds a dynamic rhythm to your movements.

Now, a common query pops up: Are tremors dangerous? Well, they can be quite the troublemakers. Handling hot beverages or anything requiring precision can pose challenges, leading to spills, burns, or complications.

Speaking of challenges, treating tremors can be tricky. While there are adaptive strategies to ease the impact, they often call for more comprehensive approaches. A hot topic is whether tremors indicate the disease's severity. Interestingly, in tremor-dominant Parkinson's, the slower progression suggests a less urgent journey for the disease.

And now, an important tip: Taming the tremor. Picture this – you're anxious, and your hand tremors amplify. Controlling anxiety can, to some extent, rein in the tremors. However, for tailored advice and more effective solutions, reach out to your closest neurologist.

Let's now unravel the complexities of bradykinesia in Parkinson's disease—a journey into the impact of slowed movements on day-to-day activities. We will be delving deeper into the intricacies of movement slowness in Parkinson's disease, exploring its effects from head to toe, quite literally. To simplify, I've categorized the impact into four facets: posture and walking, facial expressions, hand movements, and speech. Let's embark on this exploration.

Starting with posture and walking, individuals with Parkinson's often adopt a typical bent or flexed posture, giving rise to a fascinating stance. Shoulders droop, and the trunk appears crumpled, influencing walking patterns. A common observation is a shuffling gait with short steps and a narrow base, limiting arm swing. Toe drags and a higher risk of stumbling become apparent.

Moving to facial expressions, Parkinson's can manifest as a reduced facial expression, creating a mask-like face. The natural wrinkles on the forehead may vanish, and the face may lack expressive animation during conversations. Blink rates decrease, affecting eye lubrication and potentially causing dryness and scarring, impacting vision.

Now, let's focus on hand movements. Fine motor skills, such as writing or eating without spills, become challenging. *Micrographia,* a condition where handwriting starts legible but progressively shrinks, poses difficulties, especially with signatures on legal documents.

Lastly, speech in Parkinson's presents two challenges—loudness and clarity. The reduced volume makes their speechless audible, and the precision of articulation is compromised as they struggle with lip and tongue movements.

Ready to unravel another layer of the Parkinson's puzzle? Let's talk about something that might have you feeling a bit like a human statue – rigidity.

Ever had those moments when you feel like your body is channeling its inner brick wall? That's rigidity for you, a common companion in the Parkinson's journey. There are two types of rigidity. Picture trying to move your limb, and it decides to play the role of a stubborn rock, unmoving and resistant. Yes, that's the infamous lead pipe rigidity. A constant tightness, a perpetual game of tug-of-war with your own body.

Now, imagine a cogwheel – that's cogwheel rigidity for you. A little catch here, a release there, making movement feel like navigating a series of gears. It's the quirky sidekick to lead pipe rigidity. How do you know if it's Parkinson's pulling these stiff pranks on you? Well, that's where expert teams of neurologists and advanced neuro rehabilitation experts swoop in. Get yourself evaluated by a movement disorder specialist. We're here to help you decipher whether it's Parkinson's or just your muscles trying out a new role. You can reach us at www.prsneurosciences.com.

Picture this – a patient walks in, convinced there's a snake doing a non-stop tango on his body. Intriguing, right? Let's dive into the whimsical world of hallucinations in Parkinson's.

Now, don't be too quick to blame Parkinson's itself. It's like a magician's hat – sometimes, the tricks inside are side effects of the treatment, especially the dopamine supplements we dish out. Hallucinations can come in various flavors – visual, auditory, or even somatosensory, where you swear something's tap-dancing on your skin. Our star patient felt the slithering sensation 24/7, courtesy of a Parkinson 's-induced hallucination.

Studies reveal that 30 to 50 percent of our Parkinson's pals embark on this hallucinatory adventure at some point. It's like an unexpected plot twist in the Parkinson's saga, affecting not just the patient but also the supporting cast – their families.

Now, let's not forget the psychiatric buddies that often tag along. Depression might decide to be the life of the party, either as a primary guest or sneak in because Parkinson's made socializing a bit tricky. Some even get VIP passes for panic attacks and anxieties.

Let's explore a quirk that's been buzzing in the Parkinson's neighborhood – adamancy. Yes, you heard it right; that stubborn streak might just be Parkinson's knocking on the cognitive door.

Now, let's embark on the riveting journey into the cognitive realms of Parkinson's disease. It's like a four-act play, and each act has its unique twists and turns.

Act one: First up – memory. Sure, they can recount tales from the distant past like memoir pros, but ask them about today's breakfast or who they bumped into – and cue the blank stares. It's the classic case of recent memory playing hide and seek.

Act two is all about language skills – the delicate art of witty banter, jokes, and sarcasm. Picture this: you crack a joke, and instead of laughter, you get a polite ".". It's not rudeness; it's Parkinson's subtly reshaping the language landscape.

Then, we step into **act three** – visual-spatial skills. Ever walk into a room and misjudge the step, leading to a less-than-graceful stumble? Imagine that but on a daily basis. Parkinson's can play tricks on understanding object speed, depth perception, and even the fine art of navigation.

Lastly, **act four** unfolds with a flourish, revealing the impact on higher mental functions. Abstract thinking, problem-solving, adapting to change – the brain's gymnastics routine that might become a bit rusty with Parkinson's.

Now, back to the adamant question. Too much stubbornness could indeed be the brain's way of saying, "I need a little mental flexibility makeover." The frontal area, the maestro of flexible thinking, might be on a break, making way for adamant vibes.

So, if you spot this in yourself or someone close to dealing with Parkinson's, fret not! Instead of a critique, let's opt for a compassionate solution.

In this chapter, we're diving nose-first into a topic that might make you second-guess that last bite of your favorite dish – the hidden symphony of senses in Parkinson's, specifically, the underrated superhero called "smell."

Now, let's embark on a little sensory experiment, shall we? Pause your reading and grab your beloved snack or beverage – for me, it's the aromatic delight of coffee. Close those nostrils and take a sip. Voila! Suddenly, that coffee might just morph into a sweet mystery potion. What happened? Blame it on anosmia – the superhero sense of smell taking a siesta.

With Parkinson's, losing the sense of smell is like a silent ninja creeping into your culinary experiences and taking away your protective response to dangers like cooking gas leaking in the kitchen. Research tells us that a whopping 70 to 100 percent of people with Parkinson's will bid farewell to their sense of smell as the disease waltzes through their lives. Now, you might think, "Well, I can survive without smelling." True, unlike our furry friends, we humans don't rely on smell for survival. But hold your taste buds because here's the kicker – the smell is the unsung hero behind the scenes, orchestrating the symphony of taste and flavors.

Picture this: You sit down for a meal, and suddenly, your favorite dish is just a mundane mix of ingredients. Why? Because the aroma, the essence, the very soul of the dish is lost in translation. And here's the twist – as Parkinson's progresses, the aroma detective in your nose starts to retire, taking down the taste experience with it. Imagine the repercussions on your nutrition when your once-beloved dishes lose their allure.

So, here's the sniff – losing your sense of smell might be more than just an innocent casualty; it could be an early sign of Parkinson's. It's not just about missing out on the fragrance of a rose; it's about the daily battle with your dining table, the taste buds, and the delicate dance of flavors.

Let us continue because now we're flipping the switch on a fascinating topic that we have spoken about previously– the Parkinson's power button, or as I like to call it, the **"On and Off"** phases.

Now, imagine having a special switch that could toggle between being a motor maestro on the dance floor and suddenly hitting pause, leaving you frozen mid-groove. Intrigued? Well, let's unravel the enigma of these phases.

In the Parkinson's saga, our main protagonist is dopamine – or the lack thereof. Enter medications like syndopa and the dopamine sidekick, which are here to keep the party going. But, alas, you can't pop pills like candy all day.

So, here's the theatrical twist – when the medication's spell starts to fade, our Parkinsonian pals enter what we call the **"Off Phase."** It's like Cinderella's carriage turning back into a pumpkin. Suddenly, the high spirits, the smoother moves, and the cognitive wizardry all take a nosedive.

In the early stages, the **"On Phase"** might last longer, and the medication frequency isn't a daily drumroll. But as the Parkinson's plot thickens, dopamine levels drop, and you find yourself popping pills like a seasoned pro – cue the race of 'Ons and Offs' throughout the day.

Now, how do you know if you or someone you know is in the Off Phase? Picture this: the tremors rev up, slowness hits the fast lane, the risk of falling skyrockets, and your voice? It might just pull a Houdini. It's the brain's way of saying, "Hey, I need my dopamine fix!" and many of them even 'freeze' like a statue... Remember the statue game we used to play in school as kids?

Flip the script to the On Phase – within the magic window after taking your meds, the world transforms. Mood lifts, movements quicken, and it's a party with better posture and stability.

Now, you're probably thinking, "If meds work like magic, why bother with rehab or surgeries?" Ah, my curious minds, Parkinson's is a relentless artist, painting its strokes on the canvas of time. Medications might not suffice as the maestro loses control. That's where we, the rehab maestros, waltz in. Our mission? To jazz up your quality of life, even as Parkinson's tries to steal the spotlight.

But, wait, there's more – when the med party becomes too wild, leading to hallucinations, nausea, and an unruly **dance of dyskinesia**, that's when we consider neuromodulation procedures – a neuro makeover if you will.

When you're diagnosed, it's only natural to wonder, "How do the experts measure the impact of this condition?"

The **Unified Parkinson's Disease Rating Scale (UPDRS)** takes center stage. This four-section tool evaluates various aspects, from mood and behavior to daily activities and motor complications. It's considered the gold standard in Parkinson's assessments.

Now, let's not get overwhelmed. There are more tools in the toolkit. The Modified Hoehn and Yahr Scale helps stage the disease's progression, while the Abnormal Involuntary Movement Scale (AIMS) focuses on specific movements.

For cognitive evaluations, the Mini-Mental State Examination (MMSE) steps in. And when it comes to mood, depression scales provide valuable insights. Patient diaries document motor fluctuations, offering a real-life perspective.

The non-motor self-questionnaire explores olfactory losses and hallucinations. Lastly, the Quality-of-Life scales, such as the Functional Independence Measure and Modified Barthel Index, gauge how Parkinson's impacts your daily life. It might seem like a complex set of assessments, but deciphering this medical maze is our job, not yours. If you're wondering about your disease's progression or complications or simply need guidance, reach out to your nearest movement disorder specialist. In the realm of Parkinson's, there's always hope.

Contrary to popular belief, diagnosing Parkinson's isn't as straightforward as a blood test or an ECG. It requires a nuanced approach due to the initial stages often being elusive. The classical features of Parkinson's, such as tremors, rigidity, and slowness, might not manifest distinctly early on. Understanding the difference between Parkinson's disease and its mimics is crucial. The symptoms may overlap, but the diseases differ, much like fever, which is a symptom with varied causes.

If someone suspects they have Parkinson's, consulting a movement disorder neurologist or a proficient neurologist is the initial step. Patience is key, as observing and evaluating symptoms over time is essential. The doctor will navigate through the complex landscape of motor and non-motor symptoms, considering variants like Parkinson's Plus.

Diagnostic tools come into play once clinical assessments are done. An MRI scan might be recommended to rule out other issues in the brain, while an FDOPA PET scan can gauge dopamine uptake in the substantial nigra. These steps aid in confirming and understanding the severity of PD.

For those already diagnosed, seeking clarity on the disease's progression and severity is natural. However, this journey is gradual, often spanning years. Trusting your movement disorder neurologist is crucial, and they'll guide you through each step of the process. In the realm of Parkinson's diagnosis, patience, trust, and expert guidance are your allies.

I want to share a crucial aspect of managing Parkinson's disease and emphasize that surgery may not always be the immediate solution. Many Parkinson's patients seeking surgery haven't followed an optimal treatment plan. Before considering surgery, I recommend consulting a movement disorder neurologist. Like Dr. Sanjiv CC from our Bangalore team, neurologists have successfully been able to adjust medications, which improved symptoms for many patients and negated the need for surgery. Medication optimization involves personalized adjustments, considering timing, dosage, and additional medications.

A comprehensive approach to Parkinson's care includes neuro rehabilitation. A skilled team, including neuro physiotherapists, occupational therapists, speech and swallow therapists, and psychologists, can address various aspects of your condition. Neuro rehabilitation helps improve daily activities, from walking and balance to communication and daily tasks.

Joining a Parkinson's support group can provide invaluable assistance. Our support group offers guidance on modifying your living space and general advice. Embrace a proactive approach to managing Parkinson's, ensuring you lead a fulfilling life.

In the past decade, remarkable advancements have transformed the landscape of Parkinson's disease management. One notable addition to our therapeutic arsenal is Apomorphine, a mild dopamine agonist available in injectable, inhalable, and sublingual forms. Contrary to initial social media hype, it serves as an adjunctive treatment alongside the primary therapy of Levodopa.

Apomorphine is particularly valuable as a **'rescue'** therapy, swiftly alleviating sudden off-periods in patients. The injectable form provides relief for approximately one to one and a half hours. More recently, continuous subcutaneous infusion options have been introduced, though their tolerance can vary among patients, with some experiencing skin irritation.

Additionally, intestinal infusion of Levodopa, known as LCIG, has emerged as a continuous delivery system through a tube inserted into the duodenum. This approach helps manage motor fluctuations and, to some extent, dyskinesia. Meanwhile, new entrants like inhaled Levodopa and subcutaneous Levodopa infusion are gaining attention, offering alternative modalities for treatment.

It's crucial to note that these emerging treatments demand careful consideration and expertise before being recommended to the wider patient population. As we navigate the evolving landscape of Parkinson's therapies, ongoing exploration, and collaboration between patients and healthcare providers remain paramount.

Determining the optimum dosage for Parkinson's disease is a nuanced process, relying on a combination of clinical judgment and the patient's subjective experiences. The patient's symptoms and satisfaction with the current medication dosage play a pivotal role in this assessment. Clinically, we may employ tools like the UPDRS (Unified Parkinson's Disease Rating Scale) to objectively gauge the response.

The right timing of medication intake is equally crucial in Parkinson's management. Taking medications on an empty stomach early in the morning can be highly beneficial. Typically, these medications are administered in divided doses throughout the day, and while some formulations offer extended-release options, it's rare to rely solely on a single dose. The choice between immediate-release and extended-release formulations often depends on the patient's response and individual needs. In instances where a one-time dosage may not yield satisfactory results, adopting a more frequent regimen of three to four times a day might be considered. The key is to tailor the medication schedule to the specific needs and responses of each patient.

The management of Parkinson's disease involves a delicate interplay between medication and, in certain cases, surgical intervention. Initially, patients often experience a "honeymoon period" of four to five years, where they respond well to medications, complemented by physiotherapy. This combined approach can extend the favorable outcome, with some patients even maintaining satisfaction for six to eight years or longer.

For a subset of individuals, especially those experiencing a decline in medication efficacy after several years, surgical options become a consideration. Deep Brain Stimulation (DBS) is a surgical procedure involving the insertion of a pacemaker into the chest, with a wire threaded through the neck and into a specific region of the brain called the subthalamic nucleus or Globus pallidus (GPi). DBS has shown effectiveness in managing tremors, rigidity, and bradykinesia. While it may allow for a reduction in medication dosages based on individual responses, complete cessation of medication is not feasible even with DBS.

Surgical interventions also include Lesioning v3.0 procedures, where targeted areas of the brain are treated. Traditionally, lesions were performed on the opposite side to the more affected part of the body. However, recent advancements have introduced Pallidotomy or Pallido Thalamic Tractotomy on the other side after six months to a year if the clinical presentation is bilateral. It's crucial to note that medication remains a lifelong aspect of Parkinson's management, with adjustments made based on individual responses and the side effects profile.

The decision between medications and surgical options is nuanced, emphasizing personalized care to optimize patient outcomes. In surgical management for Parkinson's Disease, there's often a misconception about the potential for a cure post-surgery. As a stereotactic and functional neurosurgeon, I encounter many patients who, after undergoing surgery, express a sense of near-normalcy, stating that they feel cured. However, it's crucial to clarify that while surgical interventions aim to enhance the quality of life for an extended period, Parkinson's disease remains a degenerative condition without a definitive cure.

Before delving into the surgical options, it's essential to emphasize that not every individual with Parkinson's symptoms automatically qualifies for surgery. Rigorous screening, including the levodopa challenge test, is conducted by both movement disorder neurologists and stereotactic and function neurosurgeons to identify those who may benefit the most from surgical management.

Now, when considering surgical options, two approaches emerge, both involving a small hole in the skull to access the brain. The first method is Radio Frequency Ablation (RFA), aka Lesioning v3.0, akin to burning a misbehaving circuit in the brain. This technique, which doesn't require an implant, can yield remarkable results.

Patients often report improvements, from reduced tremors to enhanced daily functioning. Importantly, RFA is a more cost-effective alternative, making it accessible to a broader range of patients.

On the other end, there's Deep Brain Stimulation (DBS), a surgical procedure involving the implantation of a pacemaker in the brain. While DBS is equally effective, it comes with a substantial cost associated with the imported implant, ranging from 7 to 20 lakhs. The surgery's expense, coupled with postoperative programming, adds to the overall financial investment.

To decide between RFA and DBS, patients often weigh factors such as cost, long-term follow-up requirements, and their personal preferences. RFA, aka Lesioning v3.0, with its lower overall cost and minimal follow-up needs, stands out as an excellent option, especially for those who find the expenses associated with DBS prohibitive.

Both RFA and DBS offer effective surgical solutions for Parkinson's Disease. The choice between them involves considering financial constraints, follow-up commitments, and individual preferences. As we explore these surgical options further, let's address the intricacies, benefits, and potential complications associated with each procedure. In essence, I consider myself a "brain circuit surgeon" tasked with mapping functional brain circuits to alleviate the dysfunction and disability that individuals with Parkinson's Disease may experience. The aim is to enhance their functionality, enabling them to manage daily life and contribute meaningfully to society.

Now, when a patient qualifies for Parkinson's surgery and we determine that RFA is the optimal course of action, we embark on a crucial step: defining which circuit in the brain needs to be targeted. It's not a one-size-fits-all scenario; there are various circuits, each corresponding to specific symptoms experienced by the patient.

One prevalent symptom of Parkinson's is tremors. If tremor is the primary concern without accompanying features like rigidity or bradykinesia, the Ventralis Intermediate Nucleus of the Thalamus (VIM) becomes a key target. The Thalamus, a vital brain junction, houses this nucleus, and pinpointing it accurately is pivotal.

Let's delve into the specific brain circuits we target during RFA surgery. Previously, I introduced VIM (Ventralis Intermedius Nucleus of the Thalamus) as a primary target, especially when Tremor is the predominant symptom without additional Parkinsonian features. Now, let's explore two other pivotal targets: GPI (Globus Pallidus Interna) and PTT (Pallido Thalamic Tract).

GPI, a sizable nucleus, is a preferred target when addressing a spectrum of Parkinsonian symptoms, including tremors, rigidity, bradykinesia, and the on-off phenomena. Additionally, GPI becomes crucial in mitigating drug-induced dyskinesia resulting from medications like Levodopa. The surgery associated with this target is known as pallidotomy, and it has demonstrated remarkable efficacy in alleviating symptoms and enhancing the overall quality of life for many patients.

Moving forward, PTT, or the pallidothalamic tract, emerges as another valuable target. Particularly useful when planning bilateral procedures, PTT shares similarities with pallidotomy in terms of indications. Given the risk considerations associated with bilateral pallidotomy, combining it with PTT on the opposite side has proven effective, ensuring a comprehensive and balanced approach.

The planning process involves determining precise XYZ coordinates for both the target and the entry point. Now, with the surgical stage set, we transition into the operating theater. It is crucial to note that the entire procedure unfolds under local anesthesia, creating a unique atmosphere where patients can engage in conversation and provide valuable feedback throughout the surgery.

Once in the operating room, the patient is secured to the table with a rock-solid fixation system to ensure absolute stability. The local anesthesia ensures the patient feels no pain, fostering a cooperative environment. As we progress, a 14-millimeter hole is meticulously created in the skull, providing access for the electrode.

At this point, the stereotactic frame comes into play, ensuring that the electrode is guided precisely to the predetermined coordinates. The electrode's journey involves careful navigation of approximately 9.5 centimeters into the brain through a 14-millimeter burr hole. Amidst this intricate process, technology becomes the surgeon's guiding companion, continuously providing feedback through impedance, voltage, current, pulse width, frequency, and Ohm's law calculations.

The pivotal moment arrives when the surgeon confirms being on the target. A small current is applied to simulate the intended effect, and any potential side effects, such as tingling sensations or movement difficulties, are closely monitored. This interactive process ensures real-time adjustments, maintaining the utmost precision.

Once assured of being on target and eliminating any risks, the actual lesioning process begins. The targeted circuit is gradually heated to 70 degrees Celsius for 60 seconds, creating a controlled burn. The entire procedure, from electrode insertion to lesioning, involves meticulous attention to detail, with the surgeon closely monitoring the patient's response. Throughout the surgery, neurologists and rehabilitation specialists collaborate, evaluating the patient's response to specific interventions. The goal is not merely to perform a physical procedure but to witness tangible improvements in symptoms, validating the success of the surgery.

Patient satisfaction often peaks during the procedure, with many expressing the sensation that they have already taken their Parkinson's medication, even before the surgery concludes. This immediate feedback serves as a crucial indicator that the procedure has hit the "sweet spot."

The journey of RFA, aka Lesioning v3.0 surgery, is a blend of art and science, requiring the surgeon's expertise, technological support, and the patient's active involvement.

After Parkinson's surgery, patients often wonder if they can stop taking their medication. Like with chronic conditions such as hypertension or diabetes, which require ongoing medication, the same is true for Parkinson's. Surgery can help reduce medication doses, sometimes by half, which is great for improving life quality.

For a few, mainly those with tremors, stopping medication completely is possible but rare. Most people will still need some medication, but less often and in smaller amounts. The main win is a better quality of life with fewer Parkinson's symptoms.

The aim isn't to stop medication completely but to use less and live better. Surgery offers a more stable life, with less worry about Parkinson's symptoms. Recovery includes rehabilitation, where the patient's efforts are just as important as the surgeon's. Surgery is a step, but ongoing work is needed to improve symptoms.

Consider the example of Sachin Tendulkar, a cricketing legend who, after shoulder surgery, didn't merely sit back and expect miracles to happen. Despite the sutures being removed in 10 to 12 days, his return to competitive sports took nine months, during which he engaged in rigorous rehabilitation. This underscores a crucial point – the importance of rehabilitation in the overall recovery process.

As a doctor specializing in stereotactic and functional neurosurgery, I am not a magician. My skill lies in assisting patients in controlling the symptoms of Parkinson's disease. However, achieving a significant improvement post-surgery necessitates collaboration. The body, having undergone neuromodulation surgery, experiences altered circuits and firings, leading to confusion and a need for optimization.

Rehabilitation becomes indispensable in this scenario, whether or not surgery is involved. For those undergoing neuromodulation surgery, such as radiofrequency ablation or deep brain stimulation, the need for rehabilitation becomes even more pronounced. These surgeries alter the neural landscape abruptly, and the body needs guidance to adapt to these changes. A comprehensive neuro-rehabilitation program, typically involving a team of specialists including physical therapists, occupational therapists, speech therapists, language and swallow experts, cognitive and behavior therapists, and pain therapists, is vital. This team evaluates the challenges faced by the patient, creating a tailored program that addresses each aspect of post-surgical adjustment.

Patients must recognize the significance of rehabilitation, especially when opting for surgery. A minimum of three months of dedicated rehabilitation is often recommended by my team and me. Ignoring this critical phase can significantly impact the outcome of the surgery.

The risks, challenges, and financial investment made in the surgical procedure can only yield optimal results when coupled with a commitment to thorough neuro rehabilitation with a team who understands the nuances of post-op care for stereotactic neurosurgeries.

The journey to improved functioning post-surgery is a collaborative effort where rehabilitation plays a pivotal role in optimizing results. It's not just about what the surgeon can do; it's about what the patient can achieve through active engagement in the recovery process.

In the early stages of Parkinson's disease, medication can indeed offer relief, helping individuals regain a semblance of their pre-diagnosis normalcy. However, the key lies in not underestimating the importance of rehabilitation, even during these initial phases. Parkinson's is a progressive disease, and as it advances, its impact extends beyond mere movement issues.

Contrary to common belief, Parkinson's progression introduces challenges in various facets of life, encompassing difficulties in thinking, memory, bowel movements, urinary control, and postural stability.

Recognizing this multifaceted impact, a multidisciplinary rehabilitation team becomes imperative. Such a team typically comprises physical therapists, occupational therapists, speech-language pathologists, and cognitive therapists, each specializing in their domain.

Considering the diverse spectrum of challenges presented by Parkinson's – from movement disorders to issues in daily activities like eating, dressing, and toileting – a well-coordinated rehabilitation approach is essential. Let's delve into the specific roles of each specialist:

1. **Physical Therapists:** Address challenges related to movement, walking, balance, and overall physical functionality. If someone struggles with turning in bed, getting up, or maintaining balance, a physical therapist can offer invaluable assistance.

2. **Occupational Therapists:** Focus on enhancing daily living activities. Whether it's difficulties in activities like eating, brushing, or dressing, an occupational therapist intervenes to improve these aspects.

3. **Speech-Language Pathologists (SLP):** Step in when issues with swallowing, speech, voicing, or language, especially in the later stages, become apparent. An SLP plays a crucial role in addressing these specific challenges.

4. **Cognitive Therapists:** Assist individuals dealing with cognitive issues, aiding in thinking processes and memory retention.

The integration of a multidisciplinary rehabilitation team is pivotal for comprehensive Parkinson's management. While medication may alleviate some symptoms, rehabilitation ensures a holistic approach, addressing the varied challenges that arise with the progression of the disease.

To maintain an optimal quality of life, it's crucial to recognize that medication and rehabilitation are not mutually exclusive but rather work in tandem.

Moving on, I'd like to address a common sentiment that echoes through various medical conditions, including Parkinson's disease and its associated surgeries. There seems to be a collective desire for doctors to work magic, to miraculously alleviate symptoms without active involvement from the patient. It's a sentiment that is very much like a diabetic patient yearning for the doctor to manage blood sugar levels while indulging freely in sweets.

It's crucial to dispel the notion that a doctor, despite possessing skills and expertise, cannot single-handedly resolve all aspects of a patient's condition. I am not a magician; I am a doctor equipped with the ability to assist in controlling the symptoms of Parkinson's disease. However, the collaborative effort between the patient and the medical team is indispensable for achieving significant improvement.

This example illustrates a fundamental truth: recovery requires effort, commitment, and active participation from the patient. Whether it's retraining brain circuits or optimizing muscle function, rehabilitation becomes a non-negotiable component of the post-surgery journey. The body, having undergone neuromodulation surgeries like radiofrequency ablation or deep brain stimulation, experiences abrupt alterations in circuits and firings, leading to confusion.

Neuro rehabilitation becomes a must for Parkinson's disease patients, whether surgery is involved or not. However, the need intensifies when surgeries alter neural circuits suddenly. The confusion arising from different feedback, old memories, and new signals necessitates a strategic approach towards optimization.

The importance of neuro-rehabilitation cannot be overstated, particularly after undergoing surgeries for conditions like Parkinson's disease. The collaborative efforts of patients and dedicated medical teams, coupled with a commitment to a comprehensive rehabilitation program, are essential for achieving superlative results. So, let's not overlook the significance of neuro-rehabilitation at reputable centers, ensuring that the journey toward optimal functioning continues beyond the operating room.

Navigating movement disorders can be a complex journey, encompassing various conditions such as Parkinson's disease, PSP (Progressive Supranuclear Palsy), MSA (Multi-System Atrophy), and vascular parkinsonism. These terms might seem overwhelming, but there's no need for undue concern. As a neurosurgeon based in Bangalore, I work closely with Dr. Sanjiv CC, a seasoned neurologist with 30 years of experience specializing in movement disorders. Our collaborative efforts extend from thorough medical management, incorporating drugs and injections like apomorphine, to surgical considerations for drug-resistant cases. Together, we formulate a comprehensive strategy that integrates medical treatments, including injections, with physical therapy for neural rehabilitation in managing Parkinson's disease.

Our collaboration transcends surgeries; we actively participate in pre and post-operative management and contribute to global educational programs. Delivering lectures on various movement disorder topics nationally and internationally enables us to share our expertise and stay abreast of advancements in the field.

Since 2017, Dr. Sanjiv and I have successfully treated numerous Parkinson's patients using bilateral lesioning surgery and DBS procedures. Despite our meticulous care, setbacks may occur, as illustrated by a notable case involving a relative of the then Governor whose DBS needed to be explanted as she, as an uncontrolled diabetic, got her implant infected. The nuanced task of convincing and selecting the right patients involves careful consideration of various factors and applying scales in pre-surgical evaluations. During surgery, we closely monitor signs, symptoms, and potential side effects. Post-surgery, brain imaging assists in detecting issues, and we proceed with medication adjustments and rehabilitation programs.

Tackling these challenges undoubtedly demands mental preparation. Lesioning, creating a small hole in the brain, and DBS, a more intricate procedure resembling a pacemaker, are the chosen interventions. While DBS is a costly procedure, Lesioning v3.0 offers a financially feasible option, especially for patients with predominantly one-sided symptoms and financial constraints. Successful recovery often necessitates extensive and prolonged rehabilitation programming. If you find yourself confronted with these complex terms, consulting a movement disorder neurologist is the first step toward comprehensive evaluation and personalized care.

Experience During Surgery for Parkinson's and Dystonia

For conditions like Idiopathic Parkinson's Disease and dystonia, there are two main surgical options: lesioning and Deep Brain Stimulation (DBS), used when medication isn't enough.

Deep Brain Stimulation (DBS):

DBS involves putting an electrode in the brain, which stays there and connects to an Impulse Generator (IPG) in the chest. The electrode sends signals to help control symptoms.

Why "Deep Brain Surgeries"?

Deep brain surgeries target the basal ganglia, deep brain structures crucial for movement. Parkinson's affects these areas by reducing dopamine, which is essential for muscle control. It is the same for both lesioning and DBS.

When Medication Isn't Enough:

Medications can become less effective over time, which is when DBS can help. DBS uses a device like a heart pacemaker, with leads placed in the brain to deliver electrical stimulation and improve movement control.

DBS as a Solution:

DBS is a more long-term treatment, providing relief when regular medications can't help anymore. It sends electrical signals directly to the brain areas responsible for movement, reducing symptoms for many patients.

Parkinson's Disease (PD) Conclusion

As we have understood in this chapter, Parkinson's disease is a progressive neurodegenerative disorder primarily affecting movement control. Key points include common symptoms like tremors, muscle rigidity, slowness of movement, and postural instability. Its cause is linked to genetic and environmental factors, resulting in a dopamine deficiency due to the loss of nerve cells. Diagnosis relies on clinical evaluation, with no definitive blood tests or imaging studies. Management involves medications, therapies, lifestyle adjustments, and, in advanced cases, deep brain stimulation surgery. Ongoing research aims to understand the disease and develop improved treatments, with advocacy efforts, such as those by Michael J. Fox, which are crucial for awareness and funding. While challenging, advancements offer hope for better treatments and, ultimately, a cure. I know this chapter has been a long read...but here's one final story before we move on...

Stopping the 'Shakes' – a dramatic story of a poor rural lady

At Bhagwan Mahaveer Jain Hospital, a remarkable story unfolded—one that could easily be mistaken for a tale of the paranormal but was, in reality, a stark medical challenge.

A woman arrived at my consultation room, brought in by her concerned family. Night after night, her family endured sleepless hours, disturbed not by spectral whispers but by the constant jingling of her bangles and anklets. As she rested on her Katara mattress, the jewelry resonated with the rhythm of her uncontrollable tremors, casting a haunting pall over the household. The sounds were so eerie that some family members whispered of possession or curses. Yet, the true adversary was her own body's betrayal—a severe neurological disorder manifesting as intense, unrelenting resting tremors of Idiopathic Parkinson's Disease that defied all conventional treatments.

Determined to reclaim the night's peace for her family, we opted for a sophisticated approach: MRI-guided stereotactic neurosurgery targeting the Ventralis Intermedius' Vim' nucleus of the thalamus, a precise technique demanding not only medical expertise but a solid grasp of mathematics and physics.

During the procedure, the woman was awake, a testament to God's creation of the human body's extraordinary architecture; the brain, devoid of pain receptors, allowed us to operate on the patient fully conscious. After administering local anesthesia, I drilled a small 14 mm opening in her skull. Guided by advanced software, I inserted a one x4 mm monopolar electrode deep into her brain, as per the XYZ coordinates obtained from the software. The operating room, filled with bated breath, watched as I began the delicate process of stimulating and then ablating the misfiring circuits.

Then, miraculously, as I adjusted the probe and the ablation progressed, the tremors began to subside until—finally—they DRAMATICALLY stopped altogether as someone had just flipped a switch OFF inside her brain! It was a profound moment of victory, achieved on the surgical table under the harsh lights of the operating room.

When she returned for her follow-up, it was clear we had turned a corner. The tremors that had once haunted her nights were gone, and with them, the myth of the nighttime demon her family feared. They were overjoyed, grateful for the silence that had once again become a staple of their nocturnal life.

This case was more than a medical victory; it was a battle against a relentless foe, where science and determination converged to banish the tremor demon, albeit temporarily, restoring calm and normalcy to a family once gripped by fear. We will never know when Parkinson's Disease will rear its ugly head once again, but so far, so good....

6
DYSTONIA

THE DISABLING HYPERKINETIC MOVEMENT DISORDER

"I am not my body. My body is not me. I am not my dystonia. My dystonia is not me."

- Tom Seaman

Tom Seaman is an author, speaker, and coach who has written extensively about his experiences living with dystonia, a neurological movement disorder characterized by involuntary muscle contractions. Seaman shares his journey of coping with dystonia and offers insights and strategies for managing the condition through his writing and speaking engagements. His work aims to raise awareness about dystonia and provide support and inspiration to others facing similar challenges.

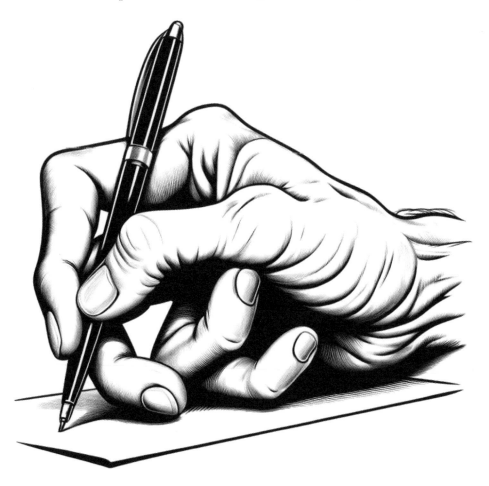

Nestled within the rustic embrace of Kuduchi, where emerald fields stretched into the horizon, Virupaksha Shekar Basagunde's story unfolded like a tragic epic. In this serene locale, Virupaksha, a resilient soul in his mid-20s, has become somewhat of a symbol of perseverance in the face of adversity. Virupaksha shares his life with a small yet tight-knit family, which includes his father, mother, grandmother, brother, sister-in-law, and her two little girls, all of whom contribute to the family's agricultural endeavors.

As the son of a family that toiled in the sun-soaked fields of Belgaum, Virupaksha was the embodiment of their dreams. Yet, fate dealt a cruel hand in 2010 when the tendrils of dystonia slithered into his world. Unbeknownst to them, this insidious adversary was about to play a sinister game, disguising itself as a myriad of ailments.

The initial whispers of dystonia manifested during Virupaksha's 10th standard, starting as an unsettling tremor in his arms. Slowly, like a venomous serpent, it coiled around his entire body, from head to toe, paralyzing them in its relentless grip.

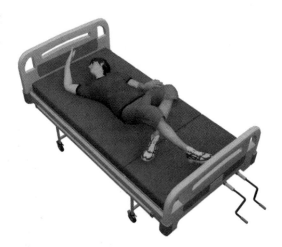

His head was pulling backward, the upper limbs shaking violently when attempting to hold a bottle or cup in his hand, and he was unable to stand and walk without support or use the toilet and clean himself up – he needed assistance 24 x 7, and his mother's only job was to help him. The quality of life of the entire family was a mess, with no hope in sight. In their desperate quest for answers, the family embarked on a pilgrimage to the mission hospital in Maharashtra, pouring their hopes and resources into a cure. However, the cruel reality struck them like a thunderbolt – their sacrifices yielded no improvement. The family, once a bastion of strength, now stood on the precipice of hopelessness.

Virupaksha, once an engineering student and a sturdy driver maneuvring a tractor through the family's fields, now found himself confined to a bed, an unwilling captive of dystonia's tyranny. The very soil that once bore witness to his agile movements became a distant memory, replaced by the haunting specter of paralysis.

Their journey for a cure led them to Qutub Makandhar Hospital in Belgaum, where the cold hands of despair tightened their grip. Dystonia, an elusive adversary, continued its relentless assault, casting a shadow not only on Virupaksha's limbs but also on his speech. His voice, once a melody echoing through the fields, became a tortured whisper.

The family's desperation deepened, and with each passing day, Virupaksha's frail form became a mere shell of his former self. In their anguish, they sought answers through CT and MRI scans, revealing the severity of his condition. Urgently directed to the nearest town, the family's beacon of hope, Dr. Shabade, referred them to a major hospital in Bangalore for a groundbreaking procedure – Deep Brain Stimulation (DBS) or brain pacemaker surgery.

Yet, the pursuit of relief through DBS became a prolonged battle marked by disappointment. The DBS results were modest, and two years of clinging on to the elusive promise of improvement left Virupaksha and his family teetering on the edge of desolation as the battery went dead, and they had no further funds to replace the battery.

On one fateful October day in 2017, hope rekindled with a flicker of light for the family. Virupaksha had finally been referred to me, and that is when I took charge, orchestrating the removal of the ineffective and dead DBS, engaging in delicate functional neurosurgery – **bilateral, simultaneous pallidotomy, a high-risk procedure.** By the second or third post-operative day, he showed a definite improvement in his preoperative retrocollis, and he was able to keep his head in a neutral position without anyone supporting it from behind. This in itself was a huge improvement, as per the family. A newfound hope emerged, and with it, the arduous journey of neuro-rehabilitation began.

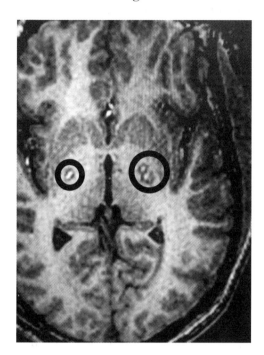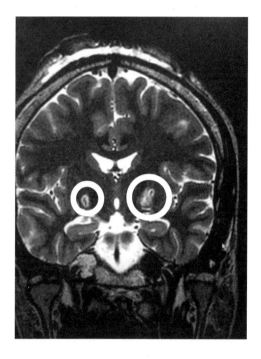

In the labyrinth of therapies and treatments, Virupaksha's family witnessed a metamorphosis. The once bedridden soul, bound by the chains of dystonia, began to slowly emerge.

Intense neuro rehabilitation began soon after the surgery. Their family was counseled that the next three to four months were crucial for Virupaksha's recovery, and intensive neuro rehabilitation was the key to that. However, the family was already out of money, and the mother cried to me in helplessness. But, like all mothers would, she wanted the best for her son. She said – I am seeing some hope now; please don't abandon us. At that point, Dr. Prathiba told them not to worry, and she did the entire neuro rehab without charging the family anything, 100% FREE of cost!

As the neuro rehab progressed, so did he, and by leaps and bounds, I must say. I remember when he came to us, there were instabilities throughout his body, but those two months of rehab changed that for him. From not being able to walk or talk, he gradually started to move around with support, eventually not needing any support at all.

The man who needed someone to hold his neck up while he spoke did not need any support, and the best part was that his speech was back! Not just murmur but intelligible speech. And he was able to feed himself. Even now, he slowly moves around his house independently (taking support of the walls) and even goes to the fields and supervises the workers! His dystonia has improved by about 50-60%, but his associated cerebellar atrophy has caused him to have imbalance issues. In spite of all this, the family is grateful.

The resilience demonstrated by Virupaksha and the unwavering support of his family exemplifies the transformative power of medical interventions and rehabilitation. While dystonia may present formidable challenges, Virupaksha's journey serves as a testament to the possibilities of recovery, reminding us that determination and advancements in medical science can bring about positive change even in the face of severe neurological conditions.

For dystonia, wearing the deceptive cloak of joint or psychological problems had momentarily obscured itself. Yet, in the crucible of Virupaksha's struggle, the truth emerged – a testament to the resilience of the human spirit and the indomitable will to unravel the mysteries hidden beneath the surface.

Dystonia, a neurological disorder characterized by involuntary muscle contractions, results in repetitive and twisting movements or abnormal postures. These movements can target a single muscle, a group of muscles, or the entire body, signifying dystonia as a spectrum disorder with varying degrees of severity. The impact ranges from mild inconveniences to severe disruptions, significantly influencing an individual's daily life and overall quality of life.

As a multifaceted disorder, dystonia manifests in diverse forms, presenting distinct challenges for both individuals and healthcare professionals in their quest to comprehend, diagnose, and manage this intricate condition. The various manifestations of dystonia are each categorized based on the pattern and distribution of muscle contractions. Here are some common types:

1. Focal Dystonia: Specific body parts are affected, such as cervical dystonia impacting the neck muscles, blepharospasm involving the muscles around the eyes, or writer's cramp affecting the hand and forearm muscles.

2. Segmental Dystonia: Adjacent body parts experience involuntary contractions, with both an arm and a leg being a common example.

3. Generalized Dystonia: Multiple muscle groups across the body are affected, significantly impairing mobility and posture.

4. Hemidystonia: Dystonic movements occur on one side of the body, affecting the arm, leg, and sometimes the face on the same side.

5. Multifocal Dystonia: Involuntary muscle contractions manifest in different non-adjacent body regions, more widespread than focal dystonia but less extensive than generalized dystonia.

6. Task-Specific Dystonia: Symptoms arise during specific activities or tasks, as seen in musicians' dystonia, which affects musicians during instrument play.

7. Idiopathic Dystonia: Cases where the cause is unknown, with genetics playing a role in some instances, though the origins remain unclear for many.

Dystonia can be either a primary condition or secondary to other medical factors, such as certain medications, brain injury leading to hypoxia of the brain, or other neurological disorders. The precise mechanism behind dystonia is not fully elucidated, but disruptions in the brain's communication with muscles are believed to underlie the abnormal and involuntary movements.

The management of dystonia often necessitates a multidisciplinary approach involving movement disorder neurologists, functional neurosurgeons, physical therapists, occupational therapists, speech and swallowing therapists, and psychologists. Treatment options encompass medications, botulinum toxin injections to mitigate muscle contractions, and, in severe cases, surgical interventions like deep brain stimulation or Lesioning v3.0.

Understanding Dystonia: Challenges in Diagnosis and Treatment

Dystonia is a complex neurological disorder characterized by involuntary muscle contractions, varying widely based on the body regions and patterns affected. Proper diagnosis and tailored treatment plans are crucial due to their diverse manifestations.

Despite its significance, dystonia often remains underdiagnosed or misidentified, particularly in less urban areas where it might be mistaken for orthopedic or psychological issues. Some even misconstrue its symptoms as supernatural afflictions. This misdiagnosis stems partly from its ability to mimic other conditions, leading sufferers down a path of ineffective treatments.

People with dystonia may experience unusual hand postures, uncontrollable neck or limb movements, and even whole-body distortions, often dismissed as stress or poor posture. Initially, they might consult orthopedic surgeons or psychologists, who are not typically trained to recognize neurological disorders like dystonia. Consequently, these professionals might overlook dystonia's neurological roots, attributing symptoms to more familiar conditions like arthritis or psychological stress.

This lack of awareness prolongs suffering and delays effective treatment. Identifying dystonia early on is challenging as many are unaware of its neurological basis. Additionally, those diagnosed may struggle with sensory perception, further complicating their ability to manage everyday tasks and receive appropriate care.

For effective management, recognizing the role of neurologists in diagnosing and treating dystonia is essential. They are equipped to understand the subtle nuances of the disorder and can offer interventions that address the root neurological causes.

Distinguishing Surgical Outcomes and Strategies for Outcome Prediction

I'd now like to draw your attention to a question most caregivers and patients of dystonia may have:

What are the differences in outcomes of surgery for dystonia vs other movement disorders, and how to predict the outcome?

Let me start by highlighting a critical distinction in outcomes between neuromodulation surgeries for dystonia and those performed for other conditions such as spasticity, Parkinson's, tremors, or rigidity. Typically, individuals undergoing surgery for conditions like tremors often experience immediate relief, sometimes achieving tremor arrest right on the operation table. The post-surgery outcomes for such cases are generally positive, with complete remission from tremors being the norm. While a persistent tremor may occasionally occur, instances of individuals not achieving complete remission are negligible, as observed in our institute.

Similarly, individuals undergoing Intrathecal Baclofen (ITB) implantation for spasticity witness rapid muscle relaxation upon drug induction, leading to improved functionality over time, particularly if voluntary control was hindered by excessive spasticity. In contrast, the scenario shifts when it comes to dystonia. The immediate changes observed on the operating table are related to a sense of muscle relaxation, indicating a temporary relief from the constant muscle contraction characteristic of dystonia.

However, the true challenge surfaces post-surgery. Unlike other conditions where the benefits are swiftly evident, individuals with dystonia grapple with the lingering presence of pre-existing maladaptive muscle synergy. In fact, it may take anywhere from 3 weeks to 3 months for the patient to experience the complete benefit from the surgery performed – so much so that the negligible results seen in the initial post-operative stages make everyone believe that the surgery might have failed.

The analogy provided likens this challenge to overriding a specific software in the brain, governing muscle behavior during task participation. This process takes time, extending up to four to six months and, in some cases, even up to a year. The critical aspect lies in monitoring patients closely during this period to assess if the dystonia component is either increasing or manifesting in new ways, such as spreading across limbs.

Moreover, the importance of post-operative rehabilitation and adherence to exercise regimes cannot be overstated. At this stage, a need for constant vigilance arises to ensure that the prescribed rehabilitation and exercise routines are followed diligently. This is crucial for rewiring adaptive muscle recruitment patterns in the brain specific to the given task, contributing significantly to the overall success and sustained positive outcomes of dystonia surgery.

Mr. Bhandari from Mangalore was once a vibrant businessman and socialite whose life took an unexpected turn. He faced a challenge that profoundly impacted his social interactions—not due to an inability to move or speak, but because of a rare condition that forced him to support his head with his hand to keep it upright. This condition, as perplexing as it was distressing, led him to my clinic. His struggle underscored the significant effects that physical limitations can have on one's social life. Diagnosed with cervical dystonia, Mr. Bhandari was at risk of severe complications, including spinal issues and potentially paralysis, if his condition went unmanaged.

The path to Mr. Bhandari's recovery involved a collaboration with Dr. Sanjiv C.C. for a surgical consultation and Mr. V. Siddharth, an occupational therapist new to our team and unfamiliar with movement disorders of this nature. Despite the initial uncertainty, Siddharth's comprehensive pre- and post-operative evaluations were instrumental. The surgical procedure of choice was a pallidotomy, targeting the brain's Globus Pallidus Interna to address the dystonia.

Post-surgery, we observed modest improvements. However, it was through Siddharth's rehabilitation program, which focused on exercises and retraining muscle memory, that Mr. Bhandari began to see significant changes. He shared that before the surgery and rehabilitation, his head would constantly pull to the right, making it impossible to keep steady for even a moment. This involuntary movement was particularly troubling during social events, like weddings, where posing for photos became a source of embarrassment due to his inability to look straight.

After the comprehensive treatment, including the pivotal surgery and dedicated rehabilitation, Mr. Bhandari experienced a remarkable transformation. He joyfully reported that he could now keep his head straight and look forward without any issues, marking a significant milestone in his recovery. This improvement in his condition not only allowed him to engage in social activities without the previous distress but also reinstated his confidence and quality of life.

However, this journey reiterated an important lesson: the path to recovery requires persistence and ongoing effort. A brief recurrence of symptoms underscored the need for continuous exercise and rehabilitation to maintain the progress achieved. Mr. Bhandari's story is a testament to resilience, the effectiveness of targeted medical interventions, and the critical role of rehabilitation. Now, enjoying his retirement, he reflects on this journey as a pivotal chapter in reclaiming his social identity and personal freedom.

In my years navigating the complex corridors of neurosurgical practice, Sadhana's case emerged as a beacon of both challenge and revelation. A young, energetic woman in her prime, Sadhana hailed from Varanasi, a city echoing with the depth of history and the distinguished honor of being PM Narendra Modi's constituency. Her journey to my clinic bypassed the conventional steps, propelling her straight into surgery without the preliminary evaluations typically conducted in the Outpatient Department (OPD). It was as if she was navigating the medical system with a map I hadn't seen. They had read and watched the extensive news coverage of my successful 'guitar surgery,' and they experienced some 'hope.'

Sadhana was grappling with an extraordinary condition called right hemi-dystonia, wherein some strange power seemed to be dragging her head and entire body to the right side the moment she tried to get up from bed or chair, so much so that she had to physically lift and prop up her head with her right hand to look forward; an unseen force relentlessly drew her to the ground with every attempt to sit, stand, or walk. This force was so overpowering that she found herself compelled to use her hands for support, battling against an invisible adversary. Coming from a Bihar locale, where women her age were often preparing for marriage, this ailment cast a shadow over her future, igniting her mother's fears that Sadhana might never find a partner.

Desperately looking for some medical miracle, they had been regularly visiting a major government hospital in Delhi, where they were repeatedly told that nothing could be done and that she would remain like that... until they saw the guitar surgery news and came rushing to my hospital in Bengaluru.

The challenge of communicating complex medical procedures and the need for extensive neuro rehabilitation was amplified by my limited Hindi, adding another layer of difficulty to our interactions. Diagnosed with right hemi-dystonia, Sadhana's condition severely disrupted the coordination and movement of her right side, infiltrating every aspect of her daily life. Siddharth, ever-committed to his role, plunged into research to untangle the complexities of this disorder that had so dramatically altered Sadhana's world. We cautiously opted for a Pallidotomy on the left side of her brain, managing expectations with a modest prediction of a 30-40% improvement.

The post-operative phase tested our patience; dystonia is stubborn, often unveiling its improvements only after weeks. This period was particularly trying as Sadhana's mother, struggling with the initial lack of visible results and the burden of financial strain, confronted me with despair and anger. Despite these challenges and in the face of her vehement objections, I waived my fees, hoping to ease their burden. But they left back to their hometown in a huff.

Remarkably, Sadhana's condition began to improve gradually over the ensuing weeks, and even without the benefit of structured neuro rehabilitation, her dystonia had diminished by more than 80% within the first eight months. This journey, fraught with slow progress and moments of despair, ultimately veered toward a hopeful horizon. However, hers was not a 'they all lived happily ever after' story.... about one year after the surgery, she developed dystonia in her right foot, which was initially mild and came on and off. However, over the next 2-3 years, this dystonia (only of the right foot, which was not there before the surgery) progressed and involved her left side. This only meant that hers was more like a progressive, generalized dystonia. God only knows what the future has in store for her.

I felt very bad and helpless...but I did offer a second surgery, which they were not very keen on. They wanted a guaranteed cure, which nobody can promise. Neurological disorders are unforgiving many a time. Unlike Essential Tremors (ET) and Focal Hand Dystonia (FHD), where precision surgery usually results in a long-term 'cure,' other dystonias are much more unpredictable. In my own series, most patients, at best, get about 50-70 % relief of symptoms and, at worst, only 20-30%. In some patients, after the initial few good years, the symptoms worsen, or new symptoms appear, marking progress in the disease. Remember that most of these surgeries only help manage the clinical symptoms of the patient and do not cure them of the underlying pathology. However, despite most of them having some level of residual symptoms, they are all happy and grateful that even such a reduction in symptoms and suffering was made possible.

7

SPASTICITY

THE NEGLECTED OR UNDERDIAGNOSED 'ELEPHANT' IN THE ROOM!

Spasticity is like trying to drive your car with the hand brakes on!

Spasticity is a 'bugbear' for every neurologist, neurosurgeon, and rehab professional globally!

–Dr. Sharan Srinivasan
Stereotactic & Functional Neurosurgeon

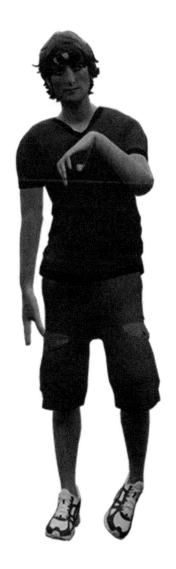

A young teenager's journey from Coma to Community! A Functional Neurosciences miracle!

In the midst of life's unpredictable whirlwind, the story of Tarun Thimmaiah, a bright 19-year-old typical middle-class Bengaluru teenager with a zest for life, took a tragic twist.

The date: 12ᵗʰ March 2020

The time: around 9:00 AM

Location: New Airport Road, Bengaluru, India

A carefree journey with four of his best buddies, after a morning game of football, in the backseat of a car, sans seatbelt, spiraled into a nightmare for his family when the driver lost control over the car and had a high-velocity collision with a road divider, resulting in a catastrophic accident. The impact was so severe that Tarun was thrown out of the car through the back windshield, landing in an open stormwater drain 20 feet away! By the time the passersby rushed towards the mangled car and then to the drain to pull him out, he had lapsed into a deep coma from a diffuse axonal injury—every family's dread and a stark reminder of the fragility of life.

Enduring an arduous 70-day vigil in the ICU and a subsequent month of rehabilitation in a major corporate hospital in Bengaluru, India, Tarun remained locked in a vegetative state, his once active frame reduced to skin and bones, weighing a mere 35 kilograms. Medical interventions, including a PEG tube, tracheostomy, and a urinary catheter, were deployed in an attempt to stabilize his condition.

Tarun Thimmaiah's journey through the shadowy depths of a coma began amidst the eerie quiet of Bangalore's streets during the first COVID-19 lockdown. The city, known for its energetic bustle, stood still as he was admitted to the hospital after a harrowing accident that left him with a traumatic brain injury. The crash that fractured his world came at a time when the entire globe was grappling with an invisible yet pervasive threat.

Throughout his ordeal, Tarun lay in a deep unconscious state, oblivious to the silent panic and desolation that had gripped the Garden City. As the first wave of the pandemic raged outside, his body waged its own battle inside the stark confines of the ICU.

After about 100 days in the hospital, in view of his persistent deeply unconscious (vegetative state), his family was informed by the treating doctors that he may not recover from this situation and they can consider taking him home, tracheostomy, PEG tube, urinary catheter and all, and nurse him at home.

Tarun Thimmaiah's battle for recovery began in the silence of a lockdown, his vibrant world dimmed by a traumatic brain injury as Bangalore, a city known for its dynamism, faced the first COVID-19 wave. Confined to the ICU, his condition remained critical, with doctors suggesting little hope for improvement.

Yet, amidst the city's quiet resilience, his father's unwavering hope led him to seek our neurosciences team's expertise. The journey ahead was marked by the dedication of healthcare workers amidst a city hushed by the pandemic, each step forward a testament to a family's enduring hope and a city's collective strength.

Tarun was eventually brought into Bhagwan Mahaveer Jain Hospital, Bengaluru, India, under my care on 3ʳᵈ June 2020. He was referred to our advanced neuro rehabilitation experts, where he was categorized as C2C BIR 1c, signifying the first segment of our unique recovery stratification system. Assessing his Rehabability Index, our rehab astrologer, we found hope—it predicted a 40-50% chance of him advancing to a more active state of C2C BIR 3a in the next 6-9 months or even longer. This sparked a rigorous therapy regimen, aiming to rouse Tarun from his prolonged comatose state.

Tarun's rehabilitation journey unfolded with the complexity of a multifaceted puzzle. The severe generalized spasticity (involving all four limbs and even his neck) contractures, the results of long-term immobility, and improper and inadequate initial rehab presented a formidable challenge. He looked like "Ashtavakra," the ancient Indian Rishi or saint, who was born with eight types of deformities. Even 1600 units of Botox, given by the movement disorders neurologist at the other hospital, hadn't benefitted him.

Seeing the severity of this and his persistent vegetative state, I was searching for an "out-of-the-box" solution to this complicated situation he was in. Why?

The longer he remained in the same clinical situation, the lower the chances of him making any meaningful recovery. As I sifted through all the files in my brain, I suddenly remembered the anecdotal evidence taught to me by my Japanese Guru, Prof. Takaomi Taira, of the possible multi-faceted benefits of Intra Thecal Baclofen (ITB) in patients with severe 'Disorders Of Consciousness' or DOC – both on the awakening as well as the spasticity. I then had a long talk about this with his parents. After explaining the science of ITB, I finally told them one thing – I always like a 'big bazaar' plan: the 'buy-one and take-one-free' offers!

Tarun's parents, who were really searching for a miracle in the lockdown mess outside, agreed. We initiated an intrathecal baclofen trial, a 2-step procedure to be done in the OT. The medical intervention for Tarun unfolded in two meticulously planned steps, beginning with an EUA—Evaluation Under Anesthesia. This step was critical to discerning the true root of Tarun's restricted movement. With muscle relaxants in effect, we could distinguish the spasticity from other factors like tightness, contractures, and deformities. The relief of spasticity-induced limitations under anesthesia would guide our next steps, while immovable constraints would signal deeper, structural challenges.

The second stage involved the precise placement of a spinal epidural catheter into Tarun's lumbar spinal subarachnoid space, threading it carefully to its target. Once secured and connected to an external infusion pump, it delivered a finely tuned dose of baclofen directly into his spinal fluid.

The trial results were transformative. Tarun's spasticity receded remarkably, heralding newfound mobility, particularly in his left-side limbs. On the third day of the trial, a moment of connection pierced the gloom—Tarun's gaze met his father's, a silent acknowledgment that spoke volumes and sparked a collective surge of hope among us.

Emboldened by this breakthrough, the family united behind the decision for a permanent ITB pump implantation. The pandemic lockdown posed a significant hurdle, delaying the acquisition of the necessary medication. But perseverance paid off, and soon, the pump and medication were ready for implantation.

Post-implantation, the transformation in Tarun was undeniable. The cloud of coma began to lift; recognition flickered in his eyes, nods became a language of agreement, and his limbs tentatively explored movement once more. Each incremental victory sang a chorus of defiance against the somber forecasts once given. Over the months that followed, with steady rehabilitation and precise pump programming, Tarun's recovery reached new heights. His speech, though still recovering, began to take shape, and he re-engaged with life, savoring the taste of home-cooked meals and reconnecting with loved ones through technology. The tracheostomy and feeding tubes, once vital lifelines, were removed, marking his return to a semblance of normalcy.

Now, Tarun's world is alive with the buzz of messages and the warmth of video calls. Emojis sprinkle his texts, each symbol a testament to regained cognitive and communicative function. His resilience mirrors the essence of Bengaluru itself—a city that embodies the fusion of tradition and innovation, just like Tarun, who redefines his life narrative with every passing day.

This is what Sneha, our youngest ANRS, has to say about her experience in treating Tarun. Tarun's journey left an indelible mark on my early days as a speech therapist. When I first encountered him in September 2020, he lay in a state of coma, unresponsive, tracheostomised, and devoid of verbal output. It was a daunting task, embarking on cognitive therapy sessions with a patient in such a condition. But with guidance from Dr. Prathiba and a determination to make a difference, I dove headfirst into the challenge.

I vividly recall the breakthrough moment when Tarun responded to a simple command—to look at and touch personal items held before him. It was a glimmer of hope in the darkness, a sign that he could understand and communicate in his own way. Armed with this newfound knowledge, I delved into augmentative alternative communication (AAC) methods, using words and pictures to facilitate interaction and expression.

As days turned into weeks and weeks into months, Tarun's progress was nothing short of miraculous. From the closing of his tracheostomy to initiating oral feeding, from single words to full sentences, he blossomed into a fluent communicator, speaking not just in one language but in several. His journey from silence to speech was punctuated by moments of joy and astonishment as he joked and conversed with newfound clarity and confidence. Yet, challenges remained, particularly in achieving speech clarity. Tarun's tongue movements were impaired, and his speech was often marred by hypernasality.

But with perseverance and a variety of techniques, including resonance exercises, we made steady strides toward improving his articulation and intelligibility. Despite lingering imperfections, Tarun found alternative ways to communicate, using his mobile phone to convey his thoughts when words failed him. It was a testament to his resilience and determination, defying the bleak prognosis that once overshadowed his journey.

For Tarun's family, witnessing his transformation was nothing short of miraculous. From being told that he may never wake up, let alone speak again, to witnessing him engage in conversations and crack jokes, it was a journey filled with hope, tears, and, ultimately, profound gratitude.

As for me, Tarun's journey reaffirmed my faith in the transformative power of therapy and the resilience of the human spirit. It was a humbling experience, one that shaped me as a therapist and instilled in me a newfound confidence in my abilities to make a difference in the lives of others.

Spasticity, Spasticity, Spasticity...

It is a term that resonates with dread and difficulty in the realm of neurology, neurosurgery, pediatric neurology, and rehabilitation worldwide. For patients, their families, and dedicated medical professionals addressing this challenge, spasticity is more than just a word; it induces restlessness, hopelessness, and sleeplessness. As the term has already popped up before, without further ado, let's delve into the intricacies of a problem that has persistently plagued the medical fraternity, caregivers, and patients alike – the perplexing phenomenon known as spasticity.

Spasticity is a common outcome for individuals who have experienced brain or spinal cord injuries. The misconception often arises that once the damaged brain heals, the paralyzed limbs should automatically and magically return to normal function. This kind of stuff only happens in movies! So, spasticity isn't just a brain thing; spinal cord injuries can join the party, too. Oh, and don't get it twisted with spasms – they're like the rebellious cousins. Spasms kick in because of super-sensitive skin, mostly in spinal cord injuries. Skin gets touchy, and suddenly, your leg decides it wants to tango without an invitation. Tricky, right?

To put it in layman's terms, imagine spasticity as attempting to drive a car with the handbrakes engaged. Picture the struggle: the brakes refuse to release, the wheels resist movement, and the strain on the system becomes immense. In the context of our bodies, envision someone placing a similar brake on either the upper limb or the lower limb, rendering movement impossible. The implications are profound – the inability to walk, turn in bed, or carry out daily activities. Now, extend this scenario to a small child, a reality for those familiar with conditions like Cerebral Palsy, a term derived from the very roots of spasticity.

For those unaware, Cerebral Palsy, often associated with organizations like the Indian Spastic Society and the Spastic Society of Karnataka, draws its name from spasticity. The impact on children with this condition is particularly poignant, emphasizing the critical need for understanding and addressing spasticity in the broader medical discourse.

Cerebral palsy, a phrase likely familiar to many, holds a significant presence in our lives, with numerous individuals possibly knowing someone in their family grappling with this condition. The distinctive gait of these children, characterized by a scissoring motion as they walk, is a poignant manifestation of the challenges posed by spasticity. The pain experienced is pervasive, with the exertion required for every step akin to traversing kilometers. While some relief can be found in certain medications designed to alleviate spasticity, their effectiveness is not universal, often accompanied by the unwelcome side effect of drowsiness.

Consider the example of baclofen, a commonly prescribed tablet. Despite its ingestion into the stomach and absorption into the bloodstream, its efficacy is limited by the blood-brain barrier. Only a mere 10 percent manage to cross this barrier, posing a hurdle in achieving the desired impact on spasticity.

Why does it happen?

Now, why does spasticity occur in the first place? It emerges as a consequence of injuries to the brain or spinal cord, encompassing a spectrum beyond physical accidents to include instances like brain tumors, spinal cord issues, infections such as TB, meningitis, encephalitis, head injuries, or strokes. As the recovery process unfolds, the affected limb initially experiences a phase of flaccidity or looseness. However, with progress, an excess of muscle tone emerges, leading to heightened tightness that begins to impede joint movements. This progression marks the onset of spasticity, categorized into beneficial and detrimental forms, depending on its impact on daily functioning. The question then arises: how do we navigate these nuances?

You may be wondering that, doc, you talked about spasticity being troublesome, and now you mention good spasticity. What's the deal? Let me clarify. When weakness is a result of brain or spinal cord damage and only partially improves, a certain level of spasticity can be beneficial. It aids in maintaining body posture and should be encouraged at this stage, facilitating better movement. However, there exists a threshold where spasticity becomes problematic, hindering smooth movements. Beyond this point, intervention becomes necessary.

Typically, 70-80 percent of patients respond to conventional medications like baclofen, tizanidine, or benzodiazepines to relax muscles. However, when spasticity is severe, rendering limbs immobile and causing distressing complications like fungal growth and hygiene issues, a more targeted approach is required. We must avoid situations where overzealous attempts to move tight joints lead to fractures, a risk that physiotherapists sometimes encounter.

At PRS Neurosciences, we adopt a three-pronged strategy for spasticity management. The first prong involves the very early identification and diagnosis and judicious use of tablets, optimizing their benefits for positive outcomes. If spasticity persists beyond the reach of medications and is localized, affecting specific body parts, we turn to botulinum toxin injections (commonly known as Botox). These injections target specific muscles, providing localized relief.

For localized spasticity, especially in one limb or part of the body, Botox injections are administered accurately and effectively. While Botox doesn't restore full movement, it significantly reduces spasticity, making movement retraining smoother and easier. It's important to note that different companies manufacture botulinum toxin injections, each one having its own impact duration, but in all situations, the effects are temporary and reversible, lasting three to six months, necessitating commitment to ongoing rehabilitation efforts.

When generalized spasticity affects larger areas, such as both legs, or involves the hands, legs, and neck, Botox injections alone may not suffice due to the need for higher doses (which makes it very expensive) and their temporary nature. In such cases, we explore intrathecal baclofen pump insertion (ITB). This involves implanting a device that continuously delivers baclofen directly into the spinal fluid. It offers a more sustained solution, but commitment to a comprehensive rehabilitation plan is crucial for lasting benefits.

Understanding the nuances of good and bad spasticity and continuous monitoring of change in function along with the response of spastic muscles allows us to tailor interventions at PRS Neurosciences, ensuring a scientific and holistic approach to improve the quality of life for individuals dealing with spasticity.

SPASTICITY vs. T/C/Ds

TCD stands for Tightness, Contracture, and Deformity.

Tightness is simple; it's tightness. It occurs when a muscle adapts and becomes shorter. However, you can bring it back to its proper length if you try to move it with your effort. Deformity, on the other hand, is at the bone level. The bone gets deformed and fuses together due to a lack of movement over time. Now, contracture involves the muscles and some other soft tissue structures. Soft tissues, apart from bones and muscles, include flexible components that aid in movement. They can get shortened and tightened, especially in tendons, which feel like a thread running in a rope. Tendons can get shortened if not given support for a long time. Tightness is easier to catch and responds well to therapy. Contracture is a bit more challenging and might require soft tissue release surgeries. These surgeries don't cure the bone but manage flexible structures to either move or stabilize the joint or restrict movement. Deformity, which involves bones, requires reconstructing a part of the bone to stabilize the joint or make it mobile. When moving a limb or joint, distinguishing between spasticity, tightness, contracture, and deformity is crucial. A novice therapist might think everything looks like spasticity, but the key is to differentiate them.

After experiencing a brain or spinal cord injury, particularly during the acute phase, it is common for limbs to initially display a state of flaccidity or relaxation. Even in conscious individuals, the transmission of signals from the brain to the muscles may be delayed, resulting in a perception that the limb is unresponsive.

However, as the brain gradually regains control over the muscles, local reflexes come into play, giving rise to spasticity—an elevation in muscle tone. This transition from flaccidity to spasticity can sometimes lead to a misconception of tightness, highlighting the importance of understanding and differentiating between these conditions in the rehabilitation process.

In instances where active movement initiation is absent, these muscles may undergo shortening, adding to the apparent tightness observed during examinations by therapists or clinicians. The differentiation between genuine tightness and spasticity becomes paramount for crafting precise interventions tailored to individuals in the recovery phase from brain or spinal cord injuries.

While assessing muscle tone, clinicians may encounter situations where the tone seems elevated, but the muscle has, in fact, shortened. This complexity poses a notable challenge for many clinicians. To navigate this challenge effectively, a thorough understanding of the optimal muscle length for accurate tone evaluation becomes crucial. This knowledge facilitates a clear distinction between heightened tone and actual muscle shortening, ensuring more nuanced and targeted approaches to rehabilitation.

The day I had first assessed Tarun, the extent of his tightness, contractures, and deformities—a result of past inadequate care—was overwhelming. I CRIED! It was then that I introduced Mahesh to our principle of 'Keeping the Body Future Ready' (KBFR), and though he agreed, the true depth of his understanding came much later. This realization hit home when we assessed.

Tarun's progress alongside another patient, a teenage girl, Vidhi, with a similar condition, who had come under my care promptly after her injury. The stark contrast in their recovery timelines was eye-opening, as Tarun had come to us after a substantial delay of 3 months. Mahesh expressed regret for the lost time and the delay he felt responsible for because he had met me one month before he made the transfer. And some of those deformities caused by the delay haunt us to this day, many years later!! Reflecting on the journey under my care, Mahesh, Tarun's father, shared this poignant insight after three months with us.

It underscored a crucial lesson: early and preventive care is the most efficient and cost-effective treatment.

At PRS Neurosciences, we exemplify the fusion of precision medicine and bespoke rehabilitation strategies, particularly when it comes to the intricate musculature of the hand, extending from the elbow to the fingertips—crucial for the fundamental action of gripping.

To accurately distinguish between spasticity and actual muscle shortening, we adopt a rigorous evaluation protocol. We assess muscle tone with the wrist in a neutral alignment to the forearm—ensuring it is perfectly straight, neither flexing downward nor extending upward. This objective positioning allows for a more precise assessment, thereby informing the targeted treatment plans for our patients grappling with the repercussions of spasticity and muscle tightness post-injury.

In long-standing conditions that may lead to muscle shortening, assessing tone with the hand in a neutral position can introduce bias. We adjust for this by flexing the wrist gently, which relaxes the muscles, and then attempt to extend the fingers. If the fingers open but with resistance, this resistance might hint at spasticity.

However, if the fingers do not open during this maneuver, this inflexibility typically suggests muscle shortening—a condition less amenable to manipulative therapies and indicative of more entrenched muscular changes. In contrast, if the fingers open somewhat but with noticeable resistance, it implies an increased tone, a direct response to spasticity.

It's imperative to delineate between muscle tightness, spasticity, and contractures for an effective treatment strategy. If tightness or spasticity is predominant, strategies such as passive stretching can elicit positive change. Conversely, contractures—characterized by more permanent changes due to immobility—might not respond well to such interventions.

Clinicians must tread with care, as misinterpreting contractures for mere tightness or spasticity could lead to unintended consequences, like tissue micro-tears, which are especially problematic for patients on anticoagulants. These micro-tears can lead to bleeding and, subsequently, calcium deposition within the tissues, potentially resulting in tendon hardening or abnormal bone growth.

Thus, deciding on interventions for fixed contractures is a matter of careful deliberation. Precision in evaluating and differentiating these conditions is vital for informed clinical decision-making. By following the Keeping Body Future Ready (KBFR) protocol at PRS Neurosciences, we proactively safeguard against such complications, ensuring our patient's road to recovery is both safe and effective.

Now, I want you to visualize a coordinate system with an X-axis and a Y-axis. On the positive quadrant of the X-axis, we have reversible spasticity or a need for reversible management. On the negative quadrant, we consider irreversible management. Similarly, on the Y-axis, we address generalized spasticity on the positive quadrant and localized spasticity on the negative quadrant. This matrix is a tool for neurologists, neurology teams, or neurosurgeons.

SPASTICITY TREATMENT ALGORITHM

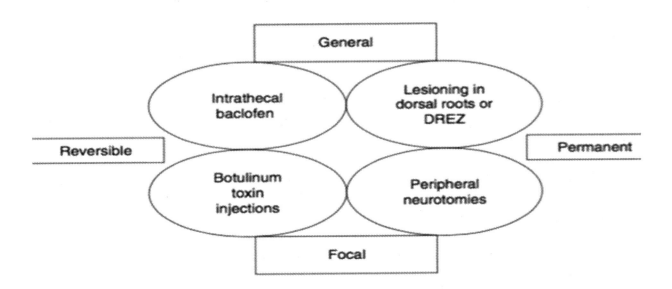

You might wonder why you should opt for reversible treatment for spasticity. *Well, there's a concept of good spasticity and bad spasticity.* Good spasticity occurs when the initial limb is completely flaccid, and to gain some movement, spasticity is necessary. Let me clarify. If you had no strength in your hand and received support to move it, initially, that support is considered good. However, as recovery progresses, reliance on that support becomes undesirable, and the spasticity needs to be modulated.

So, in the rehabilitation phase, spasticity becomes a tool. In certain cases, we don't aim to eliminate it entirely; instead, we target a specific part. This leads us to localized and reversible methods, one of which is Botox (Botulinum toxin). Botox is commonly used in cosmetic surgeries to relax muscles and reduce wrinkles. In neurological rehab, it serves to relax muscles, allowing for more manageable movements. Think of it like releasing the handbrake in a car for smoother driving. It's about letting go of the muscle tension to facilitate better movement. This approach aids in training movements more effectively. So, spasticity, when managed properly, becomes a valuable component in the rehabilitation process.

In certain cases, the approach needs to address the entire half of the body. Botox administration to each individual muscle becomes impractical in this case. We require a more comprehensive solution, a medicine with a generic effect on the entire body while specifically modulating the abnormal muscle behavior. This leans towards pharmaceutical management.

As an alternative, we've explored a procedure known as Intra Thecal Baclofen (ITB) pump implantation. In this surgery, a thin tube is inserted into the spinal cord through a lumbar puncture. This tube allows the direct release of medicine into the spinal cord. The dosage administered in the spinal cord is in micrograms (10 to the power of minus 6), significantly less than the milligrams given orally. Merely one-tenth of the dose is adequate to relax the patient.

Intrathecal Baclofen Pump (ITB) Implantation:

Switching gears to Intrathecal Baclofen (ITB) it involves a complex system. Like a petrol tank in a car, a small pump is placed in the abdomen, connected to a tube extending inside the muscle, creating a tank. This system enters the spinal cord, with the tube's ending placed at specific spinal cord levels based on the targeted muscle groups for relaxation.

When it comes to tackling spasticity in patients, there's a pretty involved process, especially when we talk about Intrathecal Baclofen Pump (ITB) implantation. This procedure aims to ease spasticity by delivering muscle relaxant Baclofen straight to the spinal cord. Let's dive into the nitty-gritty of how this all goes down.

First off, there's a check-up phase, a preoperative assessment, where doctors dig into the patient's health and how bad the spasticity is. They might throw in some high-tech imaging, like MRIs, to get a good look at the spinal cord and plan where to put the pump.

Next up is the treatment planning stage. Picture a dream team of specialists, including a brain surgeon and rehab expert, working together to create a plan that's tailor-made. They decide where to pop in the pump, how much Baclofen to use, and what kind of benefits to expect.

Then, it's all about making sure everyone's on the same page. The informed consent part is where the patient gets the lowdown on the ITB procedure – the good, the not-so-great, and other treatment options. It's like making sure everyone's singing from the same hymn sheet before diving in.

Now, onto the main event – surgical implantation. The patient goes under the scalpel, and a pump sets up shop under the skin in the belly. There's some precision work threading a catheter into the spinal cord so the pump can do its job, delivering Baclofen right where it's needed.

After the surgery, there's the programming and titration part. It's like fine-tuning a radio station. The pump gets programmed to dish out just the right amount of Baclofen in micrograms (mcg). The oral baclofen is in milligrams (mg). The calculation for you is one mcg = .001 mg, but the impact is far better owing to the direct delivery of the drug into CSF. Over a few weeks, they might tweak things to find that sweet spot between taming spasticity and keeping side effects at bay. My ANRSs, Mr. Nikhil and Mr. Ganapathy, are enrolled in this process at all steps and add valuable feedback along with the other key therapy team members, some of whom are performing far beyond their age and experience!

Post-surgery, it's all about keeping an eye out for any hiccups. The postoperative monitoring phase is crucial. Regular check-ins help catch any issues, like infections or glitches with the device. They keep tabs on how well the ITB system is working and adjust the dosage if needed. It is critical to keep a record of the refilling dates because sudden baclofen withdrawal can be unforgiving and a near-death experience!

While all this is going on, there's no ignoring the importance of rehabilitation and therapy. They go hand-in-hand with managing the pump, helping patients get the most out of the treatment, and improving their day-to-day lives.

And we're not done yet. There's the long-term follow-up to keep things in check. It's like giving the ITB system a regular check-up to make sure everything's running smoothly. They make sure the dosage is still doing the trick, and the device is on point, providing ongoing relief from spasticity.

The pump operates as a controlled drug release system. A wireless connection to a tab facilitates the programming of a 24-hour plan to control the quantity and rate of drug diffusion. Precise programming is based on the patient's daily routine, and the duration of the day or night when the spasticity or spasms are at peak are some of the factors considered while planning. At PRS Neurosciences, we have a detailed planning system to address your needs to the best. All of this is essential to avoid undesired effects. This approach provides a continuous infusion, necessitating pump refills every month based on the patient's usage.

So, whether it's Botox jabs or an ITB pump, both of these treatments involve a full-on, personalized approach. The choice between them depends on how bad the spasticity is, which muscles are playing up, and how the patient responds to different treatments. It's like tailoring the solution to fit the individual.

Kodandaram's Journey from his bed to his office: a cot to community (C2C) story

Kodandaram's path from the confinement of his bed to the independence of his office charts a narrative of resilience and medical innovation. A senior manager at Kotak Mahindra Bank, his routine was shattered by a road traffic accident that left him with a spinal cord injury—a cruel twist of fate that bound him to a hospital bed. In the wake of the accident, he was thrust into the world of medical urgency, with surgeries and scans at a private Hospital marking the beginning of his recovery. The surgery, which involved the precise placement of screws to alleviate spinal cord compression, was just the prelude to the real battle that lay ahead.

Post the spinal surgery, Kodandaram faced the demons of spasticity and pain that wracked his body, with both his legs getting folded and stuck automatically, turning nights into prolonged periods of suffering. When traditional medications brought more distress than relief, an alternative route was charted—an intrathecal baclofen trial. This procedure, a beacon in the dark, brought him the reprieve he so desperately sought. His spasms quelled, and sleep, once a distant dream, now cradled him again. Encouraged by the miraculous outcome of the trial, we proceeded to implant the actual pump. Given his heightened sensitivity to the medication, we started with a dosage as low as 25 micrograms, meticulously adjusted to meet his unique needs. This tailored approach not only managed his spasticity effectively but significantly enhanced his quality of life.

Kodandaram's remarkable sensitivity to the medication meant that a personalized dosage was key. The pump's implementation became a testament to precision in medical practice. Since the pump's installation in 2018, Kodandaram has made notable strides in his recovery. He now navigates the world with elbow crutches, a symbol of his resilience and the medical ingenuity that supported his journey back to mobility. The pump's critical role was underscored during the pandemic when the spasms returned amid drug supply disruptions, highlighting its indispensable role in his ongoing management.

The pandemic threw new obstacles in his path, but Kodandaram's journey is a testimony to perseverance. Our approach at PRS Neurosciences is a testament to our belief in continuous, meticulous care, setting us apart as we map out each step of the recovery journey. The progress is palpable, and while not every patient may reach Kodandaram's level of recovery, his story stands as a beacon of hope for many.

Now, as he gains ground each day, we continue to work towards his independence, his muscle power slowly returning. With a current functional score that reflects his significant strides, Kodandaram continues to defy the odds, his journey an embodiment of the rigorous battle against spinal cord injury—one step at a time, one triumph after another.

This journey, rich in both setbacks and victories, underscores the complexity of spinal cord injury recovery and the necessity of persistence and innovative medical approaches. Kodandaram's experience is not merely a testament to overcoming physical adversity but a narrative of rediscovering life's potential through the convergence of determined medical intervention and indomitable personal courage.

Botox for spasticity

Administering Botox for spasticity is akin to composing a bespoke symphony for each individual. At PRS Neurosciences, we abide by a fundamental tenet: without the commitment to neuro rehabilitation, there's no point in administering Botox. It's a collaboration where Botox alone benefits the caretakers more than the patient without the rehabilitation dance.

Imagine our healthcare professionals as orchestra conductors, meticulously planning each movement, securing the patient's consent, and leading up to the crescendo—the injection itself. Post-injection, our vigilant monitoring ensures the melody of recovery plays on without a hitch. Yet, it's not a one-off concert; it's an ongoing series where the tune is refined over time.

In comparison, the ITB pump is an internal reservoir of relief, offering a continuous, adjustable stream of medication tailored to the patient's daily needs—a contrast to the four-month rhythm of Botox.

The process of Botox injections at our center is a collaborative effort. The rehab team, deeply attuned to the patient's daily function, proposes which muscles to target. As a neurosurgeon, I confirm and administer the precise doses. Our approach is dynamic, and feedback is critical—it helps verify the efficacy of the dosage, which often requires a clinician's judgment within recommended ranges.

Before the needle even pierces the skin, patients are fully briefed on the benefits and risks. It's a partnership, and patients must commit to rehabilitation post-injection; Botox without active engagement is like topping up a SIM card you never use—a wasted investment.

Think of the injection as a high-stakes mission. Patients present the rebellious muscles, and I, the injector, pinpoint the exact sites for Botox delivery, with each muscle requiring its own specific entry point. My ANRS team plays a vital role, always ready to adapt the plan based on real-time assessments. After the injection, the patient enters a period of observation to ensure no adverse reactions. We provide a comprehensive list of post-injection protocols to safeguard the treatment's efficacy.

The journey with Botox doesn't stop at the injection. Follow-ups are crucial; they're scheduled to assess the symphony's harmony and make any necessary adjustments. Meanwhile, rehabilitation sessions continue unabated.

Botox treatment for spasticity is a deliberate choreography from the initial assessment, through the strategic planning and patient approval, to the injection performance and the diligent aftercare. It's a dance, with each follow-up ensuring the patient maintains the right rhythm in their recovery waltz.

Here's a Botox + Rehab success story – for post-stroke spasticity

Rajeev Jamburao's story is not just a medical case study; it's a narrative etched into our hearts, highlighting the grit and resilience of a man and his family against the tides of fate. A young, ambitious engineer from Thanjavur, Rajeev was making strides in Germany's telecommunications sector when a trip back to the cultural city known for the Brihadeeswarar Temple turned his world upside down.

No one could have anticipated that a fever and a persistent headache would cascade into a life-altering event. On a September evening in 2021, Rajeev lost consciousness. Fortuitously, his neighbor, a neurosurgeon, recognized the gravity of the situation and rushed him to Vasavi Hospital. Rajeev had suffered a stroke due to an occlusion in his middle cerebral artery, a vital vessel nourishing the brain regions responsible for movement, sensation, and cognition.

Before this tragedy, Rajeev was the family's pride, showcasing the vibrant energy of Bengaluru as he juggled a startup and a fulfilling career overseas. In a cruel twist of fate, he found himself in a battle for the most basic human functions, his wife experiencing a 'hard drive crash' of human emotions as they grappled with this new, harsh reality.

Following a 15-day coma, Rajeev awoke to a world of silence and immobility. Memory loss and paralysis plagued him—a man once known for navigating the technological and geographical landscapes of Germany now struggled with recognizing letters and objects.

Despite the overwhelming odds, Rajeev's spirit remained unbroken. His journey through the corridors of BMJH's neuro rehabilitation center, starting two years post-incident, was marked by unwavering optimism and an infectious smile that inspired our team. Under the expert care of Mr. Ganapathy Arumugham, an occupational therapist par excellence, Rajeev's case was carefully evaluated. Adverse reactions to standard medications led us down an unorthodox path—Botox therapy.

On August 4th, 2022, Rajeev received his first Botox treatment. The vial, deceptively empty to the eye, held a potent neurotoxin that promised to alleviate the relentless grip of spasticity on his muscles. Alongside this, his baclofen dosage was cautiously increased, enhancing muscle tone normalization without adverse effects. For six months, Rajeev's resolve and dedication to therapy never waned. Each session, each small improvement, brought him closer to reclaiming the independence that the stroke had stolen from him. His journey became a beacon of hope and a testament to the relentless pursuit of healing.

Rajeev's story became synonymous with motivation and resilience in our practice. Always smiling and perpetually striving, he embodied the spirit of a true 'stroke warrior.' The therapy sessions with Siddharth, filled with free advice and insightful discussions, led to further gains in Rajeev's mobility. A second round of Botox, targeting meticulously selected muscles, and the innovative use of a SAEBO-Glove were pivotal in his ongoing rehabilitation.

Today, Rajeev is a symbol of triumph over adversity. He's not just lifting weights with his right hand; he's swinging cricket bats, nurturing plants, and even taking the wheel of his car—each act a defiance of the stroke that sought to define him. Unbeknownst to him, he stands as a colossal figure inspiring those who traverse the challenging path of neurological recovery. His laughter, in the face of life's sternest tests, rings as a powerful reminder of the human spirit's capacity to overcome.

8
NEUROTECHNOLOGY
PUSHING THE FRONTIERS OF FUNCTIONAL NEUROSCIENCES

"Within the intricate tapestry of the human brain lies the future of all our potential. As we stand on the brink of new neural horizons, we realize that the power to heal, enhance, and extend the capabilities of the brain and mind is not just a possibility but an impending reality. Neuroscience will not just illuminate the mysteries of consciousness but will also pave the way for a renaissance of the human experience."

- A fictitious quote inspired by the collective wisdom of neuroscience pioneers.

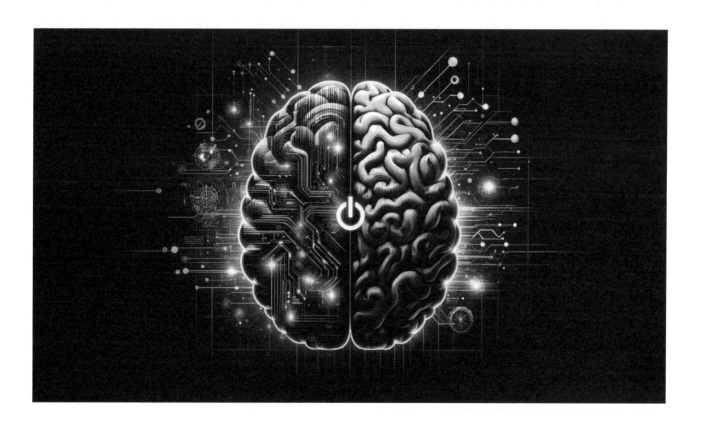

Triveni's Struggle with Spastic Paraplegia and Overcoming the Challenge

Triveni, a dedicated teacher and school principal, began her medical journey with a unique problem: she couldn't lift her right leg while sitting on a bike. This condition ultimately caused her to fall in her bathroom, marking a pivotal moment in her health journey. She became bedridden and unable to move both her legs. Seeking answers, she approached Dr. Ravi Mohan Rao, a renowned neurosurgeon, and his experienced clinical team. Through a detailed medical examination, they diagnosed Triveni with ligamentum flavum hypertrophy and severe dorsal spinal canal stenosis, conditions leading to significant spinal cord compression and progressively worsening weakness in her lower limbs.

Under Dr. Rao's surgical expertise, Triveni underwent spinal canal decompression surgery to alleviate the pressure on her spinal cord. Post-surgery, she was referred to me for intensive neuro rehabilitation. Despite initial improvements in her mobility, Triveni struggled with increasing spasticity, a condition I often liken to driving with the brakes on, the presence of which severely hindered her recovery. Due to this, she hit a DEAD END, which led to her feeling depressed. Daily crying spells were a norm when I would go on my hospital rounds. Counseling and giving her HOPE became a routine for all of us.

To address this, we opted for an Intrathecal Baclofen Pump (ITB) after oral medications proved ineffective. This device, implanted in the anterior abdominal wall and connected directly to the spinal cord, administers precise doses of Baclofen, a muscle relaxant, directly to the affected area. This targeted approach allows for better management of spasticity without the side effects commonly associated with oral medications. The installation of the ITB pump was a positive turning point for Triveni. As we fine-tuned the dosage to suit her specific needs, she saw remarkable improvements in muscle strength and a significant reduction in both pain and spasticity. The rehab team caring for her noted profound changes in Triveni's daily life. Her sleep improved dramatically, and she gained enough independence to roll over in bed and stand up with minimal support, eventually using only a walker for assistance.

Triveni's recovery transformed her outlook on life. She returned to her role as a homemaker and mother, filled with gratitude and renewed vigor. She often expresses her thanks, viewing me not just as a doctor but as a lifesaver. However, I remind her and others that while doctors possess the skills to make significant differences in patients' lives, we are not deities but dedicated professionals working to enhance the quality of life for our patients.

Triveni's journey underscores the critical role of advanced medical interventions like the ITB pump and the comprehensive care provided by teams like ours at PRS Neurosciences, highlighting how technology and compassionate healthcare can together restore independence and dignity to those suffering from debilitating conditions.

Dr. Prathiba's cognitive nuggets—one day during my hospital rounds, when I entered Triveni's room, she looked very dull; the usual 'good morning' didn't come. Her son and husband wished me, but it wasn't the usual way. I sensed something was going on, and when I asked what was happening, she held my hand and started weeping like a small baby. Her husband also had tears in his eyes. When I continued to ask what the matter was, her husband said she had been crying like this all night and couldn't sleep. Then finally she spoke up and said, "I've been putting all the efforts I can for the past 3 months, but still, I'm not able to stand. My legs move on their own at night, and it is very painful. I'm losing hope. What's the use of living like this?" A lady who was a rock-solid woman, a fighter, a teacher, a motivator, who stood by everyone in all difficult times, was talking of 'giving up'... very heart-wrenching.

But after a couple of sessions of counseling for her and her family, she sprung back to her commitment to get better and started showing good progress. After neuromodulation strategies, she was slowly able to walk with support.

Neurotechnology – Cutting-Edge Tech At The Neural Interface

Neurotechnology refers to a broad range of technical tools and methods that are designed to analyze, understand, and manipulate the nervous system, including the brain, spinal cord, and neural circuits. This technology encompasses various applications, from medical devices that monitor and influence brain activity to neuroimaging techniques that visualize the structure and function of the nervous system, as well as computational tools that model neural processes. The aim of neurotechnology is to advance our knowledge of how the nervous system works, treat neurological disorders, and potentially enhance cognitive functions.

Neural prosthetics and neuromodulation are two areas of neurotechnology that interact directly with the nervous system, but they have different goals and mechanisms of action.

Similarities:

- **Neurological Interaction:** Both interact with the nervous system to achieve a desired outcome, whether it's restoring a function (neural prosthetics) or altering nerve activity (neuromodulation).

- **Device-Based:** They typically involve implantable or external devices that interact with neural tissue.

- **Medical Objectives:** Both are used to treat medical conditions, especially those involving neurological deficits or dysfunctions.

- **Technology and Research Intensive:** They are at the cutting edge of medical technology and require significant research and development efforts.

- **Quality of Life Improvement:** The aim of both technologies is to improve the quality of life for individuals with neurological conditions.

Differences:

- **Purpose and Function:**
  - **Neural Prosthetics:** These are designed to replace or substitute for a lost neural function. For example, cochlear implants replace the function of damaged hair cells in the inner ear to provide a sense of sound to the deaf.

  - **Neuromodulation:** This technology modulates or changes neural activity. It doesn't replace a lost function but alters the existing neural circuits to achieve a therapeutic effect. Deep brain stimulation (DBS) for Parkinson's disease, for instance, uses electrical impulses to modulate the activity of specific brain regions.

- **Mechanism of Action:**
  - **Neural Prosthetics:** They often work by translating external information into a form that the brain can understand (e.g., converting sound waves into electrical signals) or by translating the brain's intentions into external actions (e.g., controlling a robotic arm with brain signals).

  - **Neuromodulation:** These devices modulate neural circuits through electrical or chemical stimulation to normalize aberrant neural activity.

- **Conditions Treated:**
  - **Neural Prosthetics:** Mainly used for sensory or motor deficits like vision, hearing, or limb loss.

  - **Neuromodulation:** Used for a broader range of conditions, including chronic pain, epilepsy, depression, and movement disorders.

- **Invasiveness:**
  - **Neural Prosthetics:** Can be either invasive (e.g., retinal implants) or non-invasive (e.g., hearing aids).

  - **Neuromodulation** Also ranges from non-invasive techniques like transcranial magnetic stimulation (TMS) to invasive methods like DBS or spinal cord stimulation.

- **Feedback and Adjustment:**
  - **Neural Prosthetics:** Typically require a period of adjustment as the user learns to interpret and use the new signals or controls the prosthetic device.

  - **Neuromodulation:** Often involves tuning and adjustments over time to maintain therapeutic efficacy as the neural tissue can adapt or become tolerant to stimulation.

Both fields are rapidly evolving, and as they advance, the distinctions may blur. For example, future neural prosthetics might include neuromodulation capabilities to enhance their functionality, and neuromodulation techniques may become so precise that they can substitute for lost neural functions in ways similar to prosthetics.

Neuromodulation surgeries encompass a range of medical procedures that alter nerve activity through targeted stimulation of nervous system components, such as the brain, spinal cord, or peripheral nerves, to treat and manage various neurological conditions.

Neural prostheses represent an emerging frontier in the field of neurotechnology, blending cutting-edge engineering with neurobiology to address some of the most challenging conditions faced in medicine today. They are devices that can replace or augment the function of a part of the nervous system that has been damaged due to injury or disease.

NEUROMODULATION

Types of Neuromodulation Surgeries:

- **Deep Brain Stimulation (DBS):** DBS involves implanting electrodes in specific brain areas and connecting them to a pulse generator implanted in the chest. This system delivers electrical impulses to treat movement disorders like Parkinson's disease, tremors, and dystonia, as well as psychiatric conditions like obsessive-compulsive disorder.

- **Spinal Cord Stimulation (SCS):** Used primarily for chronic pain syndromes, including neuropathic pain, SCS implants electrodes along the spinal cord. The electrical pulses modulate pain signals before they reach the brain.

- **Vagus Nerve Stimulation (VNS):** VNS involves the placement of a device in the chest that stimulates the vagus nerve in the neck, helping to control seizures in epilepsy and treating depression.

- **Sacral Nerve Stimulation (SNS):** SNS targets the sacral nerve to improve bladder control and has been effective in treating urinary incontinence and overactive bladder syndrome.

- **Intrathecal Drug Delivery Systems (IDDS):** These devices, often referred to as "pain pumps," deliver medication directly into the spinal fluid to manage severe spasticity or chronic pain, minimizing systemic side effects.

Indications: Patients with chronic conditions that have not responded adequately to conservative treatments may be candidates for neuromodulation surgeries. Common indications include chronic pain conditions, movement disorders, epilepsy, and certain psychiatric disorders.

Procedure Overview: Neuromodulation surgeries typically involve a multidisciplinary approach. The implantation process generally occurs in two stages: a trial phase where temporary electrodes are placed to assess effectiveness and, if successful, a second stage where permanent devices are implanted.

Benefits:

- Targeted treatment with potential reduction or elimination of symptoms
- Reversible and adjustable therapy
- Reduced reliance on oral medications and their associated side effects

Risks and Considerations:

- Potential for infection, bleeding, or hardware-related complications
- Need for battery replacements for implanted pulse generators

- Device malfunctions or need for reprogramming

What to Expect When Considering Device-based Neuromodulation Surgery?

Device-based neuromodulation surgery is a complex and highly specialized medical procedure that requires careful evaluation and preparation.

If you or a loved one is considering such a neuromodulation surgery, it's essential to be informed about what to expect throughout the process:

1. **Thorough Evaluation:** The journey begins with a thorough evaluation by a team of healthcare professionals, including neurologists and neurosurgeons. They will assess your medical history, current condition, and response to previous treatments.

2. **Discussion of Treatment Options:** Based on the evaluation, your healthcare team will discuss treatment options and determine whether a device-based neuromodulation surgery is suitable for your condition. They will explain the potential benefits, risks, and alternatives.

3. **Informed Decision-Making:** It's important to engage in informed decision-making. You should have a clear understanding of the procedure, its potential outcomes, and any associated risks. Take the time to ask questions and express any concerns. Be realistic in your expectations.

4. **Pre-operative Assessments:** Prior to the surgery, you will undergo several pre-operative assessments, which may include medical tests, imaging studies (such as MRI or CT scans), and possibly psychological evaluations, depending on the nature of the procedure.

5. **Device Selection:** If neuromodulation surgery is recommended, you and your healthcare team will decide on the type of device that best suits your condition. This could be a spinal cord stimulator, deep brain stimulator, vagus nerve stimulator, or another device, depending on the specific condition being treated.

6. **Surgical Planning:** The surgical team will develop a comprehensive surgical plan. This includes determining the precise location for device placement and the specific surgical approach. The plan will be tailored to your unique needs.

7. **Anesthesia and the Procedure:** Neuromodulation surgeries are typically performed under general anesthesia. The surgeon will make incisions as necessary to implant the device, electrodes, or leads. The device is then connected to a pulse generator or stimulator, which may be implanted under the skin, usually in the chest or abdomen.

8. **Recovery and Hospital Stay:** The length of your hospital stay can vary depending on the complexity of the surgery and the device implanted. Expect to stay in the hospital for a few days, during which your medical team will closely monitor your progress and manage any postoperative discomfort.

9. **Activation and Programming:** After surgery, the device will require programming to ensure it effectively addresses your condition. This is typically done by a specialized technician or clinician. You may need multiple programming sessions to fine-tune the settings.

10. **Postoperative Care and Follow-up:** Follow-up care is crucial. Your medical team will schedule regular follow-up appointments to monitor your progress, make any necessary adjustments to the device, and ensure it is effectively managing your symptoms.

11. **Rehabilitation and Lifestyle Modifications:** Depending on your condition and the type of neuromodulation surgery, you may need many months or even years of rehabilitation to maximize the benefits of the procedure. Additionally, your medical team may recommend lifestyle modifications to support your recovery.

12. **Monitoring and Maintenance:** Neuromodulation devices typically have a finite lifespan, so periodic replacement may be necessary. Regular check-ups with your healthcare team will ensure the device continues to work effectively.

13. **Potential Benefits and Realistic Expectations:** It's important to maintain realistic expectations regarding the outcomes of neuromodulation surgery. While many patients experience significant symptom relief, the extent of improvement can vary.

Neuromodulation surgery is a multi-step process that begins with an in-depth evaluation and involves careful planning, meticulous and precision neurosurgery, postoperative care, intensive and targeted neuro rehabilitation with frequent device programming, and ongoing follow-up.

Open communication with your healthcare team and active involvement in your care is essential to achieving the best possible outcomes from the procedure.

Outcomes and Follow-up: Patients often require regular follow-up to optimize device settings and manage any issues. Successful neuromodulation can significantly improve quality of life, alleviate symptoms, and reduce the need for medication.

Future Directions: Ongoing research in neuromodulation is exploring new targets, refining stimulation techniques, and developing less invasive methods. The field is evolving, with potential applications expanding to include treatments for conditions like obesity, addiction, and heart failure.

Conclusion: Neuromodulation surgeries offer hope for patients with debilitating neurological conditions, providing a means to manage symptoms and improve quality of life when other treatments have fallen short. As the field grows, these therapies are becoming increasingly sophisticated, offering personalized and adaptive solutions for complex medical challenges.

Story of an elderly lady who wanted to improve her Quality of Life!

Mrs. KT, a 76-year-old widow living alone in an apartment complex, is the aunt of my med school friend, now a prominent surgical oncologist, Dr. Shabber Zaveri. She has been battling a mixed type of Idiopathic Parkinson's Disease since 2007. Initially affecting only her left side, the disease progressively involved both sides of her body, including her head and face. Over the years, she consulted various neurologists and tried multiple medications, but she faced a rare complication—Levodopa, the cornerstone treatment for PD since 1968, triggered severe hallucinations and psychiatric episodes at doses beyond 110 mg daily. This unusual sensitivity prevented her from achieving the full benefits of the medication, and alternatives failed to match its efficacy.

Functionally, her condition had deteriorated to the point where she couldn't perform simple tasks like making tea. The responsibilities of her care fell on her elder sister, who, despite being over 80, lived independently in the same building.

Before consulting me, Mrs. KT was already informed about the Deep Brain Stimulation (DBS) surgery for Parkinson's Disease and was keen on undergoing the procedure. During our consultation, she expressed a strong desire to proceed with the surgery despite the risks associated with her age and psychiatric history. She even offered to sign a consent form acknowledging the potential for fatal complications, emphasizing that she preferred taking the risk over continuing her current quality of life.

Given her age and psychiatric complications, I decided against targeting the Subthalamic Nucleus (STN), which is commonly affected in DBS procedures for Parkinson's. Instead, I opted for the Globus Pallidus Interna (GPi) as the surgical target, aiming to mitigate her symptoms without exacerbating her psychiatric symptoms.

The surgery, performed in 2017, yielded significant improvements. Mrs. KT has since undergone one battery replacement and remains satisfied with the outcomes, regaining the ability to perform most of her desired activities independently. She has declined further reprogramming, content with the current settings, and the level of improvement she has achieved. This case is a poignant example of a patient-driven decision in the complex interplay of medical ethics, patient autonomy, and surgical intervention.

Deep Brain Stimulation (DBS) or Brain pacemaker

Deep Brain Stimulation (DBS) is a surgical procedure used to treat a variety of debilitating neurological symptoms—most commonly, the tremors, rigidity, and bradykinesia associated with Parkinson's disease and essential tremors.

Here's an overview of the typical steps involved in DBS implantation:

1. Preoperative Assessment: Patients undergo a thorough evaluation, which may include neurological testing, MRI or CT scans to image the brain's structure, and possibly a psychological assessment to ensure suitability for the procedure.

2. Pre-surgical Planning: Using imaging studies, surgeons plan the trajectory for electrode placement to target specific brain areas, such as the subthalamic nucleus or globus pallidus internus in Parkinson's disease.

3. Stereotactic Frame Placement: On the day of surgery, a stereotactic frame is attached to the patient's head after local anesthesia is applied. This frame helps to precisely guide the placement of the electrodes.

4. Brain Mapping: The patient may remain awake during the surgery to provide feedback, which is helpful in mapping the brain. Surgeons use microelectrode recording (MER) to identify the exact brain area that will be stimulated.

5. Electrode Implantation: Once the target area is confirmed, permanent electrodes are implanted through small holes drilled in the skull. Real-time imaging techniques, such as intraoperative MRI, can aid in accurate electrode placement.

6. Implantation of the Pulse Generator: After electrodes are in place, the patient is usually put under general anesthesia for the placement of the impulse generator (battery pack), which is typically implanted under the skin near the collarbone or in the abdomen.

7. Tunneling and Connection: A subcutaneous extension wire is tunneled from the scalp to the chest or abdominal area to connect the electrodes to the impulse generator.

8. Device Programming: Several weeks post-surgery, the DBS system is programmed and adjusted to optimal settings during follow-up visits. This process is critical as it fine-tunes the electrical impulses to maximize symptom control and minimize side effects.

9. Postoperative Care: Patients receive instructions on wound care, signs of infection, and activity restrictions following surgery. They may also need short-term pain management for surgical discomfort.

10. Ongoing Adjustments: Periodic adjustments of the DBS settings are often necessary, especially as the patient's underlying condition changes over time. Continuous follow-up with the healthcare team is essential for maintaining the benefits of DBS therapy.

11. Battery Replacement: Depending on the type of impulse generator used, battery replacements may be necessary every 3 to 5 years, which requires a minor surgical procedure.

DBS is a complex yet life-changing procedure for many patients with movement disorders. It requires careful coordination across a multidisciplinary team, meticulous surgical technique, and patient involvement for optimal outcomes.

Hitting multiple 'birds' with one stone – here with ITB

Let me tell you the story of Guru Kiran. A 6.2-foot-tall guy, 35 years old, was referred to me by Dr. Ramesh Ranganathan, a senior neurosurgeon from the Girinagar Jain Hospital. His wife came and met me first. She's about 5 feet tall, and she came and said to me, "I have a big problem. My husband is a genetically confirmed SCA type 2, which is Spino-Cerebellar Ataxia type 2. This guy is now so disabled that he's not even able to walk to the bathroom. For the last six months, he has been crawling on his knees and elbows to the bathroom. He doesn't want to take help. He doesn't want to use the wheelchair. He cannot use the walker." She was not able to convince him to do the wheelchair business. She was frustrated. They have a four-year-old who is seeing his father do this. Apart from this mess, the other big problem is his pain. His whole body has so much pain, she says, that 22 out of the 24 hours, he's 'howling' in pain. Howling is the word. He shouts so loudly in the night that the neighbors hear and come and object to her. She sounded so helpless… She'd gone to many people seeking some remedy and tried medications, but they didn't work.

Basically, nobody gave her any other solution. I had spoken to Dr. Ramesh Ranganathan about my intrathecal baclofen pump for spasticity, and he was seeing Gurukiran for spasticity. He felt maybe ITB would help. That was how she came and met me. I said, 'I need to see your husband. Please bring him along.' He did come. This guy's entire body was spastic; he was very badly spastic. He had so much pain. I asked him on the VAS scale of 0-10, where 0 is no pain, and 10 is unbearable pain, what is your pain? He said, 12! He's an IT professional, and he really meant it. Then, I explained the intrathecal baclofen pump and how it works for them. I also told them that though I'm going to put it for spasticity, there is a good possibility that the pain will come down. You know what the wife said? She said, and I quote - "I don't care if the spasticity comes down or not, but if his pain can come down, I'll be very happy." Then, I explained the trial to them. Thereafter, we scheduled him for a trial.

The trial happened... the catheter was put into his spinal subarachnoid space and placed at the D1 level. We injected 100 micrograms of the medicine. At the time, this was all done at the Bhagwan Mahaveer Jain Hospital, Girinagar. Then, we made him sit up on the operating table. The time it took from the time of injecting the medicine into the tube, 100 micrograms, in the back and making him sit up on the operating table to move him onto the trolley was about five minutes, probably. You know what he said five minutes later? He said, **"Doc, my pain is gone."** And he had a smile on his face. I was stunned to see that 100 micrograms of the intrathecal baclofen had caused this man's pain to go away. The pain, which had been so stubborn, was finally not there anymore; this was 'magical' even for me. Anyway, we did the trial. The spasticity came down, but the biggest benefit was - ZERO PAIN! And his wife was 'bought' into the surgery. She said, "Doc, I don't care about spasticity again. His pain is gone. Please put the pump." The pump got implanted, and then we programmed it. So, these were the results.

And we continued neuro rehab. We all knew that we were dealing with a degenerative condition, and he was not going to get better, and so on and so forth. Another problem that he had before the pump was his speech. His speech was so unclear that nobody could understand him, and so he had stopped speaking. His 4-year-old son craved to play with him, but he was so withdrawn because of all this that he would not spend time with his son. After about four to five months of rehabilitation, physical therapy, occupational therapy, and speech therapy, things started happening. And amazingly, we saw a couple of results.

Number one, at the top of the list, was 'no pain.' He literally had no pain. And that result of no pain has lasted till today, four years since the ITB pump was implanted. Number two, his spasticity reduced reasonably. And though he could walk with the walker a few steps, he didn't want to. He participated quite well in our efforts to manage him, turning him in bed. Earlier, getting out of bed and moving out of the chair was a struggle for his 5-foot-tall wife to move him. Now. she says that he participates in about 70 to 80% of the activities, and she is required to lend a hand only for about 20 to 30% of his movements and activities. That has made her life so much better.

Thirdly, his speech got so much better. It's much clearer, and because of that, he has started playing with his son. Big brownie points, psychologically, both for the father and the son. The fourth big thing that happened was - he had no control over his urine before the surgery. This is another problem he grappled with. Hence, he used to be in a diaper all the time, but he would still smell of 'urine.' This stopped him from mingling with anyone outside his immediate family and stopped him from stepping out for any social gatherings. And, about three months post-surgery and programming, he became continent and dry. He did not need a diaper.

One day, he called me from somewhere. He said, "Doc, guess where I am?" I could understand him on the phone. He said, "I have come out to a pub with my college friends, and I've come out for the first time in five years because I don't smell of urine." Can you imagine? I had tears of joy in my eyes!

This is the 'NASHA' of why I do these surgeries, these challenging surgeries. Because of these 'wins,' I get to hear from the patients and their families. That is what it is. Then, about eight months later, they sent me some pictures. They'd gone on a holiday to a resort. He got into a swimming pool with his son. Yes, of course, he sought assistance to get in. He just sat at the shallow end of the swimming pool; he did not want to swim. But the fact that a guy who had confined and punished himself to sitting in a corner of his house was finally willing to socially merge and get out with the family.

This had such a serious impact on not only the patient but also on the wife and son. This was the fifth impact of the intrathecal baclofen pump on a spinal cerebellar ataxic patient.

I am honored to have implanted one of the highest numbers of pumps in the country, leading to exceptional outcomes that were recognized at a major conference three years ago. The multinational company producing these pumps noted that they had not seen such impressive results before. This achievement is not solely my own but reflects the hard work of dedicated medical, surgical, and rehab teams, who collaborate closely with our patients, fine-tuning medications and therapy to enhance outcomes significantly.

Addressing the recent crisis of Intrathecal Baclofen injection Shortages

Late August 2023, a severe crisis unfolded that went largely unnoticed by the media due to its non-sensational nature and the small number of individuals affected. This crisis involved a critical shortage of medication for Intrathecal Baclofen injections, essential for managing severe spasticity. In India, only one company manufactures this medication, and due to a regulatory policy by the Drug Controller General of India requiring drug withdrawal six months before expiration, a crucial batch was destroyed prematurely in July. This led to patients facing life-threatening shortages, severe withdrawal symptoms, and the risk of death.

The shortage not only threatened patients' lives but also risked making costly medical devices, worth about eight-and-a-half lakh rupees, useless. Despite the medication costing less than Rs. 1500 per refill, it was being sold on the black market for Rs. 1.2 lakhs during the crisis.

Our efforts to find alternatives in countries like Malaysia, Thailand, and Korea were unsuccessful, and it was revealed that while the UK imports from the US, the US sources its supply from an Indian manufacturer who does not sell it in India. The situation was desperate enough that I considered filing a Public Interest Litigation in the Karnataka High Court on behalf of my patients.

Miraculously, a representative from the Indian manufacturer eventually provided us with 15 vials of the medication, bringing immense relief to our patients. This incident highlights the importance of a reliable logistical framework for medical devices, not just the presence of the devices themselves.

For those dealing with spasticity and in need of advanced intervention, our team offers one of the most effective neuromodulation systems in India, dedicated to improving your quality of life. For more information and support, please visit our website.

The latest breaking news!!

Mind control: All you need to know about Elon Musk's Neuralink implanting brain chip blurring the line between humans and machines. Neuralink's technological advancement can allow people with disabilities to control smartphones and other devices using their brains.

"The first human received an implant from Neuralink yesterday and is recovering well. Initial results show promising neuron spike detection," wrote Musk on X (formerly Twitter). Called Telepathy, the brain implant is designed to enable its user to control a computer or a smartphone—just with their thoughts.....

What are your thoughts?????

9

CHRONIC PAIN

THE FIFTH VITAL SIGN

Pain is a pain, is a pain.

Headaches are headaches, even for neurologists and neurosurgeons. Which headache should be investigated?

–Dr. Sharan Srinivasan
Stereotactic & Functional Neurosurgeon

"Pain is inevitable. Suffering is optional."

- Haruki Murakami

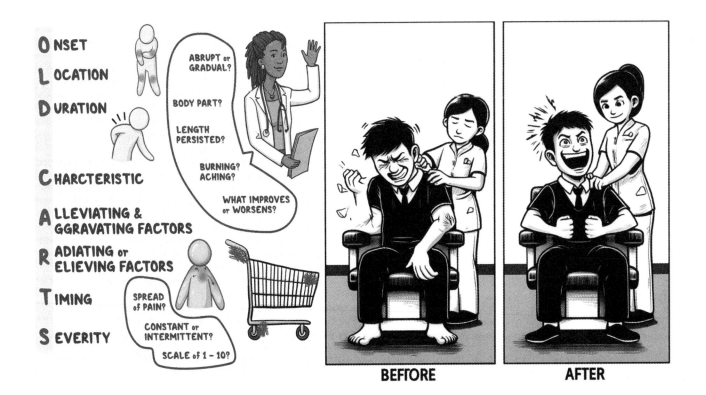

A Senior citizen who had a pain in his neck...

Now, let me start this chapter with a 'painful' story from my home...about my father.

We are currently in 2024; let me take you back to 2014: My father, who is now 84 years old, still driving and playing golf, had non-specific neck pains for many years prior; he suddenly developed sharp, shooting pain from the angle of his right jaw towards his chin. This pain was excruciating but had a very peculiar pattern – it only appeared when he bent his neck down to eat food or write or something along the lines of that.

The moment he flexed his neck forward for any reason, this pain would shoot, so much so that he would give out a loud shout, immediately stop whatever he was doing, support his chin with his right palm, and slowly lift his head up until the pain went away. It was giving his head a little bit of an upward traction! Then the pain was GONE! Very strange, isn't it? It was so, even for me.

Because it was so transient, I felt that there was no meaning in medicating him. MRI and CT scans of his neck showed that he had very severe degenerative cervical spondylosis and the right C1-C2 joint was eroded, causing the right C2 nerve root to get pinched... this was basically a case of a pinched nerve every time he moved his head down.

Many spine surgeons would have recommended surgery, but I was skeptical. After many months of suffering, he had reached such a stage that he would have to hold his plate in his left hand, very close to his chin, and eat! By this time, I had just established a pain clinic @PRS Neurosciences with an interventional pain physician, Dr. Raghavendra. He confirmed my radiological diagnosis, but he also found many myofascial 'trigger points' in the scalene muscles on the right. He did a simple 'dry needling' procedure – wherein acupuncture needles were inserted into these trigger points to release them. [Trigger points are basically 'knots' in the muscles]. And lo behold! My father's pain went away 100%. He also taught my dad some simple neck exercises that he does religiously to this day. He calls them 'Dr. Ragahvendra's exercises'! And the pains have never recurred! Can you imagine his happiness? It's been ten years now... and counting.

Here is another 'pain' story, with a happy ending... of a young international swimmer who had access to the best sports physiotherapists and yet had these long-standing neck and shoulder pains. And these were impacting her performance. She was treated by Nikhil C.H., our head of Physiotherapy and an ANRS. Here is what he had to say about her treatment.

In the shadow of an athlete's success, there often lies a tale of unseen struggle and relentless perseverance. This is the story of a young girl, a swimmer of international renown, who came to me with a problem that seemed as insurmountable as the waves she conquered in the pool—a chronic neck and shoulder pain that had haunted her for three long years.

Her journey through this pain was a silent battle fought away from the cheering crowds and the glittering podiums. She sought the expertise of the finest physical therapists across the United States, each a specialist renowned for their skill and expertise in understanding the needs of such 'high performance' elite athletes. They applied cutting-edge techniques, from electrotherapy to manual therapy, in an effort to quell the persistent ache that shadowed her every stroke. She endured multiple courses of painkillers, each offering only temporary respite. Yet, the pain, stubborn and defiant, always returned.

When she walked into the clinic, her eyes, usually bright with the competitive fire, were dulled by the frustration of endless pain. She was a month away from the national championships, and the weight of her dreams pressed heavily upon her young shoulders. As her new physiotherapist, I knew the daunting task ahead. The usual routines and therapeutic modalities would not suffice. We required a breakthrough, an 'out-of-the-box' therapy strategy, and we worked on it swiftly.

In the quiet confines of my consultation room, as we spoke of her struggles and her fears, I realized that her pain was more than physical—it was a shadow dimming her spirit. Her story was not just one of physical ailment but of a fighter facing her toughest opponent yet, not inside but outside the swimming pool. It became clear that what had been overlooked was not just a symptom to be treated but a puzzle that needed solving.

Digging deeper into her medical history and observing her movements, a revelation came to light—her neck joint displayed signs of hypermobility, causing uncontrolled movements that traditional therapies had not addressed. This was the root cause that had eluded so many before. Armed with this new insight, we embarked on a tailored program focused on "segmental stabilization." Minimal manual therapy was applied, emphasizing controlled, strengthening exercises designed specifically for her condition.

With each session, she regained not only the strength in her muscles but also the confidence in her body. I educated her about the mechanisms of her pain and equipped her with strategies to manage and eventually overcome it. Together, we explored the depths of her resilience and determination, transforming her pain into a lesson of self-awareness and control. The transformation was profound. As the days turned into weeks, she grew stronger, her movements more assured. The pain that had once seemed an indomitable foe now receded, becoming a distant memory. Her spirit, rekindled with hope and the joy of unburdened movement, soared.

The pinnacle of our journey came at the national championships. Each stroke was a testament to her courage, each lap a victory over her erstwhile torment. When she touched the final wall, not only had she reclaimed her life from the clutches of pain, but she had also surpassed herself—breaking her own national record and securing the gold medal. She is now in the race to qualify for the Olympics. I wish her all the very best.

For those familiar with our team, you know that Siddharth has been a key member at PRS Neurosciences for about seven years. For newcomers, Siddharth is our Senior Occupational Therapist and currently an Advanced Neuro Rehab Specialist (ANRS). He excels in his role partly because he deeply understands pain—not just clinically, but personally. Here's why.

Siddharth's job as an occupational therapist is physically strenuous. He spends extensive hours assisting patients with flaccid limbs, facilitating movement, and delivering remedial care.

This physical demand is coupled with the psychological strain of continuously innovating and creating new therapeutic solutions. This blend of physical exertion and mental stress led to heightened anxiety and depression, manifesting physically in his life. He started experiencing myospasms—uncontrolled muscle contractions—and faced difficulties with everyday tasks like climbing stairs. At times, his leg would unexpectedly buckle, causing him to lose balance and occasionally faint. Panic attacks further complicated his condition, making it hard to breathe and intensifying his discomfort.

The COVID-19 pandemic brought additional challenges when Siddharth needed surgery to remove renal stones, layering more pain on top of his already significant struggles. This ordeal heightened his chronic pain, with psychological stress and physical strain triggering simultaneous discomfort in his neck, shoulders, and kidneys. Despite frequent ultrasounds to monitor his condition, no new renal stones were detected, yet the pain persisted.

Recognizing the cyclical nature of his stress and pain, Siddharth focused on his psychological health to break the cycle. Counseling and self-reflection provided him with insights into his limits and strategies to manage stress effectively. Nevertheless, the pain remained unrelenting, eventually leading to a flattened cervical spine curvature and a prolapsed disc at the C7 level, which compressed his spinal cord. Once, while alone in a treatment facility, his pain escalated severely, rendering him unable to turn his neck. Despite being two hours away from any immediate medical help, Siddharth drove himself in excruciating pain to see Dr. Sadasivan Iyer, a highly respected pain physician. Siddharth received temporary relief from the pain intervention, enabling him to move his neck again. However, knowing this was not a long-term solution, he subsequently received an epidural injection for more sustained pain relief.

Over time, Siddharth has learned to manage his psychological stresses better, but the muscle issues continue, especially when he overexerts himself. His ongoing journey involves strengthening his weaker muscles, focusing on the balance between stabilizers and mobilizers, and continually assessing his posture and daily activities to prevent potential strains.

His personal experiences have not only deepened his professional expertise but also made him a testament to the challenges and resilience found in the path of recovery. It's crucial to understand that pain isn't solely physical—it's also influenced by psychological factors. To achieve lasting relief, both physical–visible and nonphysical–nonvisible aspects must be addressed comprehensively. By acknowledging and treating both the visible and invisible aspects of pain, one can strive towards a pain-free existence.

From the above three stories, you can understand that there is another 'demon' in this world, called "CHRONIC PAIN"! This is also very democratic and can afflict anyone, including you and me. I already suffer from lower back pain and right leg pain, which bothers me on and off... especially whenever I forget my back exercises for a week or two.

As I have said at the beginning of this chapter, 'Pain is a pain is a pain!'

CHRONIC PAIN: A SIGNIFICANT HEALTHCARE CHALLENGE IN THE 21ST CENTURY

As we delve into the complexities of movement disorders in this book, we confront a stark reality: chronic pain is a global healthcare crisis impacting an unprecedented number of lives. Nearly a third of the global population suffers from chronic pain, making it a leading cause of disability worldwide. A 2018 study in India highlighted that nearly 20% of its population struggles with chronic pain, with a notable increase in cases among women each year in developing countries.

Chronic pain transcends mere physical discomfort, affecting diverse groups and manifesting across various conditions like arthritis, cancer, AIDS, fibromyalgia, multiple sclerosis, and post-surgical pain. Its impact is profound, with rheumatoid arthritis, osteoarthritis, and fibromyalgia as some of the primary culprits, alongside the hidden adversaries of multiple sclerosis, malignancies, and the lasting scars of trauma and surgery.

Our observations reveal gender disparities in pain perception, with anatomical differences highlighting that males and females experience and report pain differently across various body regions. For instance, men report less foot and ankle pain than women, while women experience more intense pain in the lumbar region.

A detailed study showed that 40% of chronic pain sufferers attribute their condition to arthritis, followed by neuropathy (14%), malignancy (6%), muscular issues (15%), post-traumatic conditions (15%), and post-surgical complications (10%). These statistics underscore the diverse origins of chronic pain, emphasizing the need for comprehensive approaches to its management.

Chronic pain is more than a physical symptom; it is a barrier to normalcy, transforming daily routines into daunting challenges and often accompanied by anxiety, depression, and disrupted sleep. Understanding the nature of a patient's pain—whether a dull ache, a sharp stab, or another form—is crucial for identifying the affected anatomical structures and proposing effective treatments. In managing pain, it is essential to consider the duration and cost of treatment options, aiming to provide holistic solutions that enhance overall well-being. Strategies such as promoting good sleep hygiene, reducing stress, encouraging healthy eating, and regular exercise are vital in improving pain tolerance and helping patients return to healthy activities. Through this comprehensive approach, we strive not only to alleviate pain but also to restore the quality of life for those afflicted.

In my many discussions as a Stereotactic and Functional Neurosurgeon, I emphasize the importance of pain not just as a discomfort but as a crucial indicator of underlying health issues. Pain acts as a vital feedback mechanism, alerting us to distress within our bodies. Throughout my career, I have encountered various types of pain experienced by patients, from persistent headaches to debilitating spinal discomfort. Addressing these pains promptly is essential for improving a patient's well-being and quality of life.

One particular case involved a patient who came to me with what was initially diagnosed as migraine headaches. Further evaluation revealed that these were actually cervicogenic headaches stemming from neck muscle tension. This case underscores the necessity of accurate diagnosis and tailored treatments, illustrating how seemingly unrelated symptoms can often be interconnected.

Sharing stories like these highlights the importance of thorough evaluations to understand the root cause of pain, ensuring effective relief and avoiding misdiagnoses. I also delve into the critical role of myofascial release and trigger point therapy in managing musculoskeletal pain, especially in the neck and back areas.

The expertise of skilled physiotherapists in administering targeted therapy is indispensable in these cases. It is crucial to avoid relying solely on symptomatic relief through painkillers and to address the underlying causes directly.

During my practice, I have emphasized comprehensive examinations and detailed patient history in diagnosing complex pain conditions accurately. For instance, a patient presenting with back pain was ultimately diagnosed with post-herpes neuralgia, a discovery made possible only through meticulous physical examination. These examples underline the essential role of clinical evaluations in guiding effective treatment strategies and improving patient outcomes.

Furthermore, I stress the importance of seeking expert opinions and conducting comprehensive evaluations for precise diagnosis and treatment planning. The limitations of relying solely on imaging scans are significant;

clinical expertise in interpreting these results is invaluable. Through anecdotes and insights from my practice, I advocate for a patient-centered approach that prioritizes thorough assessments and personalized care for optimal pain management and recovery.

My discourse on pain management emphasizes a holistic approach that combines accurate diagnosis, targeted treatments, and patient-centered care. By sharing my experiences and insights, I aim to highlight the critical roles of clinical evaluation, history-taking, and expert guidance in effectively addressing various pain conditions. My comprehensive and patient-focused approach is designed to improve outcomes, enhance quality of life, and empower individuals to proactively manage their pain for better overall health and well-being.

Managing chronic pain: It is also a 'wiring' problem in the brain!

Managing chronic pain requires a comprehensive understanding that distinguishes it significantly from acute pain. Unlike acute pain, which usually has a clear cause-effect relationship linked to a specific injury or event, chronic pain is more elusive and multifaceted. It often persists without a direct or obvious cause, making it challenging to treat with traditional pain management techniques.

Chronic pain is not merely a prolonged version of acute pain but a distinct and complex medical condition. According to the *Neuromatrix Theory of Pain*, chronic pain involves sophisticated interactions between the thalamus and the cortex. These interactions can lead to changes in the brain's wiring, causing the brain to perceive pain more intensely and frequently, even in the absence of an actual physical stimulus. This theory helps explain why chronic pain can persist even after the original injury or disease that caused it has healed.

Role of a specialized 'pain' physiotherapist in the management of chronic pain

In dealing with chronic pain, manual therapies such as trigger point release and myofascial release have shown effectiveness in managing specific symptoms. These therapies focus on relieving muscle tightness and alleviating stress in the myofascial tissues—thin, strong, fibrous connective tissue that extends throughout the body to provide support and protection to the muscles and bones. Such treatments can help reduce localized pain but might not be entirely sufficient for comprehensive chronic pain management.

Dry needling is another targeted therapy often used to address persistent trigger points. This technique involves inserting thin needles into the muscles at the trigger points, leading to the release of muscle tension and pain relief. Although beneficial for many, this approach is one component of a broader therapeutic strategy.

Exercise plays a pivotal role in the management of chronic pain, particularly when muscle weakness contributes to discomfort. Strengthening exercises can fortify muscles and joints, improve body mechanics, and reduce the strain that contributes to pain. Regular physical activity not only builds strength and flexibility but also enhances endorphin production, which naturally combats pain. Moreover, exercise can prevent the reoccurrence of pain episodes by maintaining muscle tone and improving posture. Corrective exercises and adopting proper posture are crucial, especially for those who suffer from chronic myofascial pain caused by long-term poor posture. Ergonomic adjustments in daily activities and work settings are essential to ensure that posture does not continue to contribute to chronic pain.

Pain counseling is another vital aspect of a holistic approach to managing chronic pain. Chronic pain is not only a physical experience but also an emotional and psychological challenge. Pain counseling aims to address the psychological effects of chronic pain, including stress, depression, and anxiety, which can exacerbate the physical sensation of pain. Counselors specializing in pain management employ various techniques to help patients modify their attitudes toward pain, develop better-coping mechanisms, and reduce feelings of helplessness and depression.

Effective pain counseling also includes techniques such as cognitive-behavioral therapy (CBT), which helps patients reframe negative thoughts related to their pain, and mindfulness-based stress reduction (MBSR), which teaches relaxation techniques to help control the perception of pain. By integrating these psychological therapies with physical treatments, patients can achieve better control over their pain and improve their quality of life.

The management of chronic pain is thus a multidisciplinary endeavor. It combines physical therapies to address the direct symptoms with exercise to strengthen and support the body and psychological counseling to manage the emotional fallout of chronic pain. This integrated approach ensures that all aspects of the patient's pain are addressed, offering the best chance for relief and a return to normalcy.

Each patient's experience with chronic pain is unique, and therefore, treatment plans should be personalized. Healthcare providers must consider not only the physical symptoms but also the psychological impact of chronic pain on the individual. Through a combination of therapeutic exercises, manual therapies, and psychological support, patients can find meaningful ways to manage their pain and improve their overall well-being.

What are 'Trigger Points'?

Trigger points are hyper-irritable spots found within a muscle. They often feel like knots or nodules within a tight band of muscle and are not just tender to the touch but can also cause a range of symptoms. These include referred pain, which means they can cause pain in different areas of the body, not just where the trigger point is located. They can also lead to motor dysfunction, affecting movement and muscle control, as well as autonomic phenomena, which can involve changes in bodily functions that aren't consciously directed, such as sweating or blushing. Managing these trigger points often involves therapeutic techniques aimed at relieving the tension in these spots, which can help alleviate the associated symptoms.

Active Trigger Points: Characteristics and Symptoms

Active trigger points are troublesome spots in muscles that cause pain even when not being touched. These trigger points can lead to various symptoms, including:

- Aching or pain at rest.
- Consistent patterns of pain that seem to spread from one area to another.
- Possible associated symptoms like muscle weakness.
- Changes in skin temperature over the affected muscle.
- Paresthesias, which are sensations of tingling or numbness.
- Other related conditions, such as tinnitus (ringing in the ears), TMJ pain (jaw pain), headaches, eye pain, or torticollis (twisted neck).

Active trigger points can significantly affect quality of life due to their range of symptoms and constant discomfort.

Latent Trigger Points: Identification and Effects

Latent trigger points are those that don't cause pain by themselves but can become painful when pressure is applied or during certain activities. They can lead to:

- Shortened muscles, making them feel tight even when at rest.
- Muscle weakness affecting the overall strength and function.
- Limited joint movement, reducing the range of motion and flexibility.

Identifying and treating latent trigger points can help prevent them from becoming active and causing more significant pain or discomfort.

Some common referral patterns in such trigger points

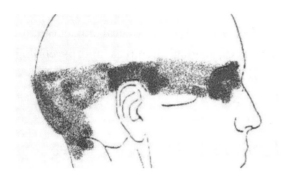 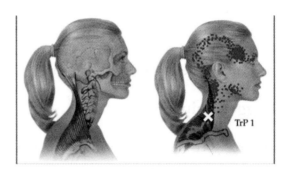

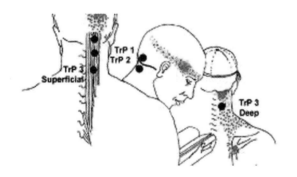 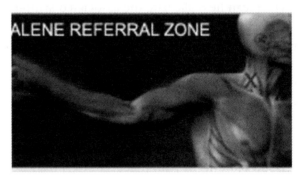

Left-sided scalene 'referral' pain can mimic a heart attack!

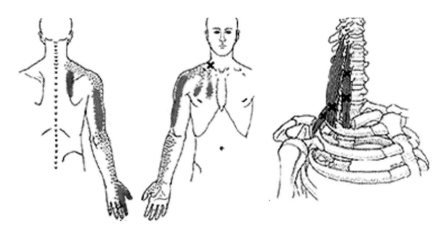

Composite pain patterns (solid red areas are the essential pain reference zones, and stippled red areas are the spillover reference zones) with locations of some

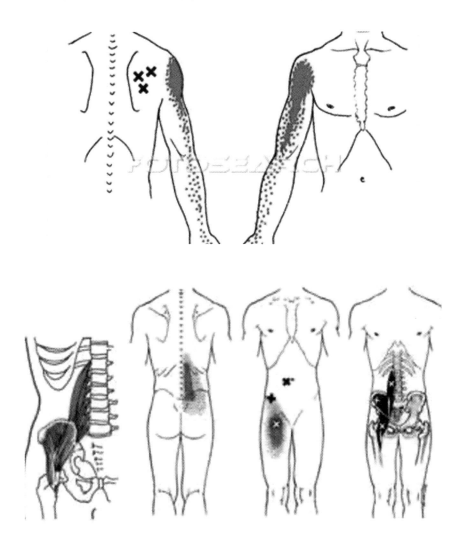

Some of the possible locations where we all can have pains due to trigger points

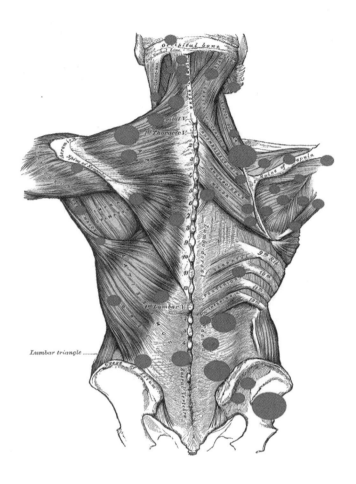

In simpler terms, managing pain is a big challenge, but we've made a lot of progress at PRS Neurosciences since 2012. Way back in the early 2000s, I had already realized the importance of chronic interventional pain services. I would try to motivate many anaesthesiologists to train and get a fellowship. Since 2012, I have had the opportunity to work with many pain physicians and a few good musculoskeletal 'pain' physiotherapists, and I have learned a lot from them.

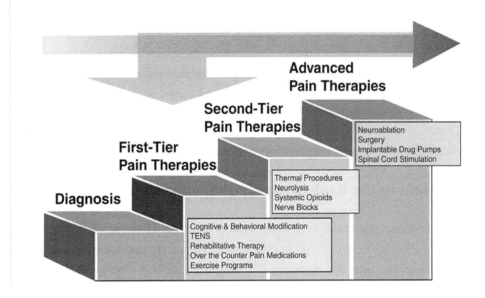

Let me summarise what I have learned: I consider myself a very conservative 'spine' surgeon, especially when compared to an orthospine surgeon. Every MRI shows some 'slipped disc,' some nerve compression, and some degeneration, including mine! If the 'aggressive' spine surgeon is performing TEN spine surgeries, I would only operate 2-3 of those. If the same people are performing TEN fusion surgeries, I would do fusion for only 3-4 of those patients. Doctors refer patients to me with a simple mandate for a second opinion – go to him; he doesn't operate unnecessarily. So, even in such a conservative situation, I feel that after my interactions, learnings, and experience with these interventional pain physicians, my spine surgeries have come down by 50%! FIFTY PERCENT!! Can you imagine? And I am so happy.

My current colleague who does all our pain interventions is Dr. Sadasivan Iyer, who is pleasant, competent, hardworking, and a great team player. I send him patients regularly, and they all come back very happy. In fact, in the month of July 2023, I had sent him 32 patients for pain interventions, my highest ever in a single month! He is not trigger-happy. If he is convinced that surgery is the right option, he sends them back.

Insights about different types of pain are crucial, but we need to be more precise in understanding and treating them. We should pay attention to where the pain is and how it responds to treatments like therapy or needling.

We also need to focus more on ergonomic assessments and exercises to prevent pain from coming back. It's essential to educate patients about maintaining their health and making necessary changes to their habits.

There's always room for improvement, and we should keep exploring new techniques to better help our patients. Let's continue working together to provide the best care possible.

It is not diabetes, cancer, or heart problems that cause people to take leave from work. Statistics have shown that a silly, stupid problem called "Low Back Pain" is the single biggest cause of 'loss of manhours' in the world today!

In one of my recent discussions on chronic pain, I explored the widespread issue of low back pain, a major cause of lost productivity across the globe. As a neurosurgeon, I've seen firsthand the impact of modern sedentary lifestyles on back health (including for myself) and stress the importance of proactive back care and regular exercise.

Low back pain involves complex pain generation mechanisms in the body, including issues with nerve roots, the spinal cord, the various joints, and muscle-related pain. Conditions like sciatica and facet joint pain illustrate the need for precise diagnosis and customized treatments tailored to an individual's specific pain sources.

Throughout my career, I've encountered various challenging cases that underscore the importance of thorough evaluation and targeted interventions.

Every pain in the back of the thigh is not 'SCIATICA'!

I remember a particular case that stood out to me. It was a 45 to 50-year-old woman who came to me with pain in the back of her buttocks, extending down to the back of her thigh up to her knee. She had been experiencing this pain for three to four months and had previously visited a neurologist who diagnosed it as sciatica.

The neurologist ordered an MRI of her spine, which showed a slipped disc at the D11 and D12 levels. Consequently, she was referred to me for surgery.

When she arrived at my outpatient clinic, she was prepared for the operation physically, mentally, emotionally, and financially. However, as she eagerly asked me when I would perform the surgery, I felt compelled to conduct a thorough examination first. After examining her, I recommended getting an X-ray of her right hip joint before proceeding with any surgical intervention.

It turned out that the X-ray revealed she had tuberculosis (TB) in her hip joint, which was the actual culprit for her so-called 'sciatic' pain, and not a slipped disk as previously (mis)diagnosed. I explained to her that she did not require spine surgery but needed to undergo treatment for tuberculosis instead. My junior assistant immediately asked me – Sir, how did you know that the D11-12 slipped disc was not the culprit? My answer was – that the so-called sciatica pain is L5 and not D11-12!

This case highlighted the importance of accurate clinical diagnosis, clinico-radiological correlation, and how symptoms like sciatica can have various underlying causes. It also emphasized the significance of proper evaluation before opting for surgical procedures to ensure the most effective treatment. This is how we can apply the CAREPa framework even with pain evaluations.

Every sciatic pain needn't be a slipped disc!

Another memorable case that I had - A 42-year-old man who happened to be the brother of an orthopedic surgeon specializing in treating slipped discs *(apart from us neurosurgeons, who I think are much better equipped in handling spine and spinal cord surgeries),* experienced recurring 'sciatic' pain for 15 years. The pain would come and go, sometimes alleviated by medication. Despite this, he never underwent an MRI scan as the pain did not seem severe enough. Eventually, out of frustration, he decided to get an MRI.

The MRI revealed a spinal cord tumor, a stark contrast to the expected diagnosis of sciatica. This unexpected discovery led to confusion and disbelief. The man's experience highlighted the complexity of medical conditions and how symptoms can sometimes be misleading, requiring thorough investigation to uncover the true underlying cause. Anyway... For the records, it was a 'non-cancerous' tumor, which I operated on and removed completely, and he is fine.

There are common misconceptions surrounding back surgery that often deter people from considering it as a viable option. However, through sharing success stories from my practice, where patients regained significant functionality post-surgery, I aim to reassure and debunk myths about back surgery. When performed by skilled professionals, surgery can be a highly effective treatment for many severe back issues.

A spine surgery dating back to the year 2010...

I was operating in one of the mission hospitals, and during that time, I didn't have any PGs under me, so the orthopedic PGs used to assist me. There was a patient with a slip disc at two levels, L4-5 and L5-S1. Considering the patient's pre-op evaluation, though his spine MRI showed slipped discs at two levels – L4-5 and L5-S1, I decided that he only needed an L5, S1 disc surgery and not for L4, 5. During the operation, the assistant asked me why I was only removing the L5, S1 disc and not the L4, five-disc. I explained that the pain was coming from the L5, S1 disc and not the L4-5 one. He asked me, "How sure are you?" To this, I gave an answer that left him stunned and in disbelief – post-operatively, if his pain is gone, I have removed the right disc, and if not, I have removed the wrong. After the surgery, once the patient woke up from anesthesia, I asked if his pain was gone. When he confirmed that the pain was gone, I knew I had removed the right disc. It was a satisfying moment knowing that I had made the correct decision in surgery without unnecessary procedures.

Moreover, I touch upon the importance of proactive healthcare and the role of spirituality in coping with illness. Encouraging a mindset focused on diagnosable conditions with accessible treatments can lead to recovery and a return to normal life, empowering individuals to take charge of their health challenges.

The magic of bed rest... masterly inactivity that has prevented many a back surgery

When it comes to recommending bed rest for my patients, I take a very conservative approach as a spine surgeon. I firmly believe in giving the body the time it needs to heal naturally before considering surgery. If a patient presents with back pain, leg pain, or any other spinal issue without weakness, I advocate for a good three to four weeks of conservative treatment involving medications and physiotherapy.

Bed rest plays a crucial role in this treatment plan. I often tell my patients that bed rest may feel like a form of 'punishment,' but it is essential for allowing the body to recover. During this period, it is important to lie down in bed and NOT SIT, as even sitting on a comfortable chair can exert pressure on the spine.

To determine if bed rest is sufficient, I advise patients to monitor their pain levels. When turning in bed, sitting up, standing, or moving around to perform daily tasks like going to the bathroom, there should be minimal to no pain. These activities serve as checkpoints to gauge the effectiveness of bed rest in alleviating discomfort and promoting healing. By emphasizing the importance of bed rest and closely monitoring pain levels during daily activities, we can give the body the opportunity it needs to heal naturally and potentially avoid the need for surgical intervention.

This discussion provides a detailed overview of the complexities surrounding back pain, emphasizing the importance of accurate diagnosis, personalized treatment plans, and an active approach to healthcare. My insights as a neurosurgeon shed light on effective management strategies, debunk myths about surgical interventions, and highlight success stories that demonstrate the critical importance of timely and appropriate interventions for achieving the best outcomes in back pain management.

CRANIO-FACIAL PAINS

The suicide disease! Trigeminal neuralgia or tic douloureux

In my discussions on the severe pain associated with trigeminal neuralgia, a nerve disorder affecting the face, I explain the unbearable intensity of the pain, which some of my patients have described as so devastating it led them to contemplate suicide. The pain, often manifesting as sharp, shooting sensations across the face, teeth, and mouth, can be so severe that it is frequently misdiagnosed, leading to unnecessary and ineffective dental treatments, including multiple teeth extractions.

I delve into the possible causes of trigeminal neuralgia, which may include compression of the trigeminal nerve by nearby arteries or veins or, less commonly, by a tumor pressing on the nerve. I emphasize the critical importance of an accurate diagnosis, urging potential sufferers to obtain high-resolution MRI scans that can pinpoint the specific nerve involvement and identify any compressive sources. Moreover, I discuss the connection between trigeminal neuralgia and herpes zoster, stressing the necessity of a comprehensive evaluation to tailor the treatment precisely to the individual's condition.

When it comes to treatment, I outline several approaches, starting with medications specifically designed to manage nerve pain, which are fundamentally different from standard painkillers. For severe cases, I discuss the potential need for interventions such as injections, radiofrequency ablation, or microvascular decompression surgery. It's crucial, I note, to seek treatment from skilled professionals who can accurately diagnose and manage the condition, akin to finding the precise nut that needs tightening to fix a leaky tap.

I also caution against jumping to conclusions about trigeminal neuralgia without a thorough evaluation, as symptoms can be similar to those of other issues like temporomandibular joint disorders or muscle trigger points. It's essential to accurately diagnose the condition to guide the correct treatment path and avoid unnecessary procedures. I also emphasize the importance of managing stress and avoiding triggers such as teeth grinding, which can exacerbate the condition.

I reiterate the distressing nature of trigeminal neuralgia but also want to reassure patients about the availability of effective treatments and the potential for significant relief. Proper medical evaluation and treatments tailored to each person's unique situation are paramount. My role as a Stereotactic and Functional Neurosurgeon is to provide patients and their families with the knowledge and means to manage this challenging condition effectively, ensuring they receive the specialized care needed to navigate the complexities of trigeminal neuralgia.

Pain is the most important sensation for us human beings. It is a harbinger of something sinister that may be cooking inside your body, and the pain may be the first symptom that leaks out the bad news! Headache, chest pain, abdominal pains, sciatic pains, etc... the list goes on and on. Pain is now called the 5th vital sign. Please DO NOT ever neglect pain... it could even be fatal.

SECTION C: ADVANCED NEURO REHABILITATION

10

Stroke

Brain Attack/Lakwa (Paralysis)

"Time lost is brain lost. Recognizing the signs of stroke and seeking immediate medical attention can make the difference between life and death and between full recovery and permanent disability."

- Dr. Thomas G. Brott
A prominent stroke neurologist and former chairman of the American Stroke Association

This quote emphasizes the critical importance of early recognition and intervention in stroke to minimize brain damage and maximize the chances of recovery.

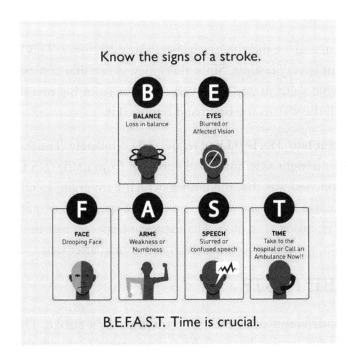

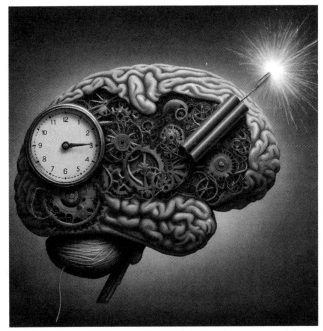

Let me start with a "BE FAST" story...

I want to emphasize the importance of the window period and thrombectomy. This is the story of a man called Chandrashekhar, a 33-year-old, obese guy with some co-morbidities not diagnosed, who used to work in one of the trustee's (Jain Hospital) garment factories. That trustee suddenly called me one afternoon around one o'clock and said this guy had collapsed in their office and seemed to have had a stroke. And that was about 20 minutes before he called me.

In my mind – WINDOW PERIOD STROKE, ask him to BE FAST! So, I asked to immediately rush him to Jain Hospital, and he brought him within 35 - 40 minutes of the stroke. We found that this guy was having a dense right-sided stroke. He was not speaking. He could just open his eyes, looking around. His blood pressure was 180/100 mmHg. He was quite obese. We did an urgent MRI of the Brain stroke protocol. MRI of the stroke protocol classically showed that he was within the window period. Only the FLAIR scan was positive. The MR Angiogram showed that there was a complete occlusion of the M1 segment of the Middle Cerebral Artery (MCA). That meant the main stem of the middle cerebral artery was occluded. He was a classic candidate for a mechanical thrombectomy. He was not a candidate for intravenous IV thrombolysis or clot-busting.

Immediately, we convinced the family. Even in a charitable hospital like ours, this is an expensive procedure and may cost anywhere between Rs. 5-7 lakhs. The trustee took the financial responsibility and asked us to go ahead. In many 'window period' strokes, though the family is willing, the finances many times do not permit them to get it done.

Then, my endovascular neurosurgeon colleague went in, and we did the mechanical thrombectomy. This is usually done under local anesthesia, often unless the patient is very restless. Since this guy was not that restless, we decided to do it under local anesthesia. As my colleague went in and removed that clot from his middle cerebral artery, from a puncture from the thigh, he went all the way to the brain and removed it.

About 10 minutes later, the clot was out, and we looked at him. His hand had recovered completely. The guy who was not able to move his hand and leg, his power of the right-side limbs had come up from grade 0/5 to grade 4/5. But his speech had not improved. So, what happened was that the umbra (which I am going to talk about later in this chapter) was affected, and the penumbra area functions were reversed. The speech took quite some time to return. He was walking around. His comprehension was okay. His expressive speech had been impacted, and he needed three to six months of speech therapy. His speech became near normal after that.

So, what is BE FAST?

Are you aware of what BE FAST stands for? It's a handy acronym to recognize the signs of a stroke. The first one is "B" for balance, which indicates issues with standing or walking straight, feeling unsteady, or the risk of falling due to balance problems. Then there's "E" for Eyes, noticing asymmetry in the eyes, double vision, blurriness, or sudden darkness affecting vision.

Moving on to "F" for Face, this involves observing facial asymmetry, drooping on one side of the face, weakness, numbness, or tingling sensations on either side of the face. "A" stands for Arms, where weakness or difficulty in raising one arm or maintaining its position is a key indicator. "S" signifies Speech, encompassing various speech irregularities like complete cessation, confused speech, or slurred speech resembling that of someone intoxicated. Lastly, "T" emphasizes Time, stressing the urgency of immediate action. Seeking medical assistance promptly is vital.

Summing it up, BE FAST urges swift action when these symptoms manifest. Whether for yourself, a loved one, or even a stranger on the road, quick recognition and response are crucial.

WHAT IS THE 'TIME IS BRAIN' THEORY?

In 1993, neurologist Camilo Gomez, M.D., coined a phrase that for a quarter century has been a fundamental rule of stroke care: 'Time is brain! ' The longer therapy is delayed, the less chance it will be successful. "It is imperative that clinicians begin to look upon stroke as a medical emergency of a magnitude similar to that of myocardial infarction (heart attack) or head trauma," he wrote.

TIME IS BRAIN–QUANTIFIED

(in a major artery occlusion)

A normal human brain is estimated to have about 100 billion neurons, and each neuron can make up to 10,000 different connections, which means that a normal human brain's capacity is 100 billion to the power of 10,000!

	Neurons Lost	Synapses Lost	Myelinated Fibers Lost	Accelerated Aging
Per Stroke	1.2 billion	8.3 trillion	7140 km/4470 miles	36 y
Per Hour	120 million	830 billion	714 km/447 miles	3.6 y
Per Minute	1.9 million	14 billion	12 km/7.5 miles	3.1 wk
Per Second	32 000	230 million	200 meters/218 yards	8.7 h

Heart is important, brain is not? The bias towards the brain!

Imagine someone in your house, be it your father, mother, or uncle, complaining of left-sided chest pain at 2:00 in the morning and urgently calling you for help. Naturally, your immediate thought is likely a heart attack. In such a situation, you wouldn't consider taking them to a gynecology-specialized hospital; instead, you'd rush them to a multispecialty hospital, probably the best in the area. You'd be frantically trying to convey, "I think my father is having a heart attack" or "My mother is having a heart attack." Urgency and prompt action become your top priorities. Despite the fact that 90% of such chest pains turn out to be non-cardiac, you recognize the critical importance of acting swiftly, as catching the 10% that could be a heart attack is paramount.

Now, consider the same scenario at 2:00 in the morning, but this time, the complaint is about a headache accompanied by slight numbness in the hand or leg. Strangely, when it comes to headaches, the common response might be to suggest taking a painkiller and going to bed, avoiding any further disturbance until morning. This contrast highlights a crucial point: the urgency and seriousness often associated with cardiac symptoms may not be immediately extended to symptoms like headaches, even when they involve neurological elements like numbness.

This observation underscores the importance of treating all potential health concerns with the same level of urgency and not dismissing symptoms that could be indicative of a neurological issue. Just as in the case of chest pain, where immediate action is essential despite the majority being non-cardiac, a similar level of concern and proactive response is warranted for symptoms like headaches, especially when accompanied by neurological symptoms. This mindset ensures that potentially serious issues are addressed promptly, enhancing the chances of positive outcomes.

The moral of the story: never neglect a headache. It could be fatal!

Let me tell you a story of a medical college student to drive this point home.

In the prime of youth, at 21, Anjali was the embodiment of aspiration and hope—a second-year medical student standing on the threshold of a promising career. Hailing from a family of medical professionals in Kerala, she was a bright spark in a lineage of healers. Her brother, a radiologist, had made his mark by running a successful diagnostic center in their hometown, with CT/MRI scan facilities, etc.

For six months, Anjali experienced intermittent headaches, a flickering pain accompanied by visual disturbances that flickered on the edges of her perception, much like the monsoon clouds that dappled the Kerala skies. Yet, she neglected her symptoms and left her condition uninvestigated—she was not an uneducated village bumpkin. She came from a family of doctors, and her brother could have done a FREE brain scan for her! She was studying in a medical college, not some other god-forsaken course. All in all, this was a clear case of "brain is not important" and hence neglected.

Tragedy struck without warning. She was having her internal assessment exams, and she lived in a hostel on campus. That morning, she had gone into the bathroom to have a shower, and since she hadn't come out for a long time, the next girl in the queue, waiting to take a shower, knocked at the door and eventually realized that something was wrong. The door was broken open, and she was found lying unconscious on the floor, with vomitus all over and around her. She was immediately rushed to the emergency and intubated.

A CT scan of her brain unveiled the unthinkable—a large aneurysm in her left internal carotid artery had ruptured, with massive subarachnoid hemorrhage (SAH). Since that medical college hospital did not have a neurosurgical backup, she was brought to our hospital in Bengaluru. By the time she was brought into our emergency 5 hours later…. she was BRAIN DEAD!

Her family, pillars in the medical community, grappled with the irreplaceable loss. The light of their lives extinguished too soon, leaving behind a trail of unanswered questions and a cautionary tale of the unpredictable nature of life. Her brother, reflecting on the paths untaken, the scans not done, found himself in the depths of introspection, his own tools of healing having fallen silent at the moment when they were needed the most. Anjali's story remains a poignant reminder of the fragility of existence and the vital importance of heeding even the softest whispers of our well-being. Her memory, etched in the hearts of those she left behind, continues to inspire an unyielding pursuit of knowledge and a commitment to the sanctity of life in the practice of medicine.

Let us now delve into the basics of a stroke. Our brains are bustling hubs, constantly active and hungry for a steady flow of energy and oxygen delivered through our blood, right? Now, when that blood flow gets disrupted, trouble brews. Think of a stroke as a roadblock, cutting off this vital supply line. This disruption means the brain cells, the neurons, aren't getting what they need, and that's when the damage starts to rear its ugly head.

Unfortunately, brain cells don't bounce back from this kind of damage. Once they're harmed, it's a lasting impact. So, a stroke? It's essentially an injury to those brain cells caused by this interruption in blood supply.

Think of a stroke as having two primary categories. First, there's the one where the blood supply to a specific brain area gets cut off—this is known as an ***ischemic stroke***. On the other side, there's the ***hemorrhagic stroke***, which happens when a blood vessel ruptures and blood leaks out.

Ischemic strokes typically have two main reasons behind their occurrence. Over time, the blood vessels carrying blood to the brain can get clogged up due to a build-up of fatty deposits, making the vessel's pathway narrower and more prone to blockages. One day, it might just close off completely, halting the blood flow to that brain area. These are called thrombotic strokes. The second reason involves blood clots formed elsewhere in the body, like in the heart's chambers. Sometimes, these clots break off and travel through the bloodstream. They might cruise through larger blood vessels, but when they hit a narrow passage, they lodge there, cutting off blood flow to the surrounding areas. This type is called an embolic stroke. Don't get confused; we're going to discuss plenty of terms here, and it might sound even more difficult than remembering your high school batchmates' names. 80% of strokes are ischemic in nature.

Now, you might have heard about a "mini-stroke," or what we call a transient ischemic attack (TIA). TIAs are quite similar to ischemic strokes but tend to recover faster, typically within 24 hours. However, they signal a serious issue with the blood vessel, significantly increasing the risk of a full-blown stroke. Even after a TIA, it's crucial to see a doctor, address any underlying problems, and modify lifestyle or risk factors to prevent a more severe stroke, which could result in lasting neurological disability. Taking proactive steps after a TIA can significantly reduce the risk of a dangerous stroke.

A hemorrhagic stroke occurs when a blood vessel within the brain bursts, leading to bleeding in or around the brain. This type of stroke is less common than ischemic strokes, which are caused by clots, but hemorrhagic strokes are often more severe. The sudden hemorrhage can increase pressure within the brain, causing damage to brain cells and resulting in symptoms like a sudden, severe headache, loss of balance or coordination, difficulty speaking or understanding speech, and vision disturbances. Immediate medical attention is critical to manage the bleeding, reduce the pressure in the brain, and minimize brain damage to give the patient the best possible chance of recovery. Treatment typically involves controlling the bleeding, reducing the pressure in the brain, and stabilizing vital signs. Long-term recovery may include rehabilitation to regain as much function as possible.

Hemorrhagic strokes can also occur from something called an aneurysm. Picture blowing up a balloon; if it has a weak spot, that's where it bulges. Similarly, in blood vessels, weak areas can expand with each heartbeat, forming what's known as an aneurysm (remember the Reader's Digest story we spoke about earlier?) —a sort of sack-like bulge. The issue here is that the wall of this bulge is quite thin and fragile, making it prone to rupture. When it ruptures, blood spills out, causing what's known as an aneurysmal rupture.

In some rare cases, there might be a pre-existing issue in the brain's blood network from birth, known as arteriovenous malformation (AVM). This looks like a cluster of blood vessels resembling a ball, and at any point, it can rupture, leading to a stroke. High blood pressure can exert so much force that it breaks a blood vessel, triggering a hemorrhagic stroke.

Now, the reasons behind these strokes usually boil down to risk factors, which we can classify into two categories: modifiable and non-modifiable. Modifiable risk factors are those we can change through lifestyle adjustments or medical interventions, while non-modifiable ones, like age and sex, cannot be altered.

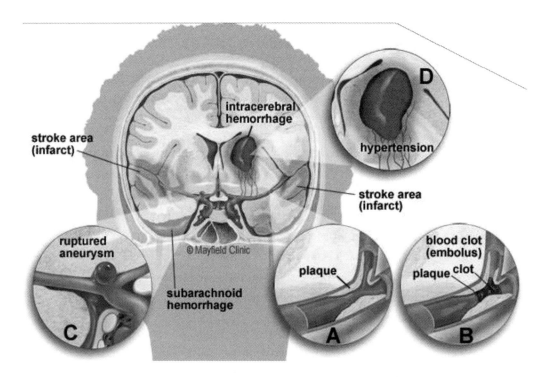

For instance, lifestyle-related modifiable factors involve issues such as being overweight or obese, excessive alcohol consumption, smoking, or drug use (such as cocaine and other synthetic drugs). On the other hand, medical risk factors include high blood pressure, elevated blood sugar levels, high cholesterol, and cardiovascular conditions like heart failure or irregular heart rhythms. Managing these factors through lifestyle changes or medical interventions can significantly reduce the risk of stroke.

Individuals above the age of 55 are at a higher risk of experiencing a stroke compared to younger adults. But it is also true that these days, the younger age group is experiencing strokes. Moreover, in terms of sex, men tend to be more prone to strokes than women. Hormonal factors also come into play; those using birth control pills or undergoing hormone therapies have an increased stroke risk.

Now, stroke prevention can be achieved through two approaches. One involves reducing the risk factors known to contribute to stroke. Lifestyle modifications such as minimizing tobacco use, reducing alcohol intake, and adopting a regular exercise routine can significantly lower the risk. The other aspect involves addressing transient ischemic attacks, or mini-strokes, which pose a risk for recurrent strokes. By managing these factors and embracing healthy lifestyle changes, the chances of experiencing a stroke can be notably decreased.

Let me tell you an **amazing, interesting** story; in fact, it is TWO stroke stories from the same family. This is not a story out of a Bollywood movie. This IS REAL. This story has two characters, a husband and a wife. First, let me tell you about the husband. The husband, Professor Sathyakrishna, was a Professor of Mathematics and former Principal of MES College, Bangalore. He was my mathematics teacher between the years 1984 to 1986 before I joined medical school. I had a very interesting run-in with him just before my second PUC, or 12th-grade exam, when we had this preparatory exam. I have this habit of answering all the questions, from top to bottom, including ALL the choices, especially in physics and mathematics subjects. I had done the same in mathematics and thereafter went on study holidays. Then I had to go back to the college to pick up my marksheets. Prof. Sathyakrishna met me, and after some time, he said - "There's some problem here. The totaling is going wrong." He showed me that he was getting 112 out of 100. I said, "Sir, it is correct, sir, because I've answered all the choice questions as well." He was livid with me. "Why are you answering the choice questions?

Do you know how much of my time you wasted?" I said, "Sir, what's your problem? I did what I did." Anyway, I'm just giving you this trivia to set more background context.

After that, I went to medical school and never met him again. One day, I got a call from a private hospital where I was a visiting doctor. I was asked to see a hemorrhagic stroke patient by the neurologist. When I walked into the ICU to see the patient, I realized it was him. I saw him. He had a left-sided brain hemorrhage. He had a right-sided weakness. He had difficulty speaking, and his weakness was about grade 2/5. Then I spoke to the family, I introduced myself, I told them who I was, that I was his student, and their family was very happy that an ex-student had come to take care of him. Thereafter, I got actively engaged in his treatment. The clot was not big enough to operate, so we managed it conservatively. As I mentioned in the past, the clot dissolved in 6-8 weeks. We got our neuro rehab team engaged. We started our usual strategies. He was in the hospital for nearly three months. He made a slow but gradual progress, and then he continued outpatient rehabilitation with us, physical therapy, occupational therapy, speech, and swallow therapy. After seven months of complete rehab, this man had improved remarkably.

His right-side weakness had improved completely. He was walking around confidently. The amazing thing was that his speech had improved to near, or I think, almost 'normal.' And guess what? He went back to teaching his favorite subject, mathematics, to students at a private tuition. To my surprise, one day, his son sent me a video on WhatsApp showing his dad doing his thing. I had tears of joy in my eyes because I felt like it was... it was 'Guru Dakshina' to one of my teachers, someone who had taught me mathematics in college. This was his story. Unfortunately, he eventually died many years later due to another brain hemorrhage. The family had rushed him unresponsive to the emergency; I saw him and realized that he was brain dead... and we chose to let nature take its course.

His story was somewhere in the year 2015-2016. Now, recently, that is 2024, in January or probably February, I got a call from his son telling me that his mother, who's the wife of my teacher, had suddenly developed a right-sided weakness and had started slurring for about half an hour. Guess what? BE FAST. It is a stroke. He had understood because of his father's experience. He called me. He had, incidentally, taken her to the same private hospital because they live very close by. But they called me from there. I said that we can't do any stroke interventions there, as it is not a 'stroke ready' hospital.

I asked them to shift her to my hospital, Bhagwan Mahaveer Jain Hospital. They immediately brought her here, much to the chagrin of that hospital – for me, commerce will never ever score over patient safety and care. She was in the window, period. We did IV thrombolysis or thrombolyzed her. Within a few hours of being thrombolyzed, her right hemiparesis started improving, her comprehension started improving, and we started very early neuro rehab for her.

She was discharged within two weeks because of the 'window period' treatment. In a week's time, she started walking to the bathroom, but her speech was still very dysphasic. She was able to understand, but she was not able to speak very well. Since she was walking around, we discharged her. Eventually, she continued to come to our outpatient services for two and a half to three months, and her speech recovered completely.

Let us now look into stroke evaluation, specifically focusing on the importance of imaging in these cases. Imaging plays a crucial role in the comprehensive assessment of strokes and the 'window period' decision-making. Why is it so vital?

Firstly, imaging aids in diagnosing the presence of a stroke, offering a clear picture of what's occurring within the brain. It provides insights into the type of stroke that's taken place, whether it's ischemic or hemorrhagic. Another significant aspect is determining the temporal stage of the stroke, essentially identifying at which phase the stroke currently exists. This information is pivotal in tailoring appropriate treatment protocols for the patient.

Moreover, imaging helps clinicians make informed decisions about the type of treatment needed, aligning with the specific type of stroke diagnosed. It's instrumental in guiding therapeutic interventions, ensuring they're precisely tailored to the patient's condition.

Lastly, imaging plays a role in detecting any potential complications stemming from the stroke, enabling medical teams to address these issues and provide comprehensive care promptly.

In a nutshell, imaging serves as a cornerstone in stroke evaluation, facilitating accurate diagnosis, treatment decisions, and monitoring for any additional complications that may arise.

Let's explore the chronological progression of stroke stages: commencing with the 'early hyperacute' phase, characterized by the initial onset of ischemic or hemorrhagic insult, swiftly progressing to the 'late hyperacute' stage, reminiscent of a delayed yet emergent manifestation of neurological deficits. Transitioning into the 'acute' phase, the clinical presentation escalates, emphasizing the urgency of therapeutic intervention to mitigate irreversible damage. Subsequently, in the 'subacute' stage, the sustained presence of symptoms underscores the need for ongoing management and rehabilitation strategies. Finally, culminating in the 'chronic' phase, a prolonged duration of symptoms solidifies the stroke's chronicity, underscoring the necessity for long-term care and support.

TYPES OF STROKES

You must understand – all strokes are not the same!

Now, strokes come in two main types, as already discussed: the "Ischemic Stroke," where it's like the brain's traffic jam with decreased blood supply, and the "Hemorrhagic Stroke," where it's more like a messy party with bleeding happening in the brain or around it. It's the ultimate "oops" moment for your blood vessels. Sometimes, brain tumors also show stroke-like symptoms!

Now, onto the imaging part! When the brain's throwing a stroke tantrum, we whip out the CT scan and MRI like our asthras. They're our trusty sidekicks in spotting what's going on inside your head on that stroke-filled adventurous road.

See, even strokes can't resist a little drama and variety in their storyline!

Ah, the CT scan, the superhero of stroke imaging – faster than a speeding bullet and more available than a cup of coffee at a hospital cafeteria! Let me paint you a picture of its quirks and perks.

So, picture this: In the world of stroke imaging, CT scans are like the fast food of diagnostics. Need results ASAP? No problem! CT scans are so speedy they make a superhero look like they're stuck in slow motion. I mean, seriously! While MRI is setting up its cozy 15 to 20-minute date, CT is already done, dusted, and on its way to grab a dessert after the date.

When it comes to spotting intracranial hemorrhages or the bad boys of strokes, CT is the Sherlock Holmes of the medical imaging universe – quick, efficient, and with a knack for spotting the troublemakers.

Now, let's talk about the quirks. CT may not have the soft touch of MRI when it comes to soft tissues, but it's like the 90's sitcom of imaging – it's reliable, it's everywhere, and it won't break the bank.

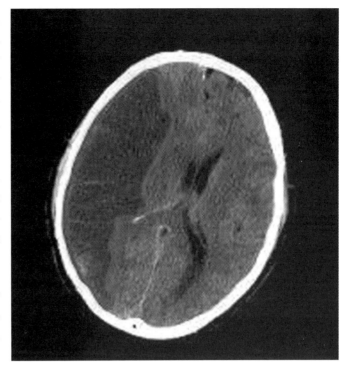

Plus, it's a lifesaver for those stroke patients who just can't keep calm and cozy in an MRI machine for too long. CT understands, and it's got their back (or brain, in this case).

But here's the catch – CT isn't the best at catching those early strokes. It's like the cool detective who solves the case fast but might miss a few subtle details. And let's not forget the X-ray exposure – CT comes with a bit of a glow-in-the-dark side effect.

So, in the world of stroke imaging, CT is the quick, reliable, and slightly flashy hero we all need – just don't forget its trusty sidekick, MRI, for those nuanced plot twists!

So, picture this: You're not in a tunnel; you're in a futuristic cocoon of magnetic wonders. No sound of whirring and clicking like a robot symphony – just a gentle hum as the magnet does its magic. And oh, did I mention that there is no need to worry about becoming a human-robot from radiation exposure? MRI is like the spa day of medical imaging – relaxing, radiation-free, and all about making you feel like a million bucks.

Now, let me give you some frightening information about the limitations of CT and MRI in very early strokes.

Did you know that for 8-12 hours after the onset of a stroke, though the patient may be having all the symptoms and signs of a stroke – the CT scan of the brain can look NORMAL??? What does this even mean?? This means that even if a CT scan is normal, it doesn't mean that there is no stroke. It only means that the brain changes have not yet reached up to a level that can be detected on a routine CT scan. Now, if this happens in a remote location, in the middle of the night, when only a radiographer/ CT technician is available (who only knows how to do a scan but cannot interpret), and you are wrongly informed that the scan is normal... what will you do? Go home, celebrate, and have a drink? Even if you have a one-sided weakness? Think??

Are you also aware that if you go to a nearby GP or a physician not well versed with stroke problems and imaging, he or she may suspect a stroke and write a prescription – MRI Brain (plain), right? He doesn't create any urgency. He only says to get the MRI and come back with the report. Seems perfectly reasonable and logical to you! Right?? WRONG!

And, like an obedient patient, you go to the diagnostic center recommended by that doctor, wait many hours in line for the MRI scan, wait a few hours longer for the report, or even wait till the next day, and then wait to see the doctor sometime during the day.... only to realize that the MRI scan is NORMAL. Does this again mean that the patient hasn't had a stroke? Even if you have one-sided body weakness? ABSOLUTELY NOT.

What am I trying to convey?

Many times, during the so-called 'window period,' even routine sequence MRIs can be normal. My goodness, then, is it all getting too confusing and complicated? Which is the right type of scan to be done to pick up an early stroke? Is such a scan even available?

Now, let's talk about the secret sauce of MRI – the sequences. It's like the different acts of a play, each with its own star. We've got the diffusion sequence, also called DWI, which is the MVP for catching strokes in their sneaky early stages. Then there's the flair and T2 sequences solving mysteries and ruling out what's going on. So, when a doctor, untrained in acute stroke management, writes 'MRI Brain,' the sequences that comprise this scan do not contain the DWI and flair sequences. Hence, the right type of MRI scan to be done is – the MRI Brain stroke protocol! This even includes an MR Angiogram of the brain's blood vessels. So, to conclude, if there are so many minute detailed nuances required to be understood just to write the RIGHT MRI prescription in an acute stroke, then imagine how many more such similar nuances there are in all the other steps in acute stroke care.

So, what is my message? In case you suspect a stroke, DO NOT go to your nearby doctor; RUSH immediately to the nearest 'STROKE READY' hospital.

Now, the grand finale – the advantages of MRI over CT. MRI is the superhero with a soft touch – it spots early strokes like a hawk and has high-resolution eyes to scrutinize every nook and cranny of your brain. It's like upgrading from an old TV to a 4K Ultra HD experience – the details, my friend, are crystal clear. And let's not forget the star power of MRI in ruling out those tricky stroke mimics. Tumors, infections – they can't hide from the magnetic spotlight. It's like having a superhero team of diagnosticians, all working together in perfect harmony.

Now, Mr. MRI isn't the life of the party when it comes to availability. Not everyone's invited to this exclusive club, as not all institutions or centers have their VIP pass to the MRI celebration. But, all stroke-ready hospitals have MRIs that work 24/7.

Wait, there's more! MRI is a bit picky about its guest list. If you've got a heart pacemaker, some metallic bling, or you're in the early stages of baby-making, sorry, but you're not on the list. Some things are just non-negotiable.

In the realm of brain stroke analysis, understanding the areas of damage is key. The "umbra" refers to the brain tissue's core region that is immediately and severely affected by the lack of blood supply during a stroke. The "penumbra" surrounds the umbra and consists of brain tissue that is at risk but might still be saved with prompt treatment. This region has reduced blood flow but maintains some metabolic activity. Identifying the penumbra can help guide effective treatments to salvage as much brain function as possible. Imaging techniques like Positron Emission Tomography (PET) and perfusion imaging with CT or MRI are crucial in distinguishing these regions and are essential for making informed decisions on stroke treatments.

Acute stroke and lunar eclipse, is there a connection?

In the theatre of the cosmos, a lunar eclipse presents a celestial play of light and shadow. Picture the umbra as the main act—the Earth's full shadow, absolute and profound, where the brain's core is in the grip of an ischemic stroke, deprived of vital blood and oxygen, akin to the moon's full embrace by the shadow, losing its bright luminescence.

Then there's the penumbra, the supporting cast, a softer, partial shadow where the moon still catches faint sun rays—this is like the brain's penumbral tissue during a stroke, impaired but salvageable, whispering for timely intervention to restore its full function, as the penumbra in the sky gently holds onto the last threads of light. Both scenarios are transient, a race against time to either save the neurological functions or witness the gradual return of the moon's glow.

Alright, gather 'round, brain enthusiasts! Let's embark on a tragicomic expedition through the cerebral landscape, where the drama of angiography meets the harsh realities of brain afflictions. Picture the brain as a bustling city with arterial roadways pulsing life to every corner.

The anterior cerebral artery is the diligent postal worker for the frontal lobes, while the middle cerebral artery is the hip courier to the brain's lateral hubs. Then there's the posterior cerebral artery and the vertebrobasilar system, lighting up the back alleys like a disco inferno.

When disaster strikes—an infarction—the scene morphs from vibrant to somber, revealing the stark impact of these unwanted guests.

The anterior cerebral artery, once a beacon of activity at the front, now dims under the shadow of tragedy, signaling a cerebral rebellion. The middle cerebral artery, the city's central conduit, lights up with distress signals, heralding a dramatic infarction. And then there's the posterior cerebral artery and the vertebrobasilar system, the brain's rear guard, which hosts a gloomy party of its own as it succumbs to the silent assault of an infarct.

Enter strokes, the ultimate disruptors—uninvited and unwelcome. They're like solo artists or a rogue parade crashing the brain's meticulous network, turning orderly traffic into chaotic standstills. Imagine a once-thriving artery abruptly declaring, 'Closed for business,' its blockage a poignant reminder of the brain's vulnerability.

In this cerebral saga of infarctions, rebellions, and parades of troublemakers, we find not just a touch of humor but a deep-seated despair. It's a narrative that swings dramatically between the absurdity of the situation and the tragic reality of its consequences. Who said neurology couldn't be both humorous and heart-wrenching? After all, in the theatre of the brain, every laugh might be shadowed by a tear, and every scientific exploration a step closer to understanding life's fragility.

Alright, fellow brain explorers, let's unravel the mysteries of strokes and their imaging escapades with a touch of whimsy!

In the CT scans, we have the **_hyperdense MCA sign_**, a brain detective's dream. Imagine the brain playing hide and seek – the left side trying to be sneaky, but oops, it's giving itself away with bright signals. Classic stroke foreshadowing at its finest!

And let's not forget the _insular ribbon sign_, where the brain is doing a mysterious dance. On one side, you've got a clear gray-white matter face, and on the other, it's like the brain decided to paint with dark signals, throwing a psychedelic party. The brain's artistic expression is at its peak!

So, there you have it, the strokes and their imaging antics, complete with embolic party crashers, thrombotic divas, and the brain's very own soap opera.

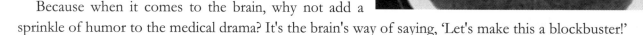

Because when it comes to the brain, why not add a sprinkle of humor to the medical drama? It's the brain's way of saying, 'Let's make this a blockbuster!'

In the initial stages of hyperacute stroke, a discernible loss of gray-white matter differentiation is evident on the left side of the brain. Upon subsequent imaging a day later, a prominent dark signal becomes apparent in the left hemisphere, accompanied by edema and compression of the adjacent parenchyma. This dark signal signifies the maturation of the infarct, particularly along the left middle cerebral artery (MCA) territory, indicative of a large acute stroke.

The consequences of this acute stroke are profound as the complete left cerebral hemisphere undergoes a transformation, appearing dark and swollen due to edema. This swelling prompts the brain parenchyma to exert pressure, potentially leading to compression on the opposite side. Surgical intervention becomes imperative to avert devastating outcomes in such cases. The removal of bone through surgery serves to prevent internal brain compression, redirecting pressure outward. This crucial step safeguards vital brain structures, ensuring the preservation of essential functions for daily activities.

In the acute stage of stroke, one of our patients, Mr. Praful, exhibited a conspicuous bright signal on the right side of the brain, consistent with findings in diffusion imaging. This brightness mirrors the hyperacute stage, emphasizing the urgency and severity of the stroke. Notable changes unfold when transitioning into the subacute phase over the next 1 to 3 weeks.

The infarct gradually reduces in size, accompanied by a decrease in density. This transformation results in a darker appearance compared to the acute stroke, signifying the ongoing healing process during this subacute period.

In the chronic stage of stroke, which manifests more than three weeks after symptom onset, distinct changes occur in the brain. The brain undergoes shrinkage, leading to the dilation of adjacent fluid-filled spaces, a phenomenon known as isomeric changes and gliosis. On CT scans, these changes are evident as dark signals, contrasting with the bright signals observed in MR imaging. This marks the chronic stage of stroke, where the brain has experienced prolonged alterations.

Examining the CT and MRI features at various intervals from symptom onset provides valuable insights. On day one, non-contrast images reveal subtle hypo-densities indicative of hyperacute stroke. By day two, conspicuous dark signals emerge on the left side, signifying acute infarction. The following week witnesses an increase in brain swelling, characterizing the subacute stage. By month two, the chronic stage manifests, showcasing gliotic changes and a chronic infarct.

However, post-treatment complications can arise. Following thrombolysis and other interventions for stroke, patients may experience bleeding within the previously infarcted region. The inherent leakiness of blood vessels in ischemic areas can lead to reperfusion injury. This phenomenon occurs due to increased blood flow to the brain post-treatment, resulting in bleeding within the cerebral hemisphere. A case example involves a patient with a right-sided stroke developing a large left middle cerebral artery infarct. Following treatment, the CT and MRI images reveal eoric areas within the infarct, indicating reperfusion injury. It is crucial to exercise caution in assessing these cases to prevent potential complications for the patient. Vigilance in recognizing and managing reperfusion injuries is imperative to ensure the patient's well-being and avoid further complications.

In the context of stroke, when we refer to a 'chronic stroke,' we mean that the symptoms developed more than three weeks ago. At this stage, the brain starts to shrink, leading to the dilation of adjacent fluid-filled spaces known as atrophic changes and gliosis. On CT scans, these changes appear as dark signals, while on MRIs, they appear as bright signals.

Perfusion imaging, performed with contrast in both CT and MRI, helps assess the blood flow within the brain. It aids in distinguishing dead tissue from salvageable tissue, which is crucial for determining the effectiveness of treatment. Specific maps, such as CBF (cerebral blood flow) and CBV (cerebral blood volume), help evaluate the viability of brain tissue. The bigger the perfusion 'mismatch,' the better the outcomes will be if interventions are done on time.

Moving to hemorrhagic stroke's causes, hypertension is a primary factor. Other reasons include cerebral amyloid angiopathy, aneurysms, arteriovenous malformations, certain drugs, vascular malformations, blood disorders, tumors, and trauma.

Imaging plays a crucial role in identifying and confirming the type and cause of stroke. For instance, aneurysms causing subarachnoid hemorrhage can be treated through coiling or clipping. Additionally, cerebral venous thrombosis, more common in young females on oral contraceptives, can lead to stroke symptoms, emphasizing the importance of prompt diagnosis and treatment. Imaging helps in assessing complications, such as fibrosis or adhesions causing CSF space blockage, leading to hydrocephalus.

It's essential to differentiate between stroke and stroke mimics, such as tumors, for accurate diagnosis. A quick consultation with specialists, immediate imaging, and regular follow-ups post-treatment are crucial for effective stroke management.

Let us now discuss the Acute Care Management of an ischemic stroke.

Often, when we hear the word "stroke," the response isn't as immediate as it is with "heart attack." To address this lack of urgency, the term "brain attack" was introduced, hoping to evoke a similar sense of urgency and prompt action. The urgency in responding to a stroke is vital, as time is crucial. Recognizing symptoms like sudden slurring of speech, weakness, numbness, difficulty in walking, or dizziness is essential.

In an acute ischemic stroke, where a blood vessel to the brain is blocked by a clot, prompt action is necessary. *The window period for intervention is up to 6 hours for supratentorial strokes and up to 24 hours for vertebrobasilar strokes.* Imaging, preferably MRI or CT, is crucial. A diffusion-weighted imaging (DWI) sequence reveals the stroke in the early stages.

Thrombolysis, using clot-busting drugs like alteplase or tenecteplase, is the standard treatment. However, if the clot is in a proximal vessel, intra-arterial thrombolysis may be necessary. In cases where the clot is large or resistant, mechanical thrombectomy becomes the next step. The success of these interventions depends on various factors, and outcomes can be dramatic but vary from case to case.

In the vanguard of endovascular neurosurgery, mechanical thrombectomy stands out as a quintessential procedure for addressing major vessel occlusions in acute ischemic strokes. This sophisticated technique involves the insertion of a catheter through the femoral artery, navigating through the body's vascular highways using advanced fluoroscopic imaging to reach the cerebral arteries. Once the site of the clot is pinpointed, a stent retriever or an aspiration device is deployed to ensnare and remove the clot, effectively restoring blood flow.

This sci-fi-like intervention harnesses real-time neuro-navigation, allowing neurosurgeons to perform what might be likened to a precision strike, akin to using spacecraft maneuverability in zero gravity to remove debris threatening a space station. The swift restoration of blood flow is critical to salvaging brain tissue at risk of necrosis, delineating zones of the brain akin to saving a starship's failing systems.

MECHANICAL THROMBECTOMY
What is this?

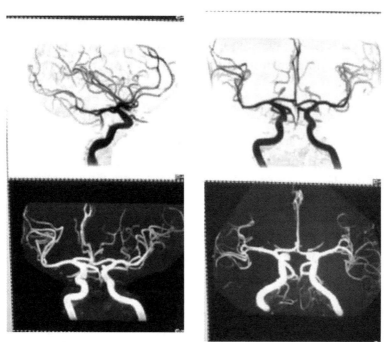

Mechanical thrombectomy not only embodies the dramatic clash between life-threatening blockages and high-tech medical interventions but also highlights a significant shift towards a future where the confluence of technology and human expertise opens new frontiers in the treatment of cerebrovascular diseases. And if the timing is right and the procedure is done well, the results are magical and dramatic.

We have seen so many patients going into the mechanical thrombectomy procedure fully stroked out, and within a few minutes of clot retrieval, over 70-80% improvement in the stroke symptoms!

Outside the window period or in cases of permanent brain damage, the approach changes. Full strokes result in complete brain damage, leading to various complications. Reperfusion hemorrhage is a risk associated with the re-establishment of blood flow, especially after clot dissolution.

The moment you hear about someone suffering from a stroke, what typically comes to mind? Often, it's a person experiencing paralysis on one side of their body, leading to a rushed hospitalization. The image that forms is one of a long stay in the ICU, with the individual never fully recovering—perhaps remaining bedridden with partial speech and motor functions.

What if I told you there's a different outcome possible? Imagine a patient completely paralyzed on the left side due to a stroke who managed to walk out of the hospital within just one week. Sounds like magic, doesn't it?

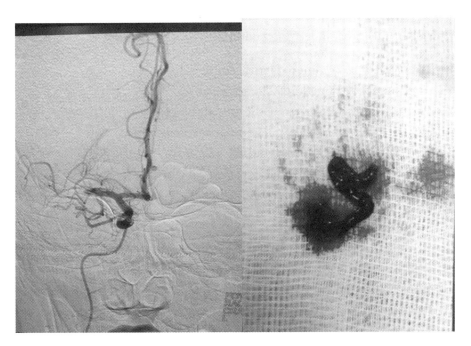

1. Brain angiogram with mechanical thrombectomy in progress

2. The clot was removed in the procedure.

This patient, a young man, arrived at our hospital—Bhagwan Mahaveer Jain Hospital in Girinagar, which is equipped for stroke emergencies—within the critical window period post-stroke. Recognizing this, our stroke team acted swiftly to perform the necessary imaging to confirm his condition. He was indeed within the window period when specific interventions were most effective. My colleague, Dr. Bhaskar, an interventional radiologist, performed a mechanical thrombectomy. Incredibly, within mere minutes of removing the clot, the patient regained movement in his limbs.

This swift recovery illustrates the profound impact of timely, appropriate treatment. If the right actions are taken at the right time by skilled specialists in a fully equipped facility, the results can be remarkable. This approach to stroke treatment, much like interventions for heart attacks, can lead to excellent outcomes.

I urge everyone to understand that strokes, which we now refer to as 'brain attacks,' are not necessarily debilitating if managed correctly. Recognizing the symptoms early on is crucial. Familiarize yourself with the B.E.F.A.S.T. acronym to quickly identify stroke signs and react promptly.

Remember, in strokes, as in many critical health situations, time is of the essence. Quickly getting to a stroke-ready hospital and consenting to the necessary treatments can lead to what may seem like miraculous recoveries.

Understanding the urgency of stroke care is crucial. Time is a brain, and every second lost can result in irreversible damage. The goal is to act swiftly, considering the risks and benefits and delivering the right treatment at the right time.

INTRA CEREBRAL HEMATOMA OR HEMORRHAGE OR ICH

Brain hemorrhage, also known as intracerebral hematoma, involves bleeding or clotting, often used interchangeably in medical terms. The key is not to get overwhelmed by different terminology; they represent variations of the same underlying conditions.

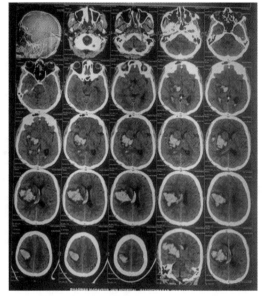

Undiagnosed hypertension is a common factor, emphasizing the importance of monitoring blood pressure. There's a subset of cases where brain hemorrhage can occur even without high blood pressure. Understanding the anatomy of the skull compartments is crucial. There are two compartments, supra-tentorial and infra-tentorial, each with right and left sides. The location of the hemorrhage within these compartments dictates the behavioral differences in patients.

Supra-tentorial and infra-tentorial hemorrhages present different risks and urgencies, with the need for quick intervention in certain situations. Serial CT scans are crucial for decision-making, whether to continue conservative treatment or opt for surgery. Post-surgery, patients might develop obstructive hydrocephalus, where accumulated fluid creates pressure on the brain. Emergency measures, like external ventricular drain (EVD), may be taken. Permanent solutions, such as ventriculoperitoneal (VP) shunting, involve redirecting fluid to the abdominal cavity.

Another type of brain hemorrhage is called CVT, Cortical Venous Thrombosis, or venous stroke.

Cerebral Venous Thrombosis (CVT) is a rare form of stroke that occurs when a blood clot forms in the brain's venous channels. This prevents blood from draining out of the brain, leading to increased intracranial pressure, which can cause headaches, seizures, neurological deficits, and, in severe cases, brain hemorrhage. CVT can affect anyone but is more commonly seen in young adults and more commonly affects women. Risk factors include genetic predispositions, oral contraceptive use, pregnancy, infections, and certain medical conditions. Treatment typically involves anticoagulants to dissolve clots and manage symptoms and complications.

Stroke (CVT) due to intake of 'periods postponing pills or Oral Contraceptive Pills'!

Once, in the heart of a festive season, like thousands of women who do so every day, a 39-year-old woman chose to delay her menstrual cycle with oral contraceptives, hoping to fully partake in the celebrations. Little did she know that this decision would spiral into a life-threatening ordeal. On the third day, amidst the festivities, she was struck by a severe headache, uncontrollable vomiting, and a drowsiness so heavy it dragged her to the brink of unconsciousness. Her left side grew weak, a condition known as hemiparesis, signaling a dire medical emergency.

In haste, she sought medical help. The first CT scan revealed a sinister shadow creeping over her right parietal lobe—a hemorrhagic venous infarct quietly unfurling its damage. Initially, doctors took a conservative approach, hoping to outmaneuver the silent crisis brewing within her brain.

But fate took a cruel turn. Eighteen hours later, her condition plummeted, her neurological functions failing her when she needed them most. A second CT scan exposed the grim truth: the infarct had ballooned into a massive hemorrhagic assault within her head.

With no time to lose, she underwent an emergency craniotomy. Surgeons worked tirelessly to evacuate the insidious blood from her brain, striving against time and the stroke that sought to claim her faculties.

Miraculously, over time, the tapestry of her brain began to mend. Bit by bit, the paralysis that once held her left side captive began to dissipate. Against all odds, she reclaimed the strength that the stroke tried to steal, her spirit unyielding. Her recovery became a testament to resilience, a narrative of hope for those who face the shadows of their own health battles.

Understanding these nuances in the treatment of intracerebral hematomas underscores the complexity of stroke care. Repetition of key phrases like "brain attack" and "stroke" aims to embed the urgency of the situation in your subconscious. Even at 2:00 in the morning, if someone informs you about a stroke, the response should be immediate and alert. Remember the importance of the Glasgow Coma Scale; in such situations, aiming for a high score is vital. Being hyperactive and responsive and ensuring prompt action, such as getting the patient to the hospital within the critical window period, is imperative.

Another distinct subtype of stroke that I want to explain to you is the aneurysmal bleed or subarachnoid hemorrhage (SAH).

For those seeking a simple explanation, a crucial point in neuroscience practice is emphasized: "If the patient walks into our emergency, the chances of the patient walking out are very high." Acting before the brain is extensively damaged is imperative. If someone reports a severe or different headache, immediate action is necessary.

Aneurysms are like manufacturing defects—a bubble or blister on a blood vessel that can grow over time and burst suddenly, a*kin to a time bomb in the brain*. One-third of patients with aneurysmal SAH die instantly, one-third collapse and may never regain consciousness or recover with disability, and the remaining one-third, who complain of the worst headache, can recover if treated early.

The universal statement often made during an aneurysmal SAH by awake patients is, "This is the worst headache of my life." It's crucial not to dismiss it casually. Treating it like a salad and going to sleep can be perilous; one may not wake up. A stroke is like a ticking time bomb in the brain, an imminent brain attack.

The diagnostic process involves a CT Angiogram scan of the intracranial blood vessels and, if needed, further evaluation with a regular brain angiogram called a 4V DSA or four-vessel digital subtraction angiography, as even a small leak might not be immediately visible. Once diagnosed, two sets of neurosurgical treatments are employed: preventing rebleeding and addressing the blood already present.

To prevent rebleeding, surgical options include clipping the aneurysm's neck or endovascular procedures, like coiling, stent-assisted coiling, or flow diverters. These techniques aim to stop blood from entering the aneurysm while preserving the parent vessel.

For the blood already present (subarachnoid hemorrhage), complications arise from vasospasm, where blood vessels constrict due to chemical irritation from dissolving blood. Vasospasms can lead to strokes and is a critical concern for neurosurgeons. Treatment involves medications like nimodipine, intra-arterial nimodipine, and, in severe cases, angiogram-guided interventions. Vasospasm usually starts by the 5th-7th day after the bleed, peaks by the 14th-15th day, and disappears by the 21st day.

Vasospasm occurs when the blood starts to dissolve and releases many chemicals which irritate the blood vessels. I have seen patients who are walking around in the ward and suddenly collapse and even die! Severe cerebral vasospasm is a nightmare even in the best of neurosurgical centers across the world. But I am happy and proud to say that whatever treatments are done for vasospasm in the best of the Western countries are done in my hospital and many others in Bengaluru and elsewhere in the country – both government and private.

The 3-week period post-bleed is crucial, during which vigilance and appropriate treatments are essential to prevent complications. Monitoring patients in a setup familiar with these nuances is crucial. Despite the challenges, timely and comprehensive management can lead to positive outcomes, with many patients returning to normal life.

Let me give you another aneurysm-related story:

Amidst the whirl of numbers and fiscal strategies, a 50-year-old finance wizard steering the financial helm of a prominent public sector undertaking encountered an unexpected snag. For four days, a non-specific headache, an uninvited guest, shadowed his thoughts, refusing to yield to the usual remedies. His status in society and access to elite medical care prompted an elective investigation—a decision made as much by privilege as by prudence.

He strode into the outpatient department, his stride as confident as it had been in boardroom battles. Yet, what awaited was a battle of a different kind. The CT scan unveiled its grim findings: subarachnoid hemorrhage, a treacherous storm brewing beneath the calm of his normotensive facade. The plot thickened with the revelation of an ACOM berry aneurysm captured in the crosshairs of a 4V DSA, an intruder lurking within cerebral territories. Time, now more precious than the fiscal year-end reports, dictated an emergency operation, craniotomy, and clipping of the aneurysm.

The precision of skilled hands and the will of a resilient spirit charted the course for what followed—an uneventful recovery, almost anticlimactic in its smoothness, akin to a well-executed audit. He emerged not just as a survivor but as a man who had triumphed over a clandestine cerebral rebellion, ready to take on the ledgers and life with equal fervor.

Stroke and Lack of Education on Health

It's disheartening to observe the lack of awareness and education regarding health issues despite the prevalence of information through the internet and technology. While people readily consume trivial content, essential educational videos often go unnoticed. This divide in attention and knowledge is a significant challenge in healthcare.

Memory Loss After Stroke and Silent Strokes

The impact of stroke on memory loss depends on the affected areas of the brain. Different circuits can be affected, causing varying degrees of memory loss. Silent strokes, although asymptomatic, can still be detected through imaging tests like MRI scans. These strokes might not manifest noticeable symptoms but can have implications for brain health.

Stroke Prevention and Importance of Drug Compliance

Preventive measures for stroke involve maintaining a healthy lifestyle, including a balanced diet, regular exercise, and avoiding risk factors like smoking. However, it's crucial to emphasize the importance of drug compliance in managing conditions like hypertension. Skipping medication doses or not regularly checking blood pressure can jeopardize the effectiveness of preventive measures.

High Blood Pressure and Stroke Risk

High blood pressure (BP) is a significant risk factor for stroke. In cases where individuals refuse medical intervention or medications, the importance of periodic monitoring and seeking professional advice is emphasized. Understanding the risks associated with uncontrolled hypertension and taking proactive measures, such as having comprehensive insurance coverage, is crucial.

Sneha Hari is our youngest ANRS! She is a speech and language pathologist by qualification but has quickly learned many of the skills required to be an ANRS. She is still a work in progress, but she is responsible and smart way beyond her years! Let's listen to her experience of treating our chronic stroke patient from the US, Nina Gulati.

"So, my first experience with Nina was not when I was her treating therapist. It was during her first admission to the hospital. So, the first time that she was there, I was not her treating therapist. But one day, I went as a substitute therapist, and when I went that day, I entered her room, where she usually had a caretaker. And that day, her caretaker wasn't there. She had stepped out for a moment, and as I entered, she looked at me, and I immediately asked her a few standard 'ice-breaking' questions that usually worked on her.

I was forewarned by my colleagues that I should expect some behavioral issues from her. As I went in there, and I spoke to her nicely, softly, expecting that she was going to behave that particular way with me, she erupted! She just started screaming. She started screaming, Mama, Mama, Mama, and kept screaming, but she didn't try listening to me. I tried my best to pacify her. I told her we'd watch TV, and I tried all of that. And within five minutes, I was out of there because she just wouldn't cooperate. She just kept crying, and I didn't know what that meant - I thought that her mother was actually there. So, that was my very first experience with Nina. So, the second time when she came in, she got shifted to the resort, and I was told that I was supposed to go and do the therapy for her and the above interaction and experience came in front of me vividly. I was a little skeptical as to how it was going to work out. And again, as it was the COVID time, travel restrictions were there, even locally.

So, on the first day, I go there, and she's in her room, and she's just looking. She has this usual way of sitting, where she keeps her hand on her face and she just looks. And she could be so adamant that she would just look, and she wouldn't even say hi, and she would just have this look on her face that will tell you - You are irritating me. Just get out of here. I don't want to talk to you, a non-verbal way of communication! Sometimes, she would say - I don't want the therapy. And I would feel so down, like, Should I really do therapy for this person? For someone like me, who has just passed out of college and this is my first job, it would be very disturbing.

This started somewhere in the first week of May. We had to do four hours of therapy with her every day. We would go in the morning. Even though two hours was my therapy time, she couldn't exactly separate out all the therapies because initially, she wasn't following the systemized, formal way of doing therapy. We had to do a lot of jugaad with her, play games on the phone, watch movies with her, play songs, talk about food, and watch funny videos on YouTube.

She had a dog, 'Theo,' who was her favorite. You tell her 'Theo,' and her face lights up! So, we'd watch funny dog videos on YouTube. And she wanted to go back home. Google Maps has this feature, especially in the US, where you can see a person's house. I'd ask her address. And so that's how I slowly started getting her into therapy.

Getting her to remember her address. I would tell her, If you tell me your address correctly, I can take it on the maps and show it to you. And she was really, really looking forward to going back home. So, I asked her, why don't you tell me your address, and then we can look at your house. So, she'd tell me the address, and we would go and see the street, and then again, her face would light up.

Those small things used to light her up, and that's how we started getting bonding. I had to spend almost a month and a half building a rapport with her. Instead of showing her pictures and asking her to identify what those are, I would try to relate them to her daily life objects. Another thing that we used to do was she loved her family. She's a woman who would do anything for the people she loves. And so, her daughter's birthday was coming, and I said, okay, we'll make a card for her.

I got all these art and craft materials, sketch pens, and colored paper. And we would spend the session coloring. So, because I had a lot of different colored papers, we introduced colors to her in that way, which made her identify the different colors. And she was a foodie. She used to love food so much. So, her reinforcement used to be that okay, Nina, you do all these activities, and we'll have a food party later. And I would say, okay, these are your goals. You complete this. We'll ask them to get Pani Puri for you. So then she would do it. But there were such instances. I still remember that she abused therapists so much, shouted at them, and made them cry, especially during her first admission. Her husband always told us how she would do the same in the US to the therapists, and hence, no rehab was possible.

So then, slowly, I guess, with Dr. Prathiba's medications and cognitive and behavioral therapy, her mood stabilized.

The turning point: I think that the biggest turning point for her was when she suddenly developed acute appendicitis, and she had to be rushed to Jain Hospital from the resort. Then she got admitted, initially treated conservatively, and six weeks later, underwent an interval appendicectomy surgery; that's when she realized that her life or therapy at the resort was way, way better than the hospital, and she would do anything to get better and go back home.

We all felt sad that she had to undergo all this suffering, but in hindsight, I feel that this was the key turning point in her recovery phase. Suddenly, a switch in her brain god flipped on, and she began taking responsibility for getting better, wanting to achieve all the rehab goals so that she could go home. So that became her goal, and she had to get better and go back home.

She started cooperating with the therapies better. I would do both her speech therapy as well as her cognitive therapy. After this incident, she had a tremendous improvement in her cognition and speech. She started talking so much. From a person who wouldn't say two words together, she started telling stories!

She started singing. She started engaging so well in the therapy. It was amazing! I was ecstatic! She would tell us stories of her childhood, and slowly, her speech became really good. Since it was the resort set up, she was not confined to a limited clinical space. Since the wheelchair was there, we would take her to the garden, under the mango tree, or near the swimming pool, and we would sit there and talk.

That's how we did the therapy without making her feel that it was therapy being done. But she knew that the first two hours used to be a combined speech and cognition session, and then the next two hours would be a combined physiotherapy and occupational therapy session by Ganapathy sir.

So, after the speech and cognitive session, she would say, okay, I need a 10-minute break. And she knew when that time was near, and then we would sit, take that break. And then, if we continued, she had no problem. So, once we got to that routine, she said she was very happy. It came to such a stage that towards the end of her admission at the resort, we could stop her speech therapy and use those four hours for her physical therapy and occupational therapy because that's what she needed more.

Her language, cognition, and speech had improved so much that she did not require the therapy anymore. And I could say that she became like a friend. And in fact, from a person who behaved like a baby and cried like a baby, by the end, she had become this person who would give you advice.

She would tell me; you should get married at this age. You should have two kids because then the children will not trouble you. They will play together, and they'll get along together, and many other things like that. So, she had become that person who started giving you life advice from a person who had come initially as a baby who was crying. So, it was a big, big transformational journey that I had with Nina, and she's still a very dear patient of mine."

Why should you care about neuroscience?

In this section, I might as well take you through my personal journey again! Well, picture this: your brain is like the CEO of your body, the control center that keeps everything running smoothly. Without it, life would be as chaotic as a squirrel in a coffee shop or, even worse, like a bull in a China shop!

Neuroscience sounds like a brainy topic, and you might feel like a fish out of water in the world of neurons and synapses. But hey, think of it as an owner's manual for your brain – the ultimate user guide to this supercomputer nestled inside your noggin (noggin is a slang word, meaning the human brain).

Imagine this scenario: You or someone you love starts showing some weird symptoms. Instead of diving into the black hole of Google health scares, a little neuroscience knowledge can be your superhero cape. You'll be like, "Hold up, brain, what's going on in there?" It's the difference between being a cool, collected detective and spiraling into a hypochondriac's nightmare.

We've got information on cancer, heart health, and even how many steps we're racking up on our smartwatches. But the brain? It's like the forgotten middle child of the family. Time to shine a spotlight on it because, let's be real, without a properly functioning brain, life would be a real head-scratcher.

So, in a nutshell, why learn about neuroscience? Because your brain is the real MVP, and understanding it is like holding the keys to the kingdom. Let's give our brains the attention they deserve and make sure they're running the show like the true bosses they are!

Ah, the age-old question – why did I decide to champion neuro rehab when most neurosurgeons are too busy slicing and dicing brains without a second thought? Well, let me take you on a journey back to my 8th-grade dreams of becoming a neurosurgeon. Fast forward, and here I am, living the dream, or as close to it as one can get... and loving every minute of it in the glorious '90s. As I embarked on my neurosurgeon training, I started encountering patients post-surgery. They survived the whole shebang thanks to cutting-edge technology and acute care support. But here's the kicker – they were left in a sorry state, semi-conscious & bedridden.

The hospital higher-ups, ever the efficiency enthusiasts, would tap me on the shoulder and be like, "Hey, buddy, these beds are not for long-term Netflix marathoners. Find a new home for your patients." Cue the heart-wrenching scenes of families asking me, "Doc, where do we take our mamaaji? He's not exactly marathon-ready right now." And there I was, stuck between a hospital bed and a hard place, feeling helpless and clueless.

My brilliant solution? I'd nonchalantly say, "Oh, just get some physiotherapy done." In reality, it was my polite way of saying, "I don't know what you do; just get out of my sight." Spoiler alert: I wasn't a fan of saying this. I hated myself every time I told the family this, but...

This is when the next reality hit home with a LONG BANG! A BIG pin just punctured my ego and said that becoming a great neurosurgeon is just not about doing surgeries, removing blood clots and brain tumors, and saving patients' lives...doing just this had suddenly stopped inspiring me. I was depressed... I realized that only 'saving' lives is not the real reason why I wanted to be a neurosurgeon. I also wanted to improve the quality of life of all these patients. Get them back on their feet, back into their lives. WOW! That seemed like another 'eureka' moment for me... until the immediate next question hit home. But HOW??? And I started asking my seniors and others around me.

That's when someone vaguely told me this word – REHABILITATION. They need good rehabilitation. This was sometime around 1997-98. That was probably the first time I actually heard this word in the context of neuro patients. Till then, for me, 'rehabilitation' was a place meant to help psychiatry patients recoup or a deaddiction center to help people addicted to alcohol and drugs.

I started probing them further... these were senior doctors who had done some kind of training or work in Western countries like the UK or the US and returned home. They told me how advanced the Western world is in the field of neuro rehabilitation, how there were dedicated facilities and teams of professionals managing such patients, how such patients were transferred to such a facility as soon as they were medically stable... etc. All this got me inspired again. I realized that there was one more dimension that I needed to address, but first, I needed to complete my neurosurgery course and become a qualified neurosurgeon. I was back in action, inspired again.

So, why neuro rehab? Because someone had to step up and bridge the gap between surgical heroics and getting patients back on their feet – literally. I figured, if I'm going to play with brains, I might as well ensure they come out dancing, right? And thus, the neuro rehab crusade began, one wobbly step at a time!

So, there I was, a young, ambitious neurosurgeon-to-be, dreaming of fixing brains and sending patients back into the world, not just patching them up and waving them goodbye.

Fast forward to the late '90s, when the term "rehabilitation" was as alien as a Martian spa day in my neck of the woods. Physiotherapy was considered cutting-edge, and anything beyond that was as rudimentary as a stick and some duct tape.

It was during this time of brainy introspection that I realized, "Hey, someone's got to dance with these damaged brain circuits and get them grooving again." The seeds of post-surgical care, way beyond the stitches business, were planted in my mind. I didn't dive headfirst into it, but I kept it simmering on the back burner of my thoughts – an unsolved puzzle itching to be cracked.

As I ventured into practice, my frustration grew. The realization hit me like a surgical light in the face – the rehab game was not up to par, and my patients were left hanging. Fast forward to 2006, and I decided to be the change I wanted to see. I took it upon myself to ensure my patients didn't just survive surgery but thrived in life post-op. Neurosurgery wasn't just about saving lives anymore; it was about guiding my patients through the entire journey, *from stitches to salsa*.

The human brain – that unsung hero in the ICU surrounded by a symphony of beeps and numbers that have nothing to do with the real star of the show. Imagine a situation where the heart rates, sugar levels, breathing patterns, and everything else are being closely monitored, and any discrepancy is immediately acted upon and corrected – but the brain NEVER gets any such attention, let alone VIP treatment.

I've been in the ICU, playing detective, and even today, in 2024, even in advanced cities like Bengaluru (and trust me, the same is true of most major cities in the world), the brain is still THE MOST neglected organ! And I keep asking my colleagues, "Why the stepmotherly attitude towards the brain, huh?"

It's like the brain's been getting the cold shoulder as if it's just a stroke and nothing more. But let me tell you, making the brain take a breather, even for two seconds, is like asking a cat to enjoy a bath – nearly impossible.

If someone loses consciousness for just one minute, it's a red flag, not a minor inconvenience. So, I've been shouting from the rooftops: "If my patient walks in with a brain issue, we've got better odds of them walking out talking. But if they're wheeled in semi-conscious or unconscious, it's an uphill battle because, surprise, surprise, brains don't come with spares."

That brings me to my favorite mantra: earlier is better. We've been yelling it worldwide, not just in India, with this nifty concept called "time is brain." Stroke? Nah, we prefer "Brain Attack" to jolt everyone into action. You say, "heart attack," and folks sprint; say "stroke," and they stroll. Go figure!

Remember, if someone's memory is playing hide-and-seek, it's not an age-related thing. We've seen legal eagles and political maestros, and even my own grandmother, in their 80s and some even in their 90s, with memories sharper than anyone. Memory issues? Investigate; don't sweep it under the age rug.

Now, onto headaches – not all headaches are migraine rockstars; some are just wannabes. Is vitamin B12 throwing a party in your memory? Fix it, and you're back in business.

Let us read the story of the radiation oncologist with a 25-year headache – now that's a marathon-level migraine! Can you believe it? He was like, "Oh, it's just a migraine, no biggie," for a quarter of a century. Self-treatment worked once in a while. Finally, out of sheer frustration, someone said, "Hey, why not throw in a scan for good measure?" Lo and behold, an uninvited aneurysm showed up in his brain, like a ticking time bomb, ready to explode anytime! Talk about a plot twist after two decades of head-throbbing drama.

But... for 25 years, he had not bothered to get imaging done for his HEAD....would he have done the same if he had left-sided chest pain??? Twenty-five years, no ECG??? NEVER! Think guys... The heart is important, but the Brain is NOT!

And then there's the tale of the 35-year-old with a case of spondylosis. They come in, looking like they've just received a terminal cancer diagnosis, and I'm like, "Whoa, who died? Oh, it's just spondylosis or spondylitis." It's like the wear and tear we all get, a little rust on the joints. I assured them, "Hey, a little TLC for your neck, and you're back in business." The relief on their faces is priceless. They thought spondy-whatever meant their life was over. Nope, just a reminder that we're not invincible, and our bodies are like vintage cars – need a bit more care, that's all.

People throw around words like spondylosis without context, and patients start mentally drafting their obituaries. It's not the disease that's deadly; it's the psychology of it all. They become the living dead, and that, my friends, is the tragic twist in this medical thing.

So, the moral of the story? Understand the context, don't let words scare you, and remember, even if your spine is being dramatic, life goes on!

A Daring Rescue: My Way on the Highway

Recall the vivid imagery of national disaster management teams during floods, particularly in places like Uttarakhand. The Bravehearts, the soldiers, and the rescuers create makeshift bridges, throw life-saving ropes, and pull people to safety.

These scenes unfold on our television screens during times of crisis, leaving us in awe of their courage and determination. We also did something similar when the Nepal earthquake happened on 26th April 2015. But that's another story... for a later date. Now, let me share with you a real-life story, perhaps not as dramatic as the movies or disaster scenarios, but one that captures the essence of bravery and quick thinking. This small yet significant tale might not have the grandeur of a Hollywood blockbuster, but it is a testament to the everyday heroes among us.

Just a few months ago, we received an urgent call, setting the stage for a real-life medical drama. The protagonist: a highly esteemed doctor from Hospet in northern Karnataka, facing a challenge that demands quick thinking and decisive action.

A VIP patient's father-in-law had just suffered a stroke. The doctor, well-versed in diagnosing such emergencies, had swiftly conducted a clinical neurological examination, revealing left-side weakness – a clear sign of a stroke. However, here's where the narrative took an unexpected turn – the CT scan appeared normal. In the realm of early ischemic strokes, a normal CT scan is not uncommon, especially in the initial stages.

Recognizing the need for an MRI and a specialized injection to reverse the effects of the stroke, the doctor encountered a harsh reality. Neither an MRI nor the crucial injection was available in Hospet. This underscored a glaring imbalance in healthcare infrastructure, revealing that where one falls sick is as crucial as when!

Undeterred, the doctor sought my counsel as the patient and the family wanted the patient to be treated by me only and hence wanted to come all the way to Bengaluru! As soon as I realized that the drive was 4.5 hours long, I told them that 'time is brain' and he needed to get to the nearest 'stroke-ready hospital, which in this case was in a city called Hubballi, 1.5 hours away. But the family refused and just put the patient in their own car and started driving towards Bengaluru. My ego got a boost, but the neurosurgeon inside me was upset...but I was helpless...

They had unilaterally, and against medical advice, made the decision to transport the patient to Bangalore, a 4.5-hour journey by road. However, the window period for stroke treatment is a critical six hours. With the travel time factored in, the patient would likely be out of the window, diminishing the chances of a successful intervention.

At this pivotal moment, Plan B was devised. Recognizing the urgency, an ambulance, accompanied by a nurse bearing the life-saving injection, was dispatched from my hospital in Bangalore towards the approaching patient. The two vehicles moved along the highway, much like scenes from a suspenseful movie, converging at Shira after two hours.

The nurse administered the injection to the patient on the highway and in the ambulance, ensuring that crucial medical intervention occurred within the critical window period. The patient was then transported to my hospital in Bangalore, where a different chapter unfolded. Instead of enduring weeks in ICU and potential unconsciousness, the patient spent a mere day and a half in intensive care. Subsequently, the recovery journey began, marked by improved consciousness and diminishing left-side weakness.

The patient himself expressed gratitude, acknowledging the doctor's daredevil decision-making and the collaborative efforts that led to this successful intervention. The entire tale is a testament to the power of quick decision-making, collaboration, and the ingenuity needed to navigate challenges in healthcare.

This story is a reminder that heroism extends beyond the cinematic realm and often plays out in real-life situations where medical professionals make split-second decisions to save lives.

In the ever-evolving landscape of healthcare, it is imperative to celebrate these unsung heroes, the ones who hold stories together and make critical decisions to ensure the well-being of those in need.

11

STROKE WARRIORS

THE FIGHT AGAINST ALL ODDS

"My stroke of insight allowed me to realize that the distance between the core of my being and the perception of myself as separate from everything else was made up of thoughts and emotion."

"As a neuroanatomist, I knew that when I lost the left hemisphere of my brain, my right hemisphere was not damaged, so I had an opportunity to experience life with my right hemisphere fully engaged."

"The stroke stripped away all of my preconceived notions and belief systems, and I was left with an overwhelming sense of clarity and peace."

"I felt like I was a cell floating in the universe, connected to everything and everyone around me."

"After my stroke, I had to learn how to walk, talk, and even swallow again. It was a challenging journey, but it taught me the power of neuroplasticity and the ability of the brain to heal and rewire itself."

These quotes capture Dr. Jill Bolte Taylor's unique perspective on stroke, neurology, and the transformative effects of her own experience.

Dr. Jill Bolte Taylor, a neuroanatomist and author of the book "My Stroke of Insight." Dr. Taylor suffered a severe stroke in 1996 and documented her experience of recovery and transformation in her book.

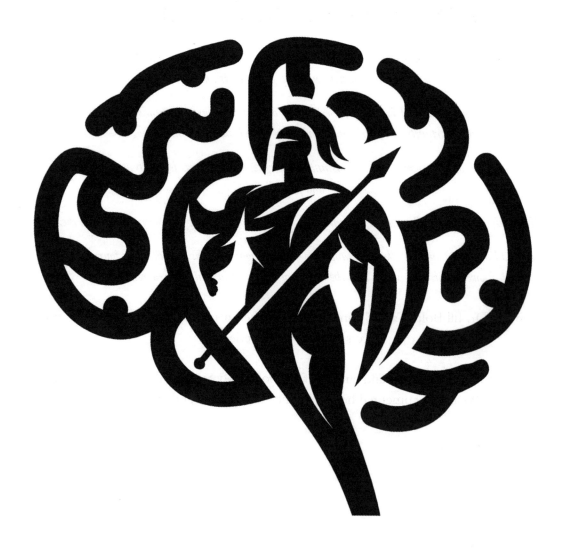

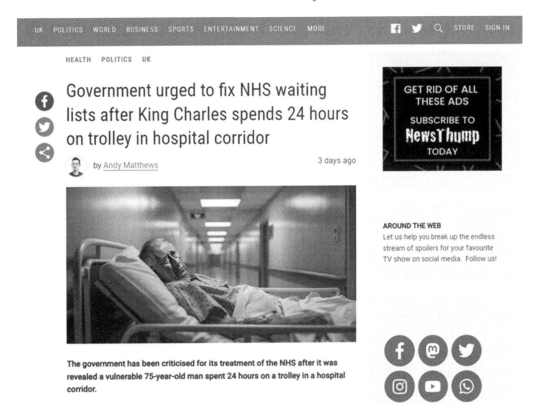

Government urged to fix NHS waiting lists after King Charles spends 24 hours on trolley in hospital corridor

by Andy Matthews   3 days ago

The government has been criticised for its treatment of the NHS after it was revealed a vulnerable 75-year-old man spent 24 hours on a trolley in a hospital corridor.

While the Western world is known for its technological advancements, it is imperative to note that India isn't too far behind. But wait… does that automatically translate to superior healthcare services in the Western world?? Hmm… it may not seem so, especially after seeing the above article. In fact, I made a YouTube short video on this topic. At the last count, it had garnered over 3,50,000 views over 1,210 comments (and counting) … you must see the video and read the comments; people from over 35 different countries have written their healthcare experiences, some are long stories… just shows how much people have been impacted, both positively and negatively. It was an eye-opener for me!

I have always wondered why we call people who get a stroke 'survivors.' Survivors are those who are forced to live without a choice! I personally believe an individual who ends up having a stroke or, for that matter, any neurological disorder should be given a choice and the right treatment environment & ecosystem to fight back! An opportunity to express their willpower to not only 'survive' but to reclaim their life, become their true self, and live like a 'warrior' with pride! We don't call them 'stroke survivors.' We call these people reclaiming their functional independence as 'stroke warriors'!

You remember Nina, our dear friend we spoke about in the first chapter, and Sneha shared her experience of fighting with her to regain her identity – she is a 'true stroke warrior'! - The one who actively participated in transforming her own life.

SEVERE GIDDINESS/VERTIGO CAN ALSO BE A SYMPTOM OF STROKE!

Here's another story! Let's drive the time machine back to 2016.

As the sun dipped behind the bustling streets of Bengaluru, a 49-year-old senior executive named Narayanaswamy found himself on a dizzying journey, quite literally. Clutching onto his sense of balance, he stumbled into the emergency department of a popular private hospital, with the cells in his head dancing with vertigo. Now, this wasn't just any executive; he was as integral to the fabric of the multinational car manufacturing company; he was literally the idli to their sambar!

With a demeanor that exuded authority, he approached the emergency staff, requesting a consultation with his trusted neurosurgeon, yours truly, poised on the tip of his tongue. However, fate had a different script in mind. The emergency doctor on call that fateful day, perhaps misinterpreting his symptoms, swiftly whisked him away into the domain of ear, nose, and throat matters.

Meanwhile, time ticked by unnoticed, much like the incessant honking on the busy streets of Bengaluru. Little did anyone realize the gravity of the situation brewing within the executive's brain. It wasn't until he began to drift into a semi-conscious state that the medical team shifted gears. Enter the neurologist, armed with suspicions as weighty as the Bangalore traffic during rush hour – an acute stroke of the vertebral-basilar artery.

But diagnosing such a condition required more than just a stethoscope and a sharp mind; it demanded the keen eye of modern medicine's sorcery. Thus, an MRI became the proverbial holy grail, albeit at a nearby diagnostic center. As the arrangements were made, time seemed to dance to its own rhythm, with every passing second akin to a mile on the city's congested roads. Remember? Time is Brain!

Eventually, the moment of truth arrived. The executive, now a passenger in the ambulance of destiny, was shuttled off to get an MRI done. The scan, a snapshot of his brain's inner workings, held the key to unveiling the secrets that had gripped him for over a day.

As the report finally surfaced, it dawned on everyone involved – it had been a race against time, a sprint against fate. Twenty-six hours since the first whispers of the stroke had echoed through his consciousness and twenty-four hours since he had embarked on this unexpected journey through the corridors of healthcare. As the MRI revealed the daunting reality of a massive cerebellar infarct, it was as if a storm had descended upon the tranquil waters of the poor executive's and his family's life. His brain, once the command center of his dynamic existence, now bore the weight of an unseen pressure, threatening to engulf him in the depths of unconsciousness.

With each labored breath, the essence of his being teetered on the precipice of existence. It was a scene straight out of a Bollywood thriller, with life and death locked in a high-stakes duel and the fate of our protagonist hanging in the balance.

I entered the operating theater, ready to confront the monstrous challenge head-on. But before I could wield my surgical prowess, there stood a formidable obstacle – the skeptic in the form of the intensivist brother-in-law, a veteran doctor of the ICU trenches.

With a touch of wit and wisdom, the brother-in-law (affectionately referred to as Dr. M) voiced his concerns, drawing from a decade of frontline experience. "Doctor," he began, his tone laced with respect and skepticism, "in all my years tending to the critical, I've yet to witness a miracle when patients are in such dire straits."

Undeterred by the shadows of doubt, I stood firm in my conviction. "Ah, but you see," I said, "I've danced with death more times than I can count and lived to tell the tale. In my realm, miracles are not just a myth – they're a reality waiting to be realized."

And so, amidst the backdrop of uncertainty, the family stood at the crossroads of hope and despair, their hearts heavy with the burden of choice. Yet, in the face of adversity, they embraced the flicker of hope that my words ignited. With a nod of consent, they entrusted their beloved executive to the hands of fate, ready to brave the tempest of surgery in pursuit of a chance at redemption.

In the corridors of the hospital, voices of doubt echoed among the white-coated figures, casting shadows of despair over the flickering ray of hope. Yet, amidst the gloom, I stood confident, providing hope to the family amidst the whirlwind.

As the weeks unfolded, and the patient remained locked in the silent embrace of coma post-surgery, a new chapter began in his journey towards recovery – the dawn of intensive neuro rehabilitation, spearheaded by us, Team PRS Neurosciences, under the brand name 'newro.'.

With a blend of innovation and determination, we rolled up our sleeves and got on our mission to unlock the dormant potential within the recesses of the patient's injured poor brain. Armed with a patented test known as the SEFA, we seeped into the depths of his cognitive abilities, revealing a stark reality encapsulated in the grim score of C2C BIR 1a – the nadir of functional ability.

In the world of neuro rehabilitation, where science meets spirituality and a pinch of Bollywood drama, we set off for our mission with all the fervor of a pro-neuro rehabilitation clinic. Armed with our secret tool, WUUB – Waking Up the Unconscious Brain, we set out to awaken the sleeping giant within the human brain.

Picture this: amidst the beeping of machines and the serious faces of doctors, there's a team of therapists armed with everything from traditional music to fragrant spices to family members' voices, all aimed at coaxing the unconscious mind back to the land of the living. It's like a scene straight out of a movie or a Hollywood series – instead of a hero battling villains, it's the patient fighting against the odds of neurological impairment.

But it's not just about stimulating the senses; it's also about keeping the body "future-ready." Enter the VOST protocol – a meticulous plan to keep aspiration pneumonia at bay. It's like preparing a sumptuous Indian breakfast – every ingredient is carefully selected to tantalize the taste buds. If one of the ingredients is added in excess quantity, the entire dish will be spoiled.

As the weeks go by, with each passing day feeling like a slow-motion sequence, like in the old Rajnikanth movie, where he walks in slow motion, our hero begins to stir. His journey from coma to consciousness is nothing short of a hit film, complete with tears of joy, hugs, and maybe even a few songs thrown in for good measure. Imagine playing Kabhi Khushi Kabhi Gham in the background. I mean, seriously!

And when he finally wakes up, it's like his movie has been shortlisted for an Oscar – with cheers, applause, and maybe even a few dance moves thrown in for good measure.

Once our stroke warrior bid farewell to the sterile confines of the hospital, he was greeted with a new chapter in his journey towards full recovery—outpatient-based intensive neuro rehabilitation. Led by the dynamic Team newro, this phase of his rehabilitation was like stepping into a dance reality show, where each move was given marks. Every session was a carefully choreographed dance of healing and progress.

With physiotherapists guiding his steps, occupational therapists helping him navigate the challenges of daily life, and speech therapists ensuring his voice regained its melody, our hero embarked on a transformation journey to win over his challenges. And let's not forget the swallow therapist, whose expertise ensured that every morsel he savored gave him energy as climbed uphill toward normalcy.

But it wasn't just about physical recovery; it was about nurturing the mind and spirit, too. Enter the pain therapist, whose soothing touch eased his discomfort. And amidst it all, Dr. Prathiba, the neuropsychologist, was there, like a wise sage, helping him navigate the maze of memory and cognition with humor and empathy.

As days turned to weeks and weeks into months, our hero's progress was nothing short of a miracle. With each milestone reached, he seemed to defy the odds with a resilience that no words can completely define. And when he finally returned to the helm of his company, it was like a scene straight out of a feel-good movie, complete with cheers, applause, and maybe even a tear or two.

But the story didn't end there. Oh no, our hero had more adventures in store. From climbing the iconic Chamundi hills in Mysuru to revving up his kinetic Honda scooter and cruising down the bustling streets of Bengaluru, and even driving his car to Mysuru, he embraced life with a newfound zest that was truly inspiring. He won the war!

Indeed, neuro rehabilitation isn't just about restoring function; it's about reclaiming life in all its vibrant colors. With Team Newro by his side, our hero proved that with determination and resilience, anything is possible.

Recovery after stroke

The recovery period after a stroke varies, and the extent of recovery depends on factors like the severity of the stroke and promptness of treatment. There is no one-size-fits-all answer, as strokes differ in their impact. Early recognition, timely treatment, extent and severity of brain circuits' damage, and adherence to medical and rehab guidance play pivotal roles in determining the recovery outcome.

Navigating the Hospital and Post-Stroke Care – know the warcraft!

Do you know what number you should dial in your city or country to call for an ambulance?

Understanding what to do when taking a family member or friend to the hospital due to a stroke is crucial. Remaining calm as a caregiver is the priority in ensuring the patient receives the best possible care. When providing information to emergency doctors, details such as whether the person fell unconscious before or after falling can significantly impact the diagnosis. In cases where a family member becomes unconscious at home, immediate ambulance assistance is emphasized. Delaying care by waiting for the person to regain consciousness could result in losing precious time. Once at the emergency department, clear communication about the events leading to the stroke is essential for the medical team to determine the course of action.

The emergency doctor may call in a neurologist to evaluate the situation further. Specific blood tests and imaging, such as CT scans and MRIs, are typically ordered. While CT scans provide valuable information, MRIs may be required for a more detailed assessment. It's advised to be prepared with extra funds to avoid delays in the investigation process.

Certain medications are initiated promptly to prevent blood clotting or break down existing clots affecting blood flow. In cases where imaging reveals blood accumulation in the brain, emergency surgery may be necessary. This could involve placing a tube to drain the blood or surgically removing the blood clot.

Impact on Consciousness and Rehabilitation

The impact of a stroke on consciousness and functionality varies depending on factors like the extent and location of the stroke. If the stroke is limited to one side of the brain, patients may regain consciousness relatively quickly. Surgery might be an option if the stroke is confined to a specific area.

Rehabilitation is a crucial aspect of post-stroke care, involving a multidisciplinary team. Physical therapists, occupational therapists, speech-language pathologists, and other specialists work together to facilitate recovery. Proper neuro rehabilitation addresses physical and cognitive aspects, including preventing complications and promoting early mobilization.

Patients with massive strokes may experience compression effects, leading to unconsciousness. The recovery process for these individuals may differ from that of those who regain awareness quickly. It's important not to compare recovery timelines between different patients, as each case is unique.

Coma and Stimulation for Recovery

Coma, often called a loss of consciousness, is rooted in the brain's ability to perceive and process sensory input. When there's an injury or stroke affecting the brain, accumulated blood or inflammation can compress the brain, leading to a state of coma. The Glasgow Coma Scale (GCS) is commonly used to assess coma based on eye-opening, verbal, and motor responses.

In rehabilitation, the Ranchos Los Amigos Scale is employed, focusing on cognitive aspects during the recovery process. The scale consists of ten stages, progressing from no response to normal functioning. The stages include no response, generalized response, localized response, agitated stage, confused state, and further stages leading to near-normal functioning.

Coma stimulation aims to activate the brain's sensory input through systematic approaches. The seven senses, including hidden ones like joint and inner ear senses, are crucial for maintaining alertness and preventing sensory deprivation. Coma stimulation involves introducing stimuli periodically and addressing visual, auditory, taste, smell, and touch senses.

Early and structured coma stimulation is emphasized, considering both fundamental and complex stimuli. It is essential to maintain a familiar environment, incorporating elements from the patient's routine before the coma. While stimulation is vital, it must be done in a systematic and periodic manner to prevent overstimulation and potential brain shutdown.

What does a patient in or emerging out of a coma look like?

Some of you fond of seeing movies or daily soaps must have seen a person in a hospital with a bandage on the forehead, well dressed, absolutely relaxed, with a facemask without oxygen supply, often healthy and chubby face with hair well kept. I want to invite the producers of daily soaps and show them how cruel a patient in a coma or, as we call them, 'in altered sensorium' be.

Many of them will have a hole in the neck to breathe (tracheostomy), a tube in the nose to feed, and a tube in the genitals to piss. They are as good as a newborn both physically and neurologically. Many of them lose over 50 % of their body weight, and many of them become unrecognizable!

They have poor awareness of both external and internal environments, do not know when to sleep and when to wake up and experience an absolute loss of orientation to time and space. Many of them who get better get super-aggressive, crying, shouting, kicking, biting, spitting, punching.

Our team of doctors, nurses, and therapists handles all this. Some of them are awake but cannot move; they are what we call "locked in!" There are some who never return from a coma despite all the efforts of the doctor, the rehab team, or the family! Returning from a coma is nothing less than a trip to hell and back! Those who successfully return from a coma leave an everlasting impression on their caregivers, which no professional can understand!

Understanding the nuances of coma stimulation and tailoring the approach to individual patients contribute to more effective rehabilitation and increased chances of positive outcomes.

Swallowing Problems and Tube Management

After a stroke, individuals often face swallowing problems, leading to dysphagia. Dysphagia can manifest at the oral or pharyngeal level, with challenges in chewing, drooling, coughing during swallowing, or difficulty propelling food back to the throat. To ensure safe eating, various tubes may be considered, such as nasogastric tubes (Ryles-tube) for short-term needs or percutaneous endoscopic gastrostomy tubes (PEG tubes) for longer-term nutritional support.

Swallowing problems can arise at different levels: oral, pharyngeal, or esophageal. These issues are addressed by speech therapists who work on rehabilitating the patient's ability to consume an oral diet. However, feeding tube management might be necessary during the recovery process as the patient recovers to achieve normal ability to eat and drink. NG tubes, inserted through the nose to the stomach, are suitable for short-term support, delivering thin liquids. PEG tubes, surgically inserted into the stomach, are used for more extended nutritional support.

Let us also talk about the assistance required for breathing. For patients initially admitted in an unconscious or coma state, ventilator support may be required. Endo-Tracheal Tubes (ETT) tubes may be utilized, but prolonged use can damage vocal folds. In such cases, tracheostomy tubes (T-tubes) are employed for breathing support while avoiding long-term complications.

In critical care scenarios where patients are on ventilator support and may require tracheostomy, care should be taken to monitor tube size, cuff status, and patient tolerance. Suctioning of the tracheostomy tube should be performed as needed, with a break of 2 to 3 hours.

Additionally, urinary catheter management is crucial for stroke and bedridden patients. Catheters are inserted and managed carefully, regularly monitoring for infection and assessing patients' sensations. Sensation checks help determine the need for catheter removal, and the overall care plan involves attentive observation for any signs of infection.

So basically, managing swallowing problems and associated tube placements involves a comprehensive approach, considering the patient's specific needs, the duration of support required, and potential long-term implications. A multidisciplinary team, including speech therapists, physicians, and nursing staff, collaborates to ensure the best possible outcomes for patients recovering from strokes or other neurological conditions.

STROKE PATIENT REHABILITATION PROTOCOL

In our approach to stroke patient rehabilitation at PRS Neurosciences, we implement a segmented protocol tailored to the specific needs of the patients at different stages of recovery.

a. Coma Management:

In the initial segment, we focus on patients in a coma or with a Glasgow Coma Scale (GCS) of less than eight. Our primary goal is to prevent secondary complications such as bedsores, chest issues, joint tightness, or deformities due to prolonged immobilization. We emphasize keeping the body "future-ready" to avoid problems during the later stages of recovery. Multimodal coma stimulation techniques involving sensory and tactile stimulations are employed to 'wake up the unconscious brain (WUUB). Family members play a crucial role in this phase, providing familiar stimuli that aid the patient's recovery.

b. Early Awakening:

As patients begin to wake up, family involvement remains essential. Patients may be in a state of minimal consciousness and may or may not be communicating. We also have strategies to help those who are regaining the ability to understand but are not yet able to connect their thoughts and actions. We call it 'cognitive motor disconnect'! A multidisciplinary team, including cognitive therapists, physiotherapists, occupational therapists, speech and swallow pathologists, vision rehab specialists, and others, works to assist patients in moving from a state of consciousness to one of orientation, and in basic movements such as rolling, opening their eyes, and turning limbs. The focus is on building tone and facilitating movements to transition from pattern movements to isolated, purposeful actions. I have seen that patients awakening from a coma and crossing their legs early have better cognitive capability.

c. Community Reintegration:

The third segment targets patients who are transitioning toward community reintegration. Once patients can sit, stand, and move in bed, we aim to prepare them for activities of daily living (ADLs). Physiotherapists play a pivotal role in training patients for tasks like turning in bed, transferring to a chair, and eventually returning home safely. Caregivers are extensively trained to ensure patients' independence, reducing fall risks and enhancing confidence.

At PRS Neurosciences, we provide comprehensive rehabilitation, instilling hope and empowering stroke patients on their journey to recovery.

Understanding physical therapy

Physical therapy is the most renowned part of neuro rehabilitation. Physical therapists are experts in understanding Osteokinematics (means joint movement) and arthrokinematics (joint surface motion.), muscle and myofascial system, the cardio-respiratory system, and the relationship of the neurological system with the muscular system. They are experts in movement sciences and anchor the responsibility of regaining the ability to move in and out of bed and access the indoor and outdoor environment. Their USP is the ability to correlate physical capacity and limitations with the opportunities and limitations posed by the environment.

The physical therapists in my team understand the problem is in the neurological system and that a specific treatment approach is needed to address these issues. The treatments for musculoskeletal issues and neurological issues are different! The physical therapist now prefers to address functional abilities rather than structural deficits, and therefore, an interesting way of retraining the injured brain or spinal cord is purely focusing on functional abilities! In my team, the physical therapist is a crucial asset. It provides care using protocols like Keeping Body Future Ready, Functional Body Levels, and Part of VOST care to prevent chest pneumonia by working closely with the Speech Language Pathologist!

Patients transitioning to the outpatient setting receive further training for gait and walking patterns. The emphasis is on correcting abnormal walking patterns early to prevent long-term complications. The goal is to instill proper walking habits to ensure patients can maintain a near-normal gait throughout their lives.

Understanding Occupational Therapy

Occupational therapy is a century-old profession, yet its essence is often misunderstood. Contrary to the assumption that it involves providing jobs, occupational therapy focuses on helping individuals regain functionality and return to their normal lives through active engagement in meaningful activities.

The term "occupation" here refers to the various daily tasks and activities that occupy our time.

Occupational therapists work in rehabilitation alongside professionals such as physical therapists, psychologists, speech therapists, and counselors. The primary goal is to facilitate the patient's recovery by emphasizing functionality and enabling them to relearn tasks they may struggle with owing to problems in performance areas, performance context, and performance components.

Common challenges addressed by occupational therapy in stroke rehabilitation include paralysis affecting the upper limb, vision-related issues, agnosia (difficulty perceiving objects), reading difficulties (alexia), and cognitive deficits impacting memory and decision-making, affecting daily life participation. Intense rehabilitation is essential to restore patients' abilities in self-care, caring for others, and productivity in daily life, including returning to work.

The specialized focus on hand function is a hallmark of occupational therapy, recognizing the significance of hands in performing fine motor activities. Occupational therapists may also create custom splints for hand-related issues and design adaptive devices such as modified utensils and tools to enhance functional independence. Occupational therapy is a dynamic and impactful profession that goes beyond misconceptions. It aims to empower individuals to lead fulfilling lives through meaningful engagement in daily activities.

Role of a Speech Language Pathologist in Stroke Management:

A Speech Language Pathologist (SLP) plays a crucial role in managing stroke and addressing issues related to speech, language, communication, swallowing, awareness, and cognition. Stroke, whether caused by a clot or a bleed in the brain, can impact these aspects, and SLPs work to understand and address these challenges.

Speech, Language, and Communication:

- Communication involves exchanging information verbally or non-verbally. Verbal communication includes producing sounds and meaningful utterances, while non-verbal communication encompasses gestures, sign language, and other non-verbal cues.
- Language refers to meaningful communication through writing or speaking.
- Speech is the verbal production of sounds and meaningful utterances.

In stroke patients, any combination of these elements can be affected. The left side of the brain is often associated with language-related issues. Stroke can result in language problems, speech problems, or both. Language may be impaired even if speech remains clear, and vice versa.

Acute Care Setting:

- In the acute care setting, where the patient may be in a comatose or unconscious state, SLPs use techniques such as auditory stimulation and speech-language stimulation to wake up the patient and improve consciousness.
- Functional communication training is initiated to ensure the patient can communicate basic needs with family, attendants, or nursing staff.

Chronic Care Setting:

- In chronic care, after the patient is discharged, SLPs continue to work with them on an outpatient basis to improve communication skills and address persistent speech or language issues.
- Techniques focus on improving comprehension, expression, or overall communication, whether verbal or non-verbal.
- Patients may struggle with one-word utterances, difficulty framing sentences, or fluency lacking meaning. SLPs employ various techniques to enhance meaningful communication.
- If patients have difficulty understanding spoken language, specific techniques are applied to enhance comprehension.

The role of SLPs in stroke rehabilitation extends from acute care to chronic care settings. Techniques include auditory and speech-language stimulation, functional communication training, and targeted interventions for comprehension and expression. SLPs work towards improving communication skills, ensuring stroke survivors can effectively express their needs and understand information in their environment.

Role of Speech-Language Pathologists in Swallowing Rehabilitation After Stroke:

Speech Language Pathologists (SLPs) play a vital role in addressing swallowing issues in Stroke patients, catering to varying levels of severity in different stages of patient recovery.

1. **Coma Stage:**

   — In the early comatose stages, SLPs work on giving gustatory stimulations as part of coma stimulation and also maintaining the swallow reflex.

2. **Swallowing Phases and Dysphagia:**

   — Dysphagia refers to difficulty swallowing and can manifest in different phases: oral, oral transfer, and pharyngeal (final) phases.
   — The oral phase includes oral preparatory and oral transfer phases.
   — The oral preparatory phase involves taking food into the mouth, chewing, and forming a bolus. Weakness or limited range of motion in muscles can lead to issues like drooling, difficulty biting, or pocketing of food.
   — The oral transfer phase involves moving the food from the mouth to the throat. Control issues during this phase can result in coughing, residue in the mouth, or early spillage.
   — The pharyngeal phase is critical to prevent aspiration (food entering the windpipe) and ensure safe passage to the stomach.

3. **Treatment Strategies:**

   — For oral preparatory issues, SLPs focus on strengthening muscles, improving muscle tone, and increasing the range of motion.
   — Oral transfer problems are addressed through awareness training and tongue-based strengthening exercises.
   — Sensory issues in the mouth are tackled using thermal and gustatory stimulation to enhance sensations.
   — Pharyngeal phase problems involve compensatory strategies and therapeutic techniques, with considerations for patient safety.
   — Instrumental evaluations like Fiber Optic Endoscopic Evaluation of Swallowing (FEES) or Videofluoroscopic Swallow Study (VFSS) help provide detailed insights into swallowing function.

4. **Complications and Indicators:**

   — Silent aspiration (food entering the windpipe without coughing) and pooling (accumulation near the windpipe) may not be evident in clinical evaluations, emphasizing the need for instrumental assessments.
   — Complications like pneumonia, wet voice, and oxygen level changes indicate swallowing issues.

5. **Rehabilitation and Timely Intervention:**

— SLPs work on both compensatory and therapeutic strategies based on the severity of the swallowing impairment.

— Compensatory strategies are introduced initially for safe swallowing, while therapeutic strategies aim to improve overall swallowing function.

— Early intervention is crucial for effective rehabilitation, preventing further complications, and promoting a return to normal swallowing function.

6. **Assessment Techniques:**

— Clinical swallow evaluation at the bedside identifies initial concerns, while instrumental evaluations like FEES or VFSS provide a more detailed understanding of the swallowing process.

— These assessments guide the formulation of personalized treatment plans for each patient.

— Addressing swallowing challenges requires a multidisciplinary team, and SLPs collaborate with other healthcare professionals to provide holistic care for stroke patients.

Understanding Cognition and Cognitive Deficits After Stroke

Before delving into cognitive deficits, grasping the concept of cognition is crucial. Cognition involves acquiring knowledge and understanding through thought, experiences, and senses. It is essential for thinking, organizing, and processing information in our daily lives.

Deficits in Cognition After Stroke:

1. **Attention Deficits:**

— Sustained attention: Difficulty focusing on a task for an extended period.
— Divided attention: Challenges in focusing on multiple tasks simultaneously.
— Focused attention: Impaired ability to concentrate, affecting tasks like listening to a lecture.

2. **Memory Deficits:**

— Various types of memory may be affected—logical, associative, short-term, long-term, and episodic memory.
— Impacts the ability to recall information or experiences.

3. **Executive Function Impairments:**

— Decision-making, planning, and problem-solving abilities are compromised.
— Difficulty in self-regulation and self-evaluation.
— Challenges in executing tasks, such as meal preparation.

4. **Perceptual and Spatial Deficits:**

   — Issues with depth perception and visual perception.
   — Apraxia and spatial neglect may occur, affecting the execution of movements and attention to one side.

5. **Behavioral and Psychological Changes:**

   — Depression and Low Mood:
   • Patients may experience sadness, low self-esteem, and lack of motivation.
   — Behavioral Changes:
   • Outbursts of anger, frustration, and crying spells can manifest.
   • Development of phobias, such as a fear of falling.

6. **Assessment and Rehabilitation:**

   — Cognitive Assessment:
   • Various tests evaluate different brain functions in different areas.
   • Identify impairments to formulate personalized treatment plans.
   — Retraining Cognitive Functions:
   • Similar to providing additional tutoring in subjects where a student struggles, retraining focuses on improving impaired cognitive functions.
   • Strategies targeting specific deficits identified during assessments.
   — Pharmacotherapy and Cognitive Behavioral Therapy:
   • Medications can help control mood fluctuations.
   • Cognitive Behavioral Therapy (CBT) and deep relaxation techniques aid in managing behavioral challenges.

Duration of Rehabilitation:

• Rehabilitation is time-consuming, spanning from 2 months to 2 years or even longer.
• Consistent efforts yield positive results, with patients often returning to work after comprehensive rehabilitation.

Care for Patients and Caregivers:

• Patients and caregivers are equally important in the rehabilitation process.
• Behavioral challenges may require patience, understanding, and distraction techniques.
• Caregivers play a crucial role in creating a supportive environment.

Neuropsychology versus Clinical Psychology

In the theater of mental health, neuropsychology takes the center of the stage, its spotlight focused on the intricacy of the brain and behavior. Like the skilled ancient Indian architects, neuropsychologists meticulously sit and remove the clogs inside human brains, detangling the threads of cognitive and behavioral impairments and weaving an understanding of the complexity of brain injuries and disorders. Meanwhile, clinical psychology casts a wider net, encompassing the spectrum of emotional and psychological disorders with the finesse of an orator. It's like the bustling markets of Bangalore, teeming with a colorful array of human experiences.

But amidst the hustle and bustle of the psychological landscape, one thing remains clear. Both disciplines share a common goal: to bring out the mysteries of the human mind, clear them, and alleviate the burdens of mental illness. Whether it's decoding the enigma of a traumatic brain injury or navigating the complicated roads of anxiety and depression, psychologists of all stripes work tirelessly to bring light to the darkest corners of the psyche.

Role of Neuropsychology in Neuro rehabilitation

In the world of neuro rehabilitation, neuropsychology is like the hero working backstage, quietly steering the ship through the waters of brain injuries. Whether it's a nasty tumble, a stroke, or a tumor resection, neuropsychologists are the magicians who decode the brain's language and help individuals bounce back from cognitive challenges like memory lapses or attention deficits.

Functional Deficits and Cognitive Rehabilitation

When it comes to brain injuries, it's like playing a game of roulette with the brain's cognitive functions – you never know which area might take a hit. From attention and memory to visual-spatial abilities and executive functions, the damage can wreak havoc on everyday life, making even simple tasks feel like climbing Mount Everest. This is where we need neuropsychologists. Only they can bring the affected person back to normal life and inspire them to confront everything in life head-on.

Cognitive therapists aim to enhance attention, memory, problem-solving skills, and executive functions in people with brain malfunctions. Like watching a phoenix rise from the ashes, individuals emerge from the depths of cognitive impairment, their abilities restored, and their quality of life vastly improved.

Understanding deficits of the visual pathways and how they impact patients' recovery after a Stroke or any other brain injury:

Now, we have praised therapists/doctors from all the departments connected with neurology. But what about the caregiver? They are really the unsung heroes! They need to be awarded the highest civilian award of Bharat – the Bharat Ratna, for sure!

Amidst the triumphs and victories, let us not forget that caregivers are the unsung heroes behind the scenes. For them, the journey is fraught with emotional challenges, a rollercoaster of frustration, and overwhelming responsibilities. But let us remember – their love and dedication shine through, lighting the path towards healing and hope. They give up all their likes and dislikes and make all sacrifices unconditionally.

Their role involves providing physical assistance to stroke survivors, from helping them with physical transfers to feeding them, helping them with their toilet and bathing chores, cleaning them up, facilitating communication, etc.

But as the disease progresses and the patient becomes more dependent, the burden on the caregiver intensifies. This burden can be categorized into objective and subjective aspects. An objective burden is like the weight of a sack of potatoes – it's the physical assistance and time required to care for the patient. Meanwhile, the subjective burden is like the never-ending drama of a soap opera – it's the mental and emotional stress experienced by the caregiver over time.

But fear not, dear caregivers! Just like adding a pinch of Haldi to your curry, we're here to offer support and guidance to help lighten your load. At the end of the day, we're all in this together—like a big, extended Indian family, navigating the ups and downs of life with humor, resilience, and a whole lot of love.

Guiding caregivers through the labyrinth of patience is akin to teaching someone to master the art of making perfectly round rotis. Our therapists undergo specialized training, akin to master chefs honing their skills, to gently coach caregivers on the importance of patience.

Caregivers experiencing stress, anxiety, or depression can benefit from psychological counseling and participation in support groups. We have introduced a couple of programs and activities that could actively reduce the intensity of work the caregiver has to put in to bring back their beloved to normal.

The study presents significant insights into the experiences of caregivers for stroke survivors, revealing that they face considerable stress across various domains, such as financial, emotional, physical, and mental well-being. This stress persists throughout the duration of care, as indicated by the follow-up assessments conducted at six months and one-year post-stroke. Notably, the caregivers in this study predominantly experienced caregiving for the first time, shedding light on the challenges faced by novices in this role.

It underscores the profound impact of caregiving on familial relationships and societal norms, with the majority of caregivers being women and immediate family members, including spouses, daughters, and sons, assuming primary caregiving responsibilities. The study also highlights the sacrifices made by family members, such as adjusting work schedules and even relinquishing employment, to provide care for their loved ones.

Moreover, the findings reveal that younger caregivers and daughters-in-law experience heightened stress levels compared to spouse caregivers, whose stress levels are relatively milder. Despite these challenges, the study provides valuable insights into the dynamics of caregiving for stroke survivors and emphasizes the need for support services tailored to the diverse needs of caregivers.

The utilization of standardized assessment tools enhances the reliability and comparability of the study's results, contributing to the body of knowledge on stroke caregiving.

The study's findings suggest that the increasing global burden of stroke, observed in both developed and developing nations, will inevitably escalate the challenges faced by caregivers. It indicates that the existing healthcare infrastructure is inadequate to cope with the social and caregiving demands associated with stroke, emphasizing the pressing need for comprehensive support systems.

Financial concerns, extended caregiving hours, and emotional stress emerged as prominent factors contributing to caregiver burden, underscoring the multifaceted nature of the challenges faced by caregivers.

The study underscores the importance of integrating caregiver support into stroke rehabilitation services, including practical nursing training and counseling sessions, to alleviate caregiver burden and enhance patient recovery.

The study advocates implementing planned research initiatives focusing on caregiver stress across multiple healthcare centers, with standardized protocols to facilitate generalizable findings and inform tailored interventions. It suggests replicating successful strategies identified in the study within clinical settings to address caregiver needs effectively alongside implementing comprehensive rehabilitation protocols incorporating psychological counseling by neuropsychologists.

Therapists play a crucial role in establishing connections with caregivers, particularly in the initial contact made by the rehab team. If team leads or unit heads understand the potential caregiver burdens, they can effectively communicate them to the team members. This understanding provides background information on the medical condition and the family situation, enabling our team to approach evaluations with greater empathy. Even if, due to time or manpower constraints, we may not always address caregiver burden effectively, establishing rapport remains vital. Communication with patients and caregivers should consider their mindset, focusing not only on the immediate problem but also on their long-term engagement in daily life or caregiving responsibilities, especially if the prognosis is bleak.

Sometimes, in our efforts to motivate patients, we may use strong words without considering their emotional impact. However, as clinicians, we carry the burden of multiple patients daily, which can sometimes lead to unintentional emotional outbursts directed toward a particular patient. Ruthless compassion is the name of the game. We also teach the caregivers to use the 'carrot and stick' policy.

It's essential to recognize that caregiver burden also affects clinicians. Thus, managing these burdens is crucial for maintaining quality care delivery.

While caring for a child typically brings joy, the narrative shifts when tending to neurological patients, introducing additional complexities and emotional strain. Unlike the joyous experience of caring for children, providing assistance to neurological patients often entails a prolonged commitment and uncertainty regarding the prognosis, thereby intensifying the burden on caregivers.

Our system can indeed help caregivers by providing them with the opportunity to take care of themselves. For instance, the ITB has allowed Tarun's, Kodanda's, and Triveni's caregivers to have some freedom, relieving their stresses and enabling them to focus on themselves and their lives. With a system yielding strong functional outcomes, caregivers will undoubtedly have more time to attend to their own needs, knowing that the burden will be significantly reduced.

Often, we overlook the importance of appreciating caregivers. We focus on assessing how they manage care but forget to acknowledge the immense value of their efforts.

I recall an experience with two patients I was treating. After some time, I decided to express my appreciation to one patient's wife for her exceptional care. Her response was heart-wrenching. She wept like a baby and eventually, after coaxing, revealed that no one had appreciated her efforts at home for the past three months. This simple acknowledgment brought her to tears. Since then, I've noticed a significant change in her demeanor. She eagerly awaited therapy sessions and actively participated, even preparing the space beforehand.

Similarly, another patient's expressing gratitude to their caregiver resulted in increased involvement and dedication from their end. It's evident that a little appreciation can go a long way in motivating and empowering caregivers, and for that matter, any human being, to continue providing exceptional care.

When they feel valued and appreciated, they often go above and beyond in their participation and efforts.

Moreover, capturing these moments of appreciation and positive experiences during therapy sessions is crucial. It adds a personal touch to their journey and distinguishes our team and facility from others. These experiences leave a lasting impression on patients and caregivers, enhancing their overall satisfaction with our services.

Every day, our goal is simple—to bring a smile to both patients and caregivers alike. It's pure bliss. And when we see the shared success with our dedicated therapists, it's like adding extra spice to an already delicious curry—simply irresistible. And as Maggie talks about their hot and spicy sauce—it's different!

From hopeless to hope... from dependence to independence....

Let me tell you another story of a 65-year-old lady called Mrs. PP. She was a known hypertensive sister of one of our senior trustees. She had a brain hemorrhage at her house, fell unconscious at home, and was immediately rushed to the nearest private hospital, where a CT scan was done, and she was found to have a brain hemorrhage. Because she had a brain hemorrhage into a water-containing cavity called the ventricles, or what we call intraventricular hemorrhage with obstructive hydrocephalus, she was immediately taken up for surgery because she was deeply unconscious. Burr holes were placed on either side; in the frontal regions, holes were made in the skull, and tubes were put inside to clear out the blood. Eventually, this happened...you know, two, three weeks in ICU, ventilator. She remained unconscious. She eventually got tracheostomized and the other usual masala. At the end of three and a half weeks, medically, she had stabilized, but she remained deeply unconscious. She was then told by the doctors there that she had stabilized medically, we had saved her life, and the mainstay of treatment now is neuro rehabilitation. That's when the patient's brother, a senior trustee of our hospital, sought me out and came and met me.

He told me a little about her condition, showed me her case summary as she was still in the other hospital, and then asked me a fundamental question. He asked Dr. Sharan and me if I thought it was worth bringing her here for treatment. Because doctors there don't seem very hopeful. Then I asked him the question – Why are you asking me this question, sir? He said, "Sir, this lady does not have money. I have to foot her bills. Please tell me, is it really worth spending any more money? Because I've already spent 15 lakhs in the other hospital." I was stunned. I told him – Sir, as far as our science is concerned, it is worth bringing her. Please bring her over. When she came over, and we evaluated her, she was a score, according to our system, of C2C BIR 1c. Deeply unconscious, hardly moving any of the four limbs and tracheostomized. From there, the rehab process started. Initially, we did the coma stimulation and kept the body future-ready strategies and other preventive strategies. Slowly, over the next few weeks, she initially started moving the right side of her limbs. Then, she slowly started waking up. Over the next three to four months, she recovered to such a degree that we were able to begin overly, close her tracheostomy tube, and pull out Ryle's tube, and she made good progress.

She started saying a few words, and then in short sentences, her cognition improved, and she reached a stage where, with support, she started walking to the bathroom at the hospital. The family was stunned because she had three children, two daughters and a son, and there was initially a lot of disagreement among themselves about what to do, how to do it, and things like that. Eventually, they fell in line after they started seeing the improvement. They were very demanding. They had a lot of questions. They were not sure whether she was going to get better. But once they saw her confidence, after she woke up, they put all their energy into making their mother better. Nine months into treatment, we had to support them with rehab at home also because they stayed on the second floor, and she couldn't come down and come to a rehab center. She currently has not yet fully recovered; she may never be normal. She's probably C2C, BIR 3a-3b. She walks with a walker at home, but she's talking reasonably well. She speaks on the phone, she watches TV, and guess what? She can even stand at the kitchen counter with her walker in tow and cook some basic stuff, including making chapatis.

It is just amazing what is possible for somebody who said this is worth bringing her to the hospital to the place she is now. I am sure many thousands of you are still out there thinking the same... or having people think the same. Please reach out to them and help them make informed decisions.

12

HEAD INJURY, AKA TRAUMATIC BRAIN INJURY OR TBI

"It's important not to give up on a patient with severe brain injury too early, as the outcome can sometimes defy initial grim prognosis."

Neurology experts' comments on early treatment decisions for TBI.

"Every brain injury is different, but every person with a brain injury requires our support."

–Dr. Sharan Srinivasan

"Brain injury is not an event or an outcome. It is the start of a misdiagnosed, misunderstood, underfunded neurological disease."

–Brain Injury Association of America (BIAA)

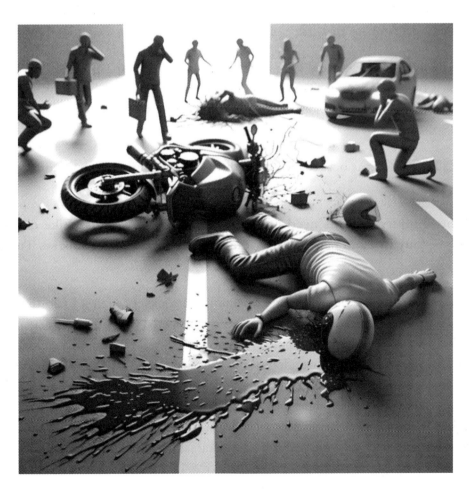

In the whirl of Anantapur, a tale unfolds that could rival an action scene in any Kollywood blockbuster. A 32-year-old in the prime of life meets with fate's twist on his two-wheeler, hurling him into a battle for survival. Since he had no helmet on his head, he sustained a severe head injury.

His entry here was as dramatic as any cinema hero's, marked by a crimson-stained bandage – a silent witness to the violent dance of metal and bone. Whisked away through dusty roads to Jain Hospital, Bengaluru, his entrance would make any Kollywood hero proud, with an action-packed backstory and a blood-soaked headband as his anti-hero's accessory.

Underneath, the story grows grimmer: a gaping wound, a skull fracture, pieces of his skull bone broken and even missing, and blood scattered on the asphalt. The plot thickens as I, the protagonist in white, unravel the mystery wrapped over his forehead. To the onlooker's horror, his frontal lobe—a pulped mass of brain —lay in my grasp, a grisly token of his ordeal. Yet, amidst this grim tableau, our hero converses, reminisces, and commands his limbs with the might of a warrior resurrected from the battlefield. His consciousness, unfazed by the carnage, perplexed the minds of mortals.

Yet, defying the grisly visuals is a miracle: he speaks, remembers, and moves! This man, ensnared in a gory spectacle, his brain's sanctum exposed, is alive and recounting his tale. The contrast is stark and bewildering— the resilience of life scripting a hopeful path amidst the chaos. It's a story of sheer tenacity, a narrative of the human spirit that refuses to bow to life's direst script.

In a twist worthy of cinema's finest, what seems like a sure prelude to tragedy becomes a testament to the enigma of human survival. A man, his mind's sanctum laid bare, conversing with the gods of life and death, while we stand as mere spectators to this dance of destiny.

Here is what seems like a hopeless and gory head injury, aka Traumatic Brain Injury or TBI; part of the patient's frontal lobe is pulped and, in my hands, and he is talking and moving his limbs. On the other extreme, we have deeply unconscious patients, without even a fracture of their skull or any cut on their heads, but deeply unconscious. Wow!

This is what we call the difference between focal and diffuse brain injuries. You will learn more as we progress in this chapter.

Do you think head injury patients need life memberships in hospitals? Like clubs? Or offers like those seen in malls— 'buy two and take one free' facilities in hospitals? I think so. To know more, read on.

One day, around 8 am, I was scrubbed up and operating on a patient with a brain tumor, and my mobile phone rang. And, as is the norm, my anesthetist, Dr. Jagadish, answered the phone and started telling the person on the other side that I was operating when he heard a familiar voice... He paused, listened for a few seconds, and realized it was Dr. Mahendra Jain, our urologist! He sounded desperate and told Jaggi that his cousin had had an accident, he had a head injury, had been unconscious since the accident, and he was bringing him to our hospital. We said OK. This guy was brought into the emergency with a coma score of 9/15, had a left-sided limb weakness, and a CT scan showed a right frontal contusion (blood clot inside the brain) and overlying acute SDH (Sub-Dural hematoma) with severe raised ICP (Intracranial Pressure).

We immediately operated on him – removed the clots, and did a DECRA surgery – decompressive craniotomy, because the brain was swollen and caused severe pressure inside a fixed skull cavity (the pressure cooker effect). The removed skull bone is not replaced on the head but kept in a pocket (for safekeeping) in the anterior abdominal wall.

After 6-8 weeks, he had made a reasonable recovery from his head injury and coma, and we replaced the skull. He had cognitive, memory, and behavioral issues and underwent intensive neuropsychological rehabilitation by Dr. Prathiba. At the end of about four months, he had made a remarkable recovery and returned to his job as a CA. So far, so good.

Incidentally, he lives near my house, and I bump into him often. But what is the amazing thing is – this guy, who has fully recovered, is back to his job as a CA (meaning he has understood whatever had happened to him), a typical 'coma to the community' story of ours, I see him in our area, riding his scooter without a helmet. I have stopped and counseled him, taken pictures and videos of him doing this, and sent it to my doc friend, but to no avail. I feel he needs our life membership plan!

One wrong turn proved fatal!

Let me educate you with a tale from the '1990s, the era of pagers and questionable fashion choices. I was training at Manipal Hospital on Airport Road in Bangalore, offering backup to the Command Hospital, an excellent place for the armed forces that didn't have a neurosurgery department. One day, an army doctor's son had a head injury from a two-wheeler accident. The lad got up from the road after the initial, so-called concussion and, in a heroic move, rode his bike home, casually mentioning his newfound headache to his dad.

Long story short, the father realized that the kid needed a CT scan, and that's where I swooped in, capes metaphorically billowing. The army doc was grateful, and I couldn't help but think, "If only he knew I'd soon be fighting not just head injuries but also the battle for proper neuro rehab." And so, the saga continued one brain at a time, with a sprinkle of humor and a dash of determination.

The army doc dad, a reader of all things medical, being a radiologist, quickly realized that his son needed a CT scan, but alas, the CT scan era had just begun in Bengaluru city, and there were just a handful of them then and command hospital was stuck in the pre-CT era. What does he do? As he exited the gate of the command hospital in an ambulance with his son, he had to make what looked at that time as a simple choice – do we go left or right? Left was into the city to a close friend, who had just established a CT scan center, or right, to Manipal Hospital. And he chose left. Little did the father realize then that the decision to go left would be fatal for his son. Imagine, does any father want to make a decision that can potentially kill their son? NEVER.

Off he goes to the city's heart, where his friend's diagnostic center is conveniently located. They slap the poor lad onto the scanner, and bam, there it is – BIG a brain clot, called an acute extradural hematoma, or what we call EDH, the kind that screams "emergency surgery needed ASAP!"

This was the pre-mobile phone era. Many of you reading this book may not even be able to imagine that such an era existed. I was on an emergency call that day, and we received a call that such-and-such patient was being brought in for emergency surgery and to be on standby. My adrenaline kicked in, and I got everything organized, and we anxiously awaited the patient's arrival.

But here's the kicker – from the moment this life-or-death decision was made to the boy's grand entrance at the Manipal Hospital's emergency, he was already pushing up daisies. Yep, you heard it right. He arrived in the emergency room with all the drama, but the lights were out. The father was gutted. *He told me that his son had just stopped breathing about 500 meters from the hospital, and he didn't know what to do. Can you imagine?* Nobody would have realized that the decision to turn left would land up taking his son's life! How cruel can such a mundane decision be... but readers, this is life in the fast lane... in fields like neurosurgery, when one momentary lapse, one wrong decision can decide between 'life and death.' The entire emergency surgery system of the hospital was ready to save his life, but God decided otherwise. Talk about a plot twist!

Now, skeptics might argue, "But hey, he was conscious, he rode his bike, he was fine!" Ah, my dear, this is where the tale turns sinister. Our hero had a classic case of the "Lucid Interval," a phenomenon where you get knocked out, shake it off, and then, well, not wake up again. Think boxing matches, where fighters get up, slug it out, and then forget to set their morning alarms.

The lesson of the day: Lucid intervals after a head injury are like red flags with sirens and flashing lights. Your brain says, "Hey, something ain't right here." So, whether you're a radiologist, a rocket scientist, or a part-time amateur detective, knowing the signs can be the real superhero cape in saving lives. As discussed in the first chapter, road traffic accidents are globally the primary cause of death. They're nastier than any pandemic and, unfortunately, are ever-growing. You can only do so much to educate people about road safety.

In fact, at the peak of the American war in Afghanistan, when there was a massive hue and cry amongst the American public about the large number of American soldiers who had died in the war, the NYT carried an editorial headed – how Americans are crying hoarse about the 3,000 odd American soldiers who die in the Afghan war, but the same people do not care about the 200,000 odd Americans who are dying every year on American roads and highways! What an irony. It is the same everywhere. People are dying like flies on highways!

Statistically, over seven million deaths have happened throughout the world due to COVID-19 over the past three years. Note the point- 7 million in 3 years… But when it comes to RTAs, over 1.3 million people die globally every single year. And the worst fact is that it is only increasing alarmingly! 1.3 million every single year!!!

COVID had a proper vaccine, but what about road traffic accidents? They do not have a vaccine, and the aftermath is usually permanent if not treated correctly at the right time.

Dear reader, whether you're a doctor, therapist, medical student, caregiver, teacher, scientist, or whatever, ensure you wear a helmet before getting on the bike. Also, ensure you've worn a seat belt, even if you're in the back seat. As I always say, accidents treat the president and the beggar alike, so influence, type of car, social status, and money are of zero value when it comes to a fatal accident. Like COVID, head injuries are also remarkably democratic!

Head injuries may happen even if you fall from heights or trip and fall inside your house. Older people, especially those on blood thinners, are particularly susceptible to falls at home, making awareness campaigns about home safety equally crucial.

And the chances of recovery are narrow. This is why you must be mindful of 'the golden hour.'

What is 'the golden hour'?

The critical period between experiencing an accident and receiving definitive care at a hospital is pivotal in determining the outcomes for trauma patients. This duration, often called the "golden hour," underscores the importance of swift and efficient pre-hospital care. The average time lost during this crucial window can significantly impact the severity of outcomes and overall survival rates.

In many urban areas, the response time for emergency services can vary significantly, typically ranging from 8 to 15 minutes, depending on traffic conditions, time of day, and the efficiency of the emergency response system. However, this is just the beginning of the pre-hospital care timeline. Once at the scene, emergency medical personnel must assess the situation, stabilize the patient, and prepare for transport, which can add another 10 to 30 minutes to the timeline. Transport time to the hospital is another critical component. In well-coordinated systems, this can be as quick as 15 to 20 minutes, but transport times can exceed an hour in less optimized systems or rural areas. During transport, medical interventions such as airway management, fluid resuscitation, and bleeding control are crucial and can significantly influence patient outcomes.

Studies suggest that the total average pre-hospital time—from the accident to arrival at a hospital capable of providing definitive care—can range from 30 minutes to over an hour in urban settings. In rural settings, where distances are greater, and healthcare resources may be sparser, this time can extend much longer, often exceeding two hours. The extended time in pre-hospital care in rural areas highlights the disparity in trauma outcomes between urban and rural populations. The longer duration not only delays essential surgical interventions but also increases the risk of complications such as infection, prolonged pain, and, in severe cases, death.

To minimize these delays, many regions are enhancing their emergency medical services by improving first responders' training, increasing the availability of ambulances, and using technology to ensure quicker and more efficient routes to hospitals. Additionally, air ambulances have become more common in accessing remote areas quickly.

In conclusion, the average time lost before a trauma patient reaches definitive hospital care is a crucial metric that influences the effectiveness of trauma systems worldwide. Efforts to reduce this time through better infrastructure, training, and technology are vital to improving patient outcomes and are a key focus of public health initiatives in trauma care.

What happens when an ambulance is not available? Autorickshaws are seen to be transporting more patients than ambulances. Is that true?

In India and similar developing economies, the availability and efficiency of ambulance services vary significantly, leading to notable disparities in emergency medical responses. Although there are formal systems like the Dial 108 for emergency services and Dial 102 for patient transport, these services often struggle with issues such as delayed response times, averaging between 41 to 47 minutes, and logistical inefficiencies such as inadequate vehicle maintenance and insufficient supervision or the commonest challenge – TRAFFIC JAMS.

This inconsistency in emergency response is exacerbated by a mismatch between the number of ambulances and the actual need, further compounded by infrastructure challenges. While the number of ambulances might meet World Health Organization standards, the functionality and accessibility of these services remain compromised.

Given these challenges, individuals in urgent need of medical care often resort to alternative means of transportation, such as auto-rickshaws. This practice highlights both the resourcefulness of the populace and the significant deficiencies within the healthcare infrastructure that need urgent attention to ensure timely medical interventions.

What is the common scenario on Indian roads? Especially in the cities...

In the din and chaos of Indian roads, where wrong-way drivers or late-night tipsy adventures are not a rarity, the 'golden hour' is a literal and figurative lifeline. The golden hour, that precious window where timely medical intervention can mean the difference between life and death, begins the moment an accident occurs, not in the sanitized corridors of a hospital.

Let me give you another tragic story here. **The message I want to give from this story is never drive on the highways after 11:00 PM.** This was my cousin. She was married. Both are IT professionals, husband and wife, working in Hyderabad. Her husband is from Bihar, and his younger brother used to work in Bangalore. His mother came to visit them from Bihar, and she came to Bangalore. So, these two decided to come to Bangalore to visit her. So, they did a full day's work, had dinner at eight o'clock, and at nine o'clock at night, and their husband and wife decided to drive to Bangalore. They thought they would save the night. So, they were driving. At three o'clock in the morning, my cousin's husband missed a parked truck on the side of the highway at night. He went into the truck from behind, *and my cousin died on the spot.* It was such a tragedy. So, when I went to their house to pay my respects to the family, the entire family was sitting there, and everybody was so upset that the truck fellow had parked there, this and that, badmouthing everyone.

You can't blame anybody because the emotions were very high. And the whole thing was, one of my aunties said, that guy, the truck fellow who parked in the road like that or half road? He shouldn't have done that and all these things. They don't have any sense. So I said – see, Aunty, people will do what they want in India. That's the reality of the process. The important thing is - they had no business being on the road at three o'clock in the morning. Because the truth is, guys, people will drink, people will drive, people will fall asleep at the wheel, and whatever is going to happen will happen. And after a full day's work, who's brain has the attention to continue to work? You tell me.

There's an article by the British Medical Journal, probably 8-10 years ago. They studied the percentage of mistakes anesthesia doctors make if they're continuously on duty. Do you know what they found? If anesthesia doctors are on duty continuously for more than 24 hours, after 24 hours of continuous duty, the percentage of their mistakes is 50 %. So, do you think this is limited to anaesthesiologists? Of course not.

Anaesthesiologists are also normal human beings like you and me and anybody else who's not a doctor, a software engineer, a professional, a politician, an engineer, whatever. Now, you may argue that many truck drivers, such as bus drivers, drive at night. Of course. But these guys are given rest. They should rest during the daytime and then do their night driving. It's their profession. That's why they have two drivers in some long-distance lorries. So that is their profession, and that's what they care for. Yes, they're also involved in accidents. But I want to communicate this big moral of the story.

Visualize the scene: a mishap on the bustling streets of Delhi or Bengaluru, a crowd gathers – a mix of curiosity and concern, yet hesitation stifles immediate action. Amid the anxious bystanders, the knowledge of calling an ambulance remains a mystery. This critical delay marks the beginning of the golden hour's countdown.

Complications abound when well-meaning onlookers, rather than aiding, become entangled in altercations with the responsible party, inadvertently hindering the swift passage of emergency services. Here, amidst the drama, valuable minutes of the golden hour ticks away as potential help morphs into silent spectators, their smartphones raised not to call for help but to capture the event for their social feeds, paralyzed by the fear of legal entanglement.

Then there's the ambulance driver, sometimes unknowingly, playing a grim lottery with the patient's fate, choosing the destination based on undisclosed incentives rather than medical necessities – another disheartening leakage of precious golden minutes.

If the patient arrives at a well-equipped hospital by some stroke of luck, the emergency team's expertise, communication efficiency, and the readiness of the neurosurgery unit become the next critical links in this chain of survival. It's a relay race against time where every handoff and decision can significantly impact the outcome.

Educating the public on basic first aid and the importance of timely medical assistance can transform bystanders into lifesavers. It's about instilling a sense of urgency and responsibility, about teaching society to prioritize humanity over curiosity.

Let's not forget the essential road etiquette—when the wail of an ambulance siren pierces through the urban hum, it's a clarion call to every driver and pedestrian. Give way, for in the hierarchy of haste, nothing is more pressing than the need to save a life. Those flashing lights and urgent sirens are not a mere inconvenience but a beacon of hope for someone fighting the most crucial battle.

So, the next time the siren's cry reaches your ears, pause, yield, and send a silent prayer for the unknown soul, hoping they win the race against the golden hour.

Sometimes, I make decisions on behalf of the family... because, many times, their brains (and even ours) stop working due to the shock of the emergency.

Let me tell you one such story of one of my earliest head injuries. The year was 2004 roundabouts. Her name is Shreya Mayur. She was not married at the time. She was riding in the back seat of a two-wheeler of her cousin. She was not wearing a helmet. They had a road traffic accident exactly opposite the hospital I used to work for. And because she was exactly opposite the hospital, she was rushed into our hospital, and I was there! Talk about luck & destiny. And she was semi-conscious. She had a Glasgow Coma score of 11/15. She was quite restless. She had been bleeding from the nose and the ears. So, she had some kind of head injury. She had a swelling on the right side of her head. So, we needed to get an urgent CT scan of her head done. Unfortunately, at the hospital, I was working at that time, the CT scan was not working. So, we had to send her to St. John's Medical College Hospital, which was the closest then, for a CT scan. I sent her in an ambulance with assistance and everything else. I was monitoring her from here.

By the time she finished the scan in St.John's, the radiologist called me and said she had a large acute extradural hematoma (EDH) and most probably needed surgery. Her GCS had dropped from 11 to 5, there only. So, at St. John's, I requested him to give her an injection of Mannitol to reduce the brain swelling and then rushed her back here. By the time she came here, she was extending to pain. She was in a GCS of 4 by 15. We had to put her on the intubation immediately, put her on the ventilator, and had to rush her to the OT to operate.

Now, by the time what had happened, the family had come, and she didn't have a father. So, the father's elder brother was like the guardian, along with her mother. And he was very upset with me because I had shifted her to the OT by the time he came, and he came to talk to me in the changing room. And he said, "NO, I want to take her to a bigger hospital because this is a smaller hospital." I said – Sir, she's already in the OT. If you take her out of the OT, you're going to get a dead body by the time you go anywhere else. She's very bad. I'm not going to send her anywhere. Leave her to me. I'm going to operate.

I fired that uncle, made him sit outside, and went inside to operate *'Jabardasti.'* He looked at me. He didn't know what to say. He said, "Okay". And I operated on her. We removed the extradural hematoma. She went through a craniotomy. And then, for two weeks, she was unconscious, slowly getting better. And then, eventually, after about a month or six weeks, she recovered completely. She's now happily married. She's got two children. We have become great friends now. We haven't seen each other's families. We call each other occasionally, and that's how the family is now.

TYPES OF HEAD INJURIES (FOCAL VS. DAI)

As we have already discussed, head injuries are a wide and complicated category of trauma that can result in a wide range of consequences, both immediate and long-term. Learning and understanding the different types of head injuries is crucial for accurate diagnosis, effective treatment, and prognostic considerations.

Let us look into the two primary classifications of head injuries: focal injuries, which localize damage to specific areas, and diffuse axonal injuries (DAI), which involve more widespread damage across neural pathways.

1. **Focal Head Injuries:**

Focal head injuries are traumas that are confined to a specific spot of the brain. These injuries typically result from a direct blow or force applied to the skull, leading to severe damage in a specific area. Let's use a real-life example to make it easier for you- you all love hanging photo frames in your room, right? Imagine punching a hole in the wall using a hammer and nail. You keep the metal nail at your desired position and hit it with a hammer. A hole in the wall will be right where you fixed the needle. Just like that, when your head gets hit by something, there will be damage, specifically to where the injury happened. The severity and symptoms associated with focal injuries depend on the location and extent of the damage. Common types of focal head injuries include:

a. **Contusions:**

Like bruises or clots in the muscle, contusions are blood clots within the brain. They occur when your head is struck hard or stops suddenly, as in a fall or a vehicle accident. Small blood vessels inside the brain may burst due to this collision, resulting in bleeding and swelling. Consider your brain as a squishy jelly enclosed in a hard shell, your skull. There is jelly rattling around inside your skull when you have a contusion, which damages it. This damage can impair the function of that area of your brain, similar to when you bump your arm and it hurts or isn't functioning well for a while.

b. Traumatic Hematomas – EDH and SDH

Hematomas are similar to little blood collections outside of blood vessels in the body. Regarding your head, hematomas can be classified into two primary types: (i) epidural hematomas and (ii) subdural hematomas.

i. When blood builds up between the skull and the hard outer layer of the brain (called the dura mater), an epidural hematoma (EDH) occurs. It resembles blood clotting in the area between your brain's outer layer and the hard shell of your skull. This may occur if your head is struck suddenly, such as during a fall or a hit. Blood clots can exert pressure on the brain, resulting in various symptoms associated with brain function. On a CT scan, it looks like the South Indian dish, idly.

ii. Blood clots between the layers of the tissue protecting your brain and the brain's surface cause subdural hematomas (SDH). It feels like blood accumulating in the spaces between your brain's protective covering layers. Similar to epidural hematomas, this can also result from head trauma. Depending on where and how much pressure is applied to the brain, it can induce various neurological symptoms. This is very common in the elderly and those who take blood thinners. Such patients also suffer from a variant of the SDH called sub-acute or chronic SDH. ***The famous Indian spiritual Guru Sadguru was recently operated for this.***

Both types of hematomas are serious because they can press on your brain and affect its normal functioning, potentially causing symptoms like headaches, confusion, weakness, or even loss of consciousness.

c. Skull Fractures

When something hits your head hard, it can cause the bones in your skull to crack or break. This is called a skull fracture. It's like when you drop something hard, and it breaks into pieces. Relate it to a nice crystal glass.

Sometimes, these fractures happen without any injury to your brain, but they can still indicate a lot of force involved. Other times, they can be linked to injuries inside your brain, like bleeding or bruising.

So, if someone has a skull fracture, it's a sign that they've experienced a significant impact on their head, and it's important to check for any potential brain injuries, too. Skull fractures can occur on the convexity (of the top of the skull) or the skull base (indirectly indicated by bleeding from the nose, ears, and mouth).

2. Diffuse Axonal Injury (DAI):

In contrast to focal traumas, diffuse axonal injury (DAI) is a more extensive and diffuse type of brain damage. This kind of injury happens when the head is subjected to a powerful rotating force that tears or shears many nerve fibers, or axons, throughout the brain. DAI is frequently observed in high-impact incidents, like serious auto accidents or a fall. In contrast to localized damage, DAI impacts several brain regions at once and is linked to more serious outcomes. Acceleration-deceleration forces that cause the brain to move inside the skull are the mechanisms causing DAI, which inflict extensive damage to neuronal connections.

Treatment options

Let us now understand the various treatment options/methods for both conditions mentioned above:

1. Focal Head Injuries:

For focal injuries, treatment is precisely aimed at the damaged zone, where specific brain areas are impacted. Options include surgeries to remove blood clots (hematomas) or to decrease the pressure on the brain caused by swelling (contusions). Alongside these interventions, patients often receive medication to control the brain's swelling and prevent secondary issues like seizures. Recovery plans for focal injuries require a nuanced approach to ensure the best outcomes.

2. Diffuse Axonal Injury (DAI):

DAI is characterized by widespread brain damage and requires a broad-based treatment approach. Primary care involves maintaining critical life functions, like breathing and circulation, and managing intracranial pressure.

Prognosis and Rehabilitation

1. Focal Injuries:

The outlook for someone with a focal injury depends on several factors, including where in the brain the injury is, how bad it is, and how quickly treatment begins. With effective, prompt care and rehabilitation efforts, some patients with focal injuries can significantly recover. However, others may experience ongoing challenges and require long-term support.

2. Diffuse Axonal Injury (DAI):

Patients with DAI often face a tougher road to recovery. The prognosis is typically more guarded due to the extensive and diffuse nature of the injury. Because DAI can disrupt multiple brain functions, individuals often face a lengthy and complex rehabilitation process. Rehab efforts are geared towards enhancing patient abilities and compensating for deficits, striving to improve the quality of life for those affected.

Diffuse Axonal Injury (DAI) - The 'Poltergeist' of Brain Injuries

DAI stands out in the spectrum of traumatic brain injuries for its elusive and pervasive nature, often staying hidden until its effects become more apparent. It occurs when sudden forces cause tearing of the brain's axonal fibers, resulting in a scatter of injuries.

The Silent Intruder: Understanding DAI

1. Mechanisms of Injury:

DAI often results from high-velocity impacts or shaking that subject the brain's axons to forces they cannot withstand, leading to widespread neurological damage.

2. Widespread Neural Damage:

Unlike focal injuries, DAI is not contained in one area but involves the axons throughout the brain. It disrupts critical networks for cognitive and motor functions and poses significant challenges in diagnosis and management.

3. Invisible and Pervasive:

DAI can initially be deceptive, showing little evidence of the chaos it has wrought, akin to the hidden nature of a poltergeist. It's critical to monitor patients closely after an injury for any signs indicating the presence of DAI.

4. Delayed Manifestations:

Symptoms can develop slowly, making DAI akin to an unseen force that reveals its presence and impact over time. Recognizing DAI calls for a vigilant, methodical approach post-injury to identify and address the extensive repercussions it can have on the individual's neurological health.

Clinical Manifestations:

1. Cognitive Impairments:

Diffuse Axonal Injury (DAI) can precipitate a spectrum of cognitive deficits, encompassing memory loss, attention difficulties, and impaired executive functions. As a result, individuals grappling with DAI may encounter challenges in decision-making and problem-solving, significantly impacting their daily functioning and interpersonal relationships. These cognitive impairments not only pose hurdles in navigating day-to-day tasks but also exert profound emotional and social ramifications, necessitating comprehensive support and rehabilitation interventions tailored to address the multifaceted needs of those affected by DAI. Unfortunately, cognitive and perceptual deficits render people without physical impairments unfit to return to daily life, work, and leisure and make them dependent.

2. Motor Deficits:

Diffuse Axonal Injury (DAI) causes significant damage to brain networks, which can lead to motor deficits that affect balance, coordination, and fine motor abilities. Only a 'functional Independence' evaluation can determine the deficits. These deficits have to be connected back to the areas of the brain that control them. This is an example of CAREPa- Re Framework. Intense rehabilitation efforts focused on regaining functional independence are often necessary to address these deficiencies. People with DAI work to retrain their motor skills, overcome physical obstacles, and regain control over their daily tasks through specialized therapy and exercises. For those coping with the motor after-effects of DAI, such rehabilitation initiatives are critical to their recovery and quality of life.

3. Sensory Disturbances:

Diffuse Axonal Injury (DAI) can impair sensory processing, leading to changes in hearing, vision, or spatial awareness. This may manifest as difficulties in correctly interpreting sensory inputs, which makes it more difficult for a person to manage their environment efficiently. These sensory disturbances can significantly influence day-to-day functioning and quality of life. Thus, specific interventions and support are needed to lessen their effects and help the affected person adapt to their new sensory environment.

Diagnostic Challenges:

1. Hidden on Imaging:

Diffuse Axonal Injury (DAI) can be difficult to diagnose since it often goes undetected in traditional imaging investigations such as computed tomography (CT) scans. Due to their subtle nature, axonal injuries require sophisticated tools to reveal the diffuse damage occurring within the brain, such as magnetic resonance imaging (MRI) with particular sequences. Through advanced imaging technologies, healthcare professionals can comprehensively comprehend the scope and dispersion of DAI, leading to more precise diagnoses and well-informed treatment choices.

2. Clinical Suspicion:

When dealing with severe injuries that do not exhibit any obvious abnormalities on initial imaging scans, diagnosing diffuse axonal injury (DAI) often depends on a high index of clinical suspicion. Given the enigmatic nature of DAI and the possibility of delayed symptom manifestation, medical practitioners need to remain watchful. Healthcare practitioners can rapidly identify indications suggestive of DAI and conduct appropriate diagnostic investigations by continuously monitoring patients and being aware of subtle clinical indicators. This allows for timely intervention and optimal patient outcomes.

The Impact on Individuals and Families:

1. Long-Term Consequences:

Diffuse Axonal Injury (DAI), or for that matter any TBI, is a pervasive and diffuse injury that often has long-term effects on those who are affected. These people could experience persistent difficulties with their day-to-day activities, requiring continuous assistance and modifications to lessen the effects of their wounds. These ongoing challenges may affect different facets of life, such as the cognitive, motor, sensory, and emotional domains; therefore, comprehensive and ongoing interventions specifically designed to meet the diverse needs of those living with DAI's aftereffects are imperative. Healthcare providers and caregivers can help individuals coping with the long-term impacts of DAI adapt and improve their quality of life by offering continuous support and creating a supportive environment.

2. Emotional and Psychological Toll:

Dealing with Diffuse Axonal Injury (DAI), or for that matter any TBI, aftermath goes much beyond accommodating physical restrictions. DAI exacts a high emotional and psychological cost that significantly affects affected persons as well as their families. These costs include emotions of frustration, depression, or personality changes. These psychological difficulties can make the recovery process extremely difficult, and strain relationships with others, which emphasizes the significance of holistic care approaches that take into account the emotional and psychological needs of individuals affected by DAI in addition to their physical needs. Healthcare providers and support systems may assist people and their families in managing the emotional upheaval of life after DAI by identifying and meeting these complex emotional requirements. This promotes resilience and makes meaningful recovery journeys possible.

Rehabilitation and Management

1. Multidisciplinary Approach:

A comprehensive and multidisciplinary approach is necessary for managing diffuse axonal injury (DAI), or for that matter, any TBI, wherein different healthcare specialists work together synergistically to address the wide spectrum of deficiencies related to this disorder. With their in-depth knowledge of brain pathology and function, neurologists are essential in directing the course of diagnosis and treatment. To promote the best possible recovery and independence in daily activities, occupational therapists and physical therapists use their specific knowledge to help restore motor and functional deficits. Neuropsychologists provide techniques to deal with cognitive deficiencies and psychological difficulties, as well as insight into the emotional and cognitive components of DAI. By working together, we can provide DAI patients with comprehensive care that considers all aspects of their disease, increasing their chances of recovery and improving their quality of life.

2. Rehabilitation Programs:

Personalized therapies are provided by tailored rehabilitation programs, which are the cornerstone of managing Diffuse Axonal Injury (DAI), or for that matter, any TBI, and its diverse array of deficiencies. A major component of these programs is intensive physical and occupational therapy, which aims to improve motor abilities and promote functional independence. Individuals impacted by DAI or TBI strive to restore agility, mobility, and coordination through focused workouts and therapies, eventually enhancing their capacity to perform daily life activities. Another important concurrent element is cognitive rehabilitation, which targets memory, attention, and executive function deficiencies. Cognitive rehabilitation uses various methods and approaches to maximize cognitive capacities and improve general cognitive functioning.

By combining these approaches, tailored rehabilitation programs empower individuals with DAI to achieve their fullest potential and regain a sense of control over their lives.

Neuro rehabilitation plays an essential role in the overall progress of neurosurgical and neurological patients. We've observed significant improvements in patients after undergoing neuro rehabilitation. It's important to note that this isn't a generalized form of physiotherapy; it involves specific aspects tailored to each patient's needs.

For instance, patients who have undergone tracheostomy require speech therapy and swallowing assessments to minimize the risk of aspiration. Aspiration occurs when a patient accidentally swallows food into the windpipe instead of the food pipe, leading to chest infections and further complications.

This sets off a cycle of events, ultimately leading to deterioration in the patient's overall consciousness level and possibly requiring ICU admission. Proper assessment and systematic evaluation are crucial for these patients to ensure they receive the appropriate treatment and care.

This is another head injury story – from coma back to work! An end-to-end C2C story.

This is probably 2014 or '15 story. I got a call around 6:30 - 7:00 AM one morning from my close friend, Purnima Nambiar. She told me that Sharan, my cousin, Praveen Nambiar, had had an accident last night around 3:00 when he was coming back from the airport in a taxi and going towards his house. The car was hit by another car near Raj Bhavan near the GPO. You can imagine what the situation is. So, this can happen to any of us. It was a bad crash. He had been unconscious at the time of the accident. The cops picked him up because he was 'unknown,' and they were on patrol and rushed him to the nearest government hospital, Bowring Hospital, where he was lying for a couple of hours. And because he was very sick, he needed to go to a hospital with neurosurgical care, which they didn't have, and so on. She immediately came to know. She saw his health there and said, "He needs to be shifted. Can I bring him to Jain Hospital?" And she rushed him to Jain Hospital. When he came to Jain Hospital, he was deeply unconscious. His coma score was above 6-7/ 15. He was not breathing very well, so we immediately intubated him and put him on the ventilator.

The CT scan showed what we call a severe diffuse axonal injury, which didn't need any surgery. He was put on a ventilator, and we were managing conservatively. So, two and a half weeks on the ventilator. Because of this delay in the government hospital in intubating him, he aspirated and developed aspiration pneumonia. We treated all of that. Eventually, because of prolonged ventilation, he needed a tracheostomy. His GCS didn't improve much. Remained 6,7,8,- 6,7,8, - 7, 8 by 15 for many weeks. Slowly, we weaned him off the ventilator, and about three and a half weeks after that, we shifted him to the ward. Maybe a week or ten days into the ward, he opened his eyes, looked around, and got some basic consciousness level. He was a senior Vice President with Citibank, working in Bangalore. Once he woke up, he started trying to identify his wife and daughter and slowly started responding to all of us. So, by the time the neuro rehabilitation was in full flow, with all our usual waking up the unconscious brain, keeping the body future-ready, the swallow therapies, tracheostomy care, and getting his modified barium swallow done to see how safe his swallow was, and speech therapy and everything was going on.

He had a left-side weakness, which was more obvious by about the second week and slowly improving. Once he woke up and started telling his name and communicating, we realized he didn't recognize his wife or daughter. He thought his wife was a colleague. He didn't know who the daughter was; he was stuck in some world, and it was a struggle. One day, the wife came and told me, "Doc, I thought he was recognizing me. Today, I realized he thought I was his colleague in the office." He does not even remember his wife, and she cries. Then I told Dr. Prathiba & she did caregiver counseling. She made her understand how this whole thing goes in people with head injuries. It was a work in progress, painful, traumatic, mentally, psychologically. Dr. Prathiba's cognitive retraining team came in. The behavioral team came in. He used to be happy-go-lucky, speaking whatever he wanted. Slowly, we mobilized him. Then came a stage because he was able to walk to the bathroom. We sent him home. He needed to continue outpatient rehab because he needed all departments, which are physical therapy, occupation therapy, speech, language, swallowing, memory, cognition, behavior, and all of that.

Let's hear about his cognitive rehabilitation journey from Dr. Prathiba.

When I saw Praveen for the first time in the hospital, he wasn't in any state to recall his name or identify his family members anybody. He looked very confused, but he kept talking about his office. Anything I asked him, question, who is this? Who is that? He kept saying things related to his work and his office. He thought his daughter was his secretary or office staff. His wife was one of the staff. He kept thinking like that. His wife was disheartened because he wasn't identifying her, her daughter, or any family member. She was disheartened.

But I think it hardly took any time for him to come out of his so-called physical ailment. He did not have a problem with walking or doing his own ADL and things like that. Physically, he looked very all right. Cognitively, he was a mess. He was confused. He was disoriented. He had no clue what people were talking to him. The only thing he kept responding to was about the work. Not that his speech was not all right. He was speaking well but was completely irrelevant and disoriented.

That is where we realized he had software issues, not the hardware issue. So, he was walking around talking as though everything was all right, but cognitively, he was dysfunctional. That is when I spoke to the wife for a very long time and understood that he kept talking only about work the whole day. Anything anybody spoke, he kept telling about his work. He thought the whole environment was his workplace. So, I took this as a cue and decided to enter into his life through the work process. So, when we spoke to him, we started asking him about work. Slowly, we started entering his life, and he started relating to us. Then, when the assessments were done, he kept thinking he was doing something at the office. We continued to say it was office work and kept doing the assessments. Finally, there were a lot of impairments. Though there were impairments, we continued to do the cognitive rehabilitation through his work language. It took almost a month for him to stabilize, start orienting himself, recognize his wife and daughter as they are, and recognize his family members. Slowly, he started identifying.

He also started to understand that he had a problem and he was undergoing some treatment. But it took, I think, to say, a very long time for him to recollect what was told. So, the memory circuits and the attention circuits were not working. So, with the intense cognitive retraining, almost for six months, he started slowly relating to what was happening, what was happening to him, what was happening to the family, how disheartened they were, and what the impact of his accident on the family and himself. That is when he took it seriously to undergo rehab, before which his family had to force him to bring him to rehab. But after that, he volunteered to say that I wanted to improve. I want to go back to work. These were the statements from him. Then, after over a year of intense training, when we did an assessment, I think out of the 17 different tasks that we had assessed him on, he cleared off almost 15 of them. This was over a year. And there were two or three impairments left, but he was so functional that he could almost live a near-normal life.

After attending a couple of interviews, he found some shortcomings in the memory and behavior circuits. Otherwise, on the whole, he was looking all right. He sounded all right. He also cleared some of his interviews and got back his job. Though he did not return to his original job in the same office, he got a job almost equivalent to that, or I could say a little better than what he was doing with the functionality he gained over one and a half years.

One important thing in the cognitive retraining, the CBT that I used, was that he was very spiritual. And I think, as we all understand, the Shlokas help a lot with cognitive functions. That is one proof that I got with Praveen, that he returned a memory of all the Shlokas, whether it is Vishnu Sahasranama or Gayatri Mantra, all those things. He would get back to that. Initially, he couldn't remember them, but he started reading them. Finally, he got to a state where he could recite them without looking at the book. I think that was an additional impact that the cognitive retraining had, as was what we were doing.

From this, I understood that the Shlokas played a big role. So, anybody who had some Shlokas or mantras recital in their previous life. That is when they were all right and used to these things. Getting them to start reciting or remembering these things is good, which adds dimension to cognitive retraining. And Praveen was proof of that. Praveen is back to work now, back to his family life, enjoying his family life, enjoying his work. And he's very prompt when calling on any occasion to wish for birthdays or festivals. He's in touch with me. It feels so good when your patient is in touch with you, almost near normal cognitively.

In conclusion, traumatic brain injuries can be prevented through safety measures: helmets during sports and cycling, vehicle seatbelts, and fall-proof living spaces, especially for the elderly. Management is equally critical: seek immediate medical attention for head injuries, even minor ones. Early treatment can mitigate long-term effects. Remember, the brain is your command center; protect it like the precious resource it is. Always consult healthcare professionals and trusted medical websites for comprehensive information and resources.

Educate yourself and others, especially children, on how to play safely. Remember, it's not just about wearing a helmet; it's about making smart choices to avoid injury in the first place. Rash-driving is a risk to yourself and your co-passengers, people walking on the road, your family, friends, and your employer! Think before experimenting with your life next time by driving recklessly! Or even worse... drinking and driving!

Now let us take a look at the stories of some more individuals who were brought back to life from TBI at PRS Neurosciences:

Vidhi Mulani- the story of one of our youngest friends.

A story from a coma to college!

Vidhi came from Mumbai to Bangalore to chill and have fun with her cousins during her college vacation. Bangalore, being the tech hub, is vibrant throughout the day, but that isn't anything new to a Mumbaikar. Vidhi and her cousins decided to visit Nandi Hills instead of roaming through commercial and church streets this time. After watching the beautiful and bright sun rising from amidst the clouds, they thought they could return home and snuggle under a blanket to compensate for the sleep they lost while waiting for Mr. Sun.

Happily, they started their bikes and kept moving, and then suddenly, a truck, which was completely out of control, ran over Vidhi's bike. The poor young lady was thrown away from the vehicle in a matter of a few seconds. She suffered a severe head injury. But what makes her case unique is the fact that her injury was confined to only one side of her body and that her brain circuits declared war inside the brain, resulting in a high body temperature. Dr. Krishna Prasad, a neurosurgeon on our team and a visiting consultant at the hospital where Vidhi was taken, says this.

"Vidhi Mulani, I can't forget that patient because one fine morning, I received a call from a local hospital in Yelahanka, where they had admitted a young lady patient, around 17 or 18 years old, involved in a road traffic accident near the Nandi Hills. I rushed to the hospital to find her in a very severe neurological condition.

Regarding the Glasgow Coma Scale (GCS), she scored E1VTM4. The scan they had performed showed a large subdural hematoma. When I discussed the situation with her relatives, mainly her cousin and another friend of her cousin who had brought her to the hospital, they were shocked by her condition and the accident.

Furthermore, the patient's parents were in Mumbai, adding to the situation's complexity. However, as a neurosurgeon, I emphasized the importance of time and explained the need for early surgical intervention to them. Despite their initial hesitation, I urged them to decide promptly for the patient's well-being. *I even had to practically beg them to give consent for the surgery as they couldn't decide, and the patient was in a critical condition.*

Eventually, they agreed, and we proceeded with the surgery immediately.

After the surgery, I explained to them that surgical intervention alone was not enough; it was a critical step in saving her life in the early stages. I warned them about the challenges she might face in the postoperative period, including the risk to her life. I emphasized the need for a comprehensive rehabilitation program once she recovered from the surgery.

Given her youth and the timely interventions, I expressed hope that she would respond well to a prolonged and consistent rehabilitation program. Fortunately, she showed significant improvement postoperatively, which was reassuring.

Once she was stable, we arranged for her to undergo further treatment at our rehabilitation center. Our neuro rehabilitation team at Mahaveer Jain Hospital discussed her case, and the family came down to evaluate the setup. They were satisfied with what they saw. Consequently, she was transferred to our facility for ongoing neuro rehabilitation."

We at PRS Neurosciences decided to take our screwdrivers and spanners out and train the tiny neurons within Vidhi's brain to behave. Gradually, we could prevent blood clotting, eventually bringing her back to consciousness. With all the therapy and training sessions, Vidhi regained her communication ability. She underwent thorough rehab and relearned how to brush her teeth, eat with her hand, and even spoon and fork, and began to live her life to the fullest. Like Nina Gulati, Vidhi also loves to see herself through the camera. Her recovery path was difficult, but she has resumed her studies and occasionally makes Instagram reels and funny videos with her friends.

Dear reader, I want you to understand that neural damage isn't a life sentence. It may not be completely curable. However, getting yourself back on your feet is never impossible. Life can be tough, but if you're determined, you can row your boat through this lake, surpassing all the heavy winds. Look for hope, and you shall find it!

Dorai mama – my Pati's younger brother!

Here is Dorai Mama's story. This was more than a decade ago. He is my grandmother's younger brother, a fit as a fiddle 89-year-old man! One day, early in the morning, he fell at home in the bathroom and had a hemorrhage. He had two sons, one of whom worked for a renowned IT company. He called me in the morning and informed me about this unfortunate event. He was rushed to the hospital immediately and was found to be at a Glasgow Coma score of 7, which is pretty serious. He was diagnosed with a left hemorrhage contusion. He was immediately moved to the ICU of a famous hospital.

There is a stigma around the rehabilitation of aged people in hospitals- I overheard the doctor ask an insensitive question – "the patient is 89 years old. Do you still want to save him? Why do we have to put him on the ventilator? I think we should send him back." Now, before you consider this question offensive and mean, let me tell you something- usually, when it comes to aged people, it is always better to let them spend time with their family instead of fighting for life in the ventilator, provided the patient is actually in pain or suffering or has a chronic health condition.

In our case right here, the man might be 89 or 90, but what matters is the fact that he did not have any other health disorders or was not even under medication for any sort of chronic illness. He could be saved if we could put in the effort.

I spoke to my uncle's older son, who is a doctor practicing in the USA, and unfortunately, he, too, came up with the same question: "Do you think he's gonna make it through?" His own son decided to give up on him. I was shocked to hear this response. Parents spend a whole fortune to educate and raise their kids, which is the kind of response they receive in return.

Now, being a neuro-astrologer, I took responsibility for my uncle's case and decided to continue to treat him and not do what his older son wanted me to do – palliative care, considering his so-called advanced age. I informed his wife and sons that I may be able to get him out of the coma, but he may find it difficult to name objects and people. This promise was made while he was still in a coma.

I walked them through the expected recovery trail and kept them updated after each surgery and therapy session. Months later, my uncle regained consciousness, but just as I had predicted, he lost his ability to name things. His family was shocked to see everything happening, just as I told them it would.

Four months later, he could walk like a healthy young man. He lived independently for another ten years and succumbed to old age at 97. He was an avid cricket fan and was always in touch with everyone. He doesn't remember the names, but he recognizes all of us. Interestingly, the first son, who refused to care for his father, left before him. After all, destiny has its own fully functional brain, right?

Story of Krishna – never give up attitude... keep trying until you succeed!

So, let me give you the lowdown on Krishna. This guy's been through more twists and turns than a rollercoaster. Imagine cruising along in life at 18, minding your own business, and then bam! An accident hits you like a ton of bricks. Yep, that's Krishna's story.

Fast forward eight years, and here he is, sitting in our therapy room, telling us his tale of pain and recovery. I'm no miracle worker, but I think I've got a few tricks up my sleeve. So, I dive into his treatment plan like a seasoned detective, trying to untangle the mystery of his ailments.

First, his legs were tighter than a drum, and the poor guy couldn't stretch them without wincing. So, we at PRS Neurosciences introduced him to a little something we like to call neuro rehabilitation. Picture this: the therapist Krishna Prasad (therapist), Krishna the young boy, and a foam board. Sounds like the setup for a comedy stage show, right? Well, balancing on that foam board was harder than juggling flaming torches. Practice makes perfect, and after a few sessions, Krishna was wobbling less and standing tall. He was later taken care of by our therapist, Mehar.

After a month or so, Ashwathy (therapist) stepped up, taking over from Mehar as Krishna's therapist. And let me tell you, Ashwathy's been putting in some serious work. Fast forward four months, and Krishna's not just standing on that foam board; he's playing catch with a football like a pro. Talk about progress!

Now, let's talk about his social life. You know you've hit rock bottom when even the auto drivers on the street start giving you advice. That's life. People love to dish out wisdom, whether you ask for it or not. But back to the main event – Krishna's therapy journey. It wasn't all smooth sailing, but we powered through like champs. And you know what? Seeing him leave my therapy room with a spring in his step and a smile on his face – that's the kind of victory that makes it all worthwhile.

What sets our therapy team apart is that we're not just a bunch of lab coats – we're pals. Krishna's always felt at ease with us, like he's just hanging out with friends rather than being stuck in a stuffy doctor-patient scenario. And trust me, that makes all the difference regarding motivation. Before that accident, Krishna turned his world upside down. Krishna was a sports fanatic—football, table tennis, badminton—you name it, he was into it. But then life threw him a curveball, and he had to rebuild from scratch.

Picture this: six months post-accident, and Krishna's taking his first wobbly steps. But it wasn't all smooth sailing. With the pandemic throwing a spanner in the works and proper physiotherapy hard to come by, his progress hit a bit of a snag. That is until he found his way to us at PRS Neurosciences, under yours truly, Dr. Sharan's care.

We kicked things into high gear, with Krishna diving headfirst into physiotherapy exercises like a champ. And let me tell you, his dedication paid off. In just five and a half months of intensive therapy, he's made leaps and bounds of progress.

So, here's to Krishna, the comeback kid who's proving that with the right team in his corner and a whole lot of determination, there's no obstacle he can't overcome. Cheers to the journey ahead!

13

SPINAL ODYSSEY

NAVIGATING THE WORLD OF SPINAL CORD INJURIES

"A hero is an ordinary individual who finds the strength to persevere and endure despite overwhelming obstacles."

Christopher Reeve

Spinal cord injury should not happen Even to Your Worst Enemy! It is unforgiving!

Dr. Sharan Srinivasan
Stereotactic & Functional Neurosurgeon

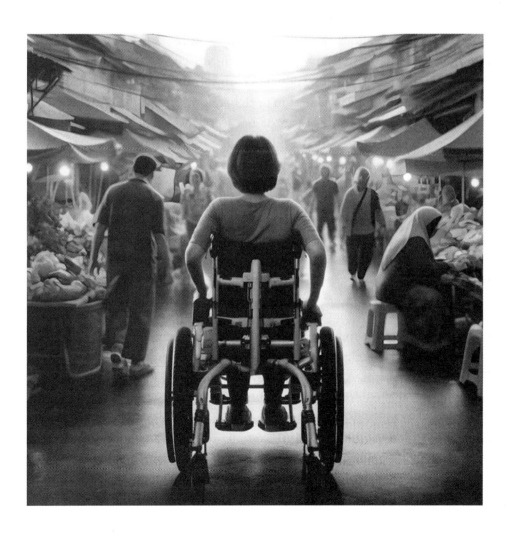

Nikhil CH is an ANRS @PRS Neurosciences. A passionate and dedicated neuro-physiotherapist by qualification, he, like the other ANRSs in our system, has undergone rigorous clinical neurological training beyond just being a therapist. He is also a key PRS Neurosciences leadership team member, constantly striving to achieve the best possible results for all our patients.

Here is what Nikhil has to say about one of his toughest patients.

Conquering both TB and paraplegia! A powerful and inspirational 'cot to community' story

Prologue

As a clinician, I carry with me countless stories of struggle, pain, and, ultimately, triumph. Each patient's journey is unique, etched deeply in my memory, shaping my experience and approach as a neuro rehab professional. Among these, the story of Ms. Savitha, a 42-year-old banker, is a profound testament to the human spirit's resilience and the intricate dance between hope and despair in the face of adversity.

Phase 1: The Onset

The first time I heard of Ms. Savitha was through her medical files—a dry recount of symptoms that hardly captured the gravity of her situation. She was like many others in her profession, spending long hours before a computer, which she believed was the cause of her persistent neck and shoulder pain. As the pain escalated into severe discomfort, she initially met an orthopedic surgeon who treated her as a case of non-specific pains and put her through a course of medications and physiotherapy. On retrospective analysis, though she did have some subtle weakness in her distal upper limbs, it had been missed. Two to three weeks into this, her pains worsened significantly, and they began radiating down her arms, trunk, and legs. It became impossible to ignore. She could now also experience a definite weakness in both her upper limbs, mainly distally. She was immediately referred to the neurologist, who got an MRI scan of her Cervico-Dorsal spine, and this revealed a possible diagnosis of TB of her C8 and T1 vertebral bodies with extradural pus and granulation tissue that was compressing her spinal cord. She was immediately referred to Dr. Sharan, and his evaluation revealed a dire diagnosis: tuberculosis of the spine. At the time of his evaluation, she already had asymmetric weakness in both her lower limbs and some weakness in the grip of both hands. This necessitated an immediate spine surgery to remove the infected segments and stabilize her spine. The surgery was successful, and the initial recovery was promising as she regained strength and mobility.

Phase 2: The Fall

However, recovery is seldom a straight path. Despite warnings from the therapy team, on post-surgery Day 5, Ms. Savitha's determination to reclaim her independence led to a premature attempt to get out of her hospital bed without supervision. The fall that ensued was catastrophic, causing a spinal bleed and leaving her completely paralyzed from the upper chest down. A repeat MRI revealed a large blood clot at the operated site with severe spinal cord compression, and she underwent an emergency redo-surgery – to remove the clots and decompress her spinal cord. The confusion and fear in her eyes when I first met her in this condition were heart-wrenching. She could not comprehend the severity of her situation—how a simple standing act could drastically alter her life.

Phase 3: A Glimmer of Hope

In these dark times, Dr. Sharan introduced us to the **Rehabability Index (RI)**, *a tool called the "Rehab Astrologer."* It predicted that Ms. Savitha could achieve a 'cot to community' score of C2C SCIR3b recovery state within 6 to 9 months, indicating a potential for at least an assisted mobility stage. This prediction was a lifeline, a thread of 'hope' in a seemingly bleak future.

Phase 4: The Slow Climb

Encouraged and emboldened by the RI's forecast, we began the painstaking process of rehabilitation. It started with the faintest signs—pain in her legs, a twitch here and there. Each small victory was a monumental effort, celebrated with quiet satisfaction and renewed determination. Her posture began to improve; her hands slowly regained strength, though she still depended on her elderly father for turning in bed, sitting up, and feeding. Progress was slow, and there were days when doubt clouded our hopes. But we persisted, driven by the possibilities that lay in each incremental improvement.

Phase 5: Contemplating Mobility

One day, over two months post her second surgery, she hadn't shown any significant motor recovery yet. Caught between optimism and practical concerns, I discussed with Dr. Sharan whether we should introduce a wheelchair for Ms. Savitha's mobility… in my mind, I was thinking, 'I don't think she will recover and not quickly.' His conviction was unshakeable. "We will wait," he said, confident with his surgical skills and the RI's predictions. As days turned into weeks, the cramps in her legs evolved into deliberate movements.

Phase 6: Regaining Independence

The road to recovery, especially after a 'double whammy' event like this, is often fraught with challenges and uncertainty. For Ms. Savitha, regaining her independence was a testament to human resilience and the power of dedicated therapeutic support.

The initial stages of her physical rehabilitation involved reintroducing her to standing and walking within the controlled environment of parallel bars. This setup provided her with the necessary support to bear weight on her legs without the risk of falling.

Each session within the bars was a mix of anxiety and achievement, as she focused intensely on each movement, her hands gripping the bars tightly. The first few attempts were tentative; her legs trembled, and fear was evident in her eyes—fear of a repeat fall was so paralyzing that it had drastically changed her psychology. She would hold onto the bars or me as if her dear life depended on it! But with each day, as her confidence grew, and her grip on the bars loosened.

Progressing from the parallel bars to using a walker marked a significant milestone. The walker offered less stability than the bars, pushing her to rely more on her strength. The transition was challenging. She stumbled occasionally, each misstep a sharp intake of breath for both of us. Yet, these stumbles were crucial learning moments, each teaching her body to regain control and balance. During this phase, the atmosphere was tense but also charged with hope. Every small advance was celebrated, and every setback was analyzed and learned from.

As her strength and confidence improved, Ms. Savitha graduated to using elbow crutches. This was a critical step towards achieving walking independence, as it required physical strength, significant coordination, and balance. The crutches demanded more from her than the walker; they required her to maintain her posture, balance her weight, and coordinate the movements of her arms and legs simultaneously. The sessions were grueling, often exhausting, yet she persevered.

Finally, the day came when Ms. Savitha was ready to walk without any mechanical support. It was a momentous day filled with anticipation and trepidation. Her first steps were hesitant, each taken with a profound awareness of what was at stake. As her therapist, I watched closely, ready to intervene at the slightest hint of imbalance. However, step by step, her confidence built, and her strides became more assured. The room, usually filled with the clinical sounds of therapy, echoed with her triumphant laughter and the applause of the therapy team.

Beyond the confines of the rehabilitation center, Ms. Savitha faced the real world with its uneven terrain and unpredictable obstacles. Training extended to outdoor environments—walking across the grass, navigating the treacherous Bengaluru footpaths and escalators in a mall, and dealing with the uneven surfaces of a park. Each environment presented new challenges, and she tackled them with the skills and resilience she had honed over months of hard work.

Her final achievement was reintroducing more dynamic movements, such as jogging, into her routine. Initially, the idea of jogging seemed unthinkable to her. But as she had conquered each previous step, she approached jogging with the same tenacity. Starting on a treadmill with safety harnesses, she gradually moved to jogging outdoors, her every step symbolizing not just physical recovery but a return to the vibrancy of life.

Ms. Savitha's journey from the devastation of paralysis to jogging in the park is a powerful narrative of the human spirit's capability to overcome adversity. This 'cot to community' story underscores the role of dedicated healthcare professionals and the critical importance of a patient's courage and perseverance. Her story is not just about walking; it's about reclaiming a life disrupted by sudden illness and finding the path forward, step by step.

Epilogue: Reflections on Recovery and Innovation

Reflecting on Ms. Savitha's journey, Dr. Sharan's innovation, the Rehabability Index (RI), was crucial. This predictive tool helped build a sense of belief in us to tailor our rehabilitation strategies with greater precision and confidence, providing a clear roadmap for recovery based on data-driven insights. The RI indicated that despite her severe condition, walking independently was a probable outcome for Ms. Savitha. Dr. Sharan's active involvement in applying his invention in a real-world clinical setting demonstrated a perfect blend of scientific rigor and compassionate care. His dedication optimized Ms. Savitha's recovery process and brought hope and clarity to her and her family during a challenging time.

The RI has also spurred broader discussions within the medical community about the potential of predictive tools to revolutionize patient care, especially in rehabilitation settings. It exemplifies how technological advances can complement personalized patient care, enhancing clinical outcomes and patient experience. This story underscores the powerful synergy between human resilience, clinical dedication, and innovative tools in navigating the complex recovery journey.

From patient to a colleague- the story of our front desk executive, Monish

Usually, parents must chase their children before their final exams and make them sit and study. But here we have this student who proactively decided to have a combined study at his friend's place. I vividly recall the day Monish, a bright young student, entered our clinic. He underwent a life-altering accident while preparing for his exams. He fell off the balcony of his friend's place, and unfortunately, there was a construction happening next door, and a rod pierced his spine.

The acute spinal injury had snatched Monish's ability to walk, and the lack of blood circulation in his lower body caused a significant challenge. It was heart-wrenching to witness his agony, compounded by the financial strain of affording the required treatment. Fortunately, Monish found his road to our clinic through one of his friends. Dr. Prathiba, with her unwavering dedication, provided him with invaluable counseling, easing some of the burdens he carried.

However, fate gave Monish another blow during surgery to address his initial injury. The resulting spinal cord injury further added to his physical limitations. Despite these setbacks, Monish's determination remained unmoved.

Our team at PRS Neurosciences kept him company round the clock, providing treatment and hope. Through months of rigorous therapy, Monish showed considerable improvement. Once dormant, the flicker of movement in his legs now hinted at a chance of recovery. We ensured we would not charge even a single penny for his treatment as we understood their financial condition.

His transformation is amazing! From being dependent on his family for even the most basic tasks, he can do everything with renewed, modified independence!

He learned several tips and tricks for dealing with life's situations and the life skills necessary to overcome his physical challenges. He left the clinic and later appeared for his exams. The intellectual young man cleared every subject with flying colors, but little did he know about the surprise waiting for him.

One day, Dr. Prathiba called him and offered him a job at PRS Neurosciences. With that, a new chapter of his life was unlocked. He was on cloud nine. Monish joined our team as a front office assistant without a second thought.

In his role, Monish serves as the welcoming face of our clinic, offering support to patients online and over the phone. His commitment extends beyond administrative tasks; he coordinates patients' seamless transition from referral hospitals to PRS Neurosciences, ensuring they receive the holistic care they deserve.

Monish's journey from patient to colleague is about the spirit of resilience and community that defines PRS Neurosciences. He has overcome adversity and become integral to our mission to restore hope and dignity to those in need.

At PRS Neurosciences, we understand that rehabilitation goes beyond just the physical aspect. We believe in nurturing the body and mind, instilling strength, hope, and a sense of direction in every individual who walks through our doors.

For Monish, every patient arriving at PRS Neurosciences reminds him of his journey. Though he may not directly encounter critical cases, the mere presence of those seeking help triggers memories of his struggles. Yet, within this flood of emotions, there's a profound sense of gratitude for the opportunity to pay forward the kindness and support he received.

In our clinic, Monish has found more than just a job. He's discovered a second family, a community of individuals who treat him not as a former patient but as an equal. The friendly atmosphere and genuine respect he receives from his colleagues make his work environment a place of comfort and belonging.

As Monish continues to thrive in his role, he remains a beacon of hope for those navigating their paths to recovery. His journey is a testament to the transformative power of perseverance, compassion, and the unwavering support PRS Neurosciences provides. Together, we stand committed to guiding others toward a life beyond disability, empowering them to embrace challenges and redefine their futures with courage and resilience.

According to us, the long-standing disabilities of SCI or Spinal Cord Injury can be so devastating that we should not even 'curse' our worst enemy with that! The brain and the spinal cord make up the central nervous system. The brain controls thoughts and interpretations of the external environment through our senses and physical movements.

The spinal cord is the main source of communication between the body and the brain. This is why spinal cord injuries disrupt information between the brain and other body parts. The main cable connecting the server and the entire network is being damaged! Imagine! No signals reaching the end users.

Unfortunately, our central nervous system still functions on a 'wired' model and hasn't yet shifted to a 'WiFi,' 'Bluetooth,' or 'cloud-based' model!

The spinal cord and the brain make up the central nervous system. The brain is the command center for your body, and the spinal cord is the pathway for messages sent by the brain to the body and from the body to the brain.

Like a slender, fragile vine made of highly sensitive tissue and A BILLION NEURONS, your spinal cord is like a living extension of your brain running through your spine. The spinal cord partners with the brain to send information around the body as electrical signals. It tells the body what the brain wants and the brain what the body is feeling, sending out all the vital nerve signals *that allow you to do everything from picking up a pen to walking across a room, voluntary movements like picking up a spoon or opening a door, but the involuntary movements (those made without your conscious decision) of the diaphragm (breathing), bowels, and bladder.*

The spinal nerves carry electrical signals from the brain to the skeletal muscles and internal organs through the spinal cord. They also carry sensory information like touch, pressure, cold, warmth, pain, and other sensations from the skin, muscles, joints, and internal organs to the brain via the spinal cord.

The spinal cord is a column of nerves that connects your brain with the rest of your body, allowing you to control your movements. Without a spinal cord, you could not move any part of your body, and your organs could not function. This is why keeping your spine healthy is vital if you want to live an active life.

Why is the spinal cord so important for our health?

Your Spinal Cord is important because, without it, your brain and body couldn't communicate with each other. The spinal cord is the pathway for impulses from the body to the brain and from the brain to the body. These impulses are different signals our brain sends and receives from our bodies.

What does the spinal cord do?

The spinal cord carries out the following major functions:

1. Electrical communication. Electrical signals are conducted up and down the cord, allowing communication between different sections of the body and with the brain since the cord runs through different levels of the trunk section.

2. Walking (also known as locomotion). Several muscle groups in the legs are coordinated to contract repeatedly during walking. Although putting one foot in front of the other while walking may seem simple, it must be carefully coordinated by several groups of neurons known as central pattern generators in the spinal cord! These neurons send signals to the muscles in the legs, causing them to extend or contract, producing the alternating movements involved in walking.

3. Serves as a center for initiating and coordinating many reflex acts.

SCI—Spinal Cord Injuries, regardless of the level, can be devastating. Although there are many clinical-anatomical-radiological classifications of SCI, what is needed for rehab professionals is a formatted, clear, well-elucidated, step-by-step program that helps to predict outcomes.

The newro model for SCI Rehabilitation is called "Cot to Community (C2C)" - a multi-dimensional, SCIM-III (Spinal Cord Independence Measure) and ASIA (American Spinal Injury Association) based (AIS - ASIA Impairment Scale) model that is categorized into four stages (and ten levels), and uses our proprietary CAREPa-Re® Framework, as under:

1. **100% bedridden/completely dependent +/- ventilator (either invasive or CPAP)**

   a. On ventilator/ CPAP/ O2
   b. On tracheostomy, but no ventilator/ O2
   c. No respiratory support of any kind

2. **Mobile on WC (inside home) – but with max-mod dependence or limited ambulation with walker/ crutches/calipers, etc.**

   a. Max assist
   b. Mod assist
   c. Min assist

3. **Mobile/Ambulant outside home/in community**

   a. Assisted with outdoor ambulation
   b. Supervised +/- community ambulation (wheelchair)
   c. Modified independence community ambulation but without a wheelchair

4. **100% reintegrated or 100%QoL**

Each stage is further strategized based on the following:

1. Neurological issues – depending on the level and current severity of the SCI

    -Motor
    - Sensory
    - Autonomic
    - Bowel/ Bladder
    - Respiration
    - Sexual/menstrual
    - Miscellaneous

2. General Condition (GC) related issues – like DVT, nutrition, pressure sores, etc
3. Functional capabilities/ disabilities – basic to complex (back into their normal life before the SCI)
4. Psycho-social issues
5. Seating/ Mobility/ Locomotor issues
6. Quality of Life (QoL) issues

    - Personal
    - Family
    - Community
    - Avocation
    - Leisure/ sports/ entertainment

7. Financial issues
8. Reintegration issues.

THE NEWRO MODEL OF COT TO COMMUNITY (C2C) FOR SPINAL CORD INJURY REHABILITATION

The newro model of C2C for Spinal Cord Injury Rehabilitation (SCIR) defines the possible journey of a patient from a state of being completely bedridden to reintegrating them back into their community. This model is applicable for people who have incurred damage to the spine and spinal cord due to:

1. Infections like – transverse myelitis, TB, etc.
2. Traumatic causes
3. Degenerative spinal diseases
4. Miscellaneous causes like – spine and spinal cord tumors (extradural, intradural extramedullary, intra-medullary), vascular causes (spinal AVMs, spinal cord infarcts, etc.).

The C2C Model clearly outlines the pathway of how the patient progresses from a stage of severe flaccid, areflexic weakness (paraplegia, quadriplegia, paraplegia, etc.) through the various stages of recovery, eventually and possibly reaching the stage of complete functional recovery and/or reintegration back into society/ return to a job (modified independence).

Awareness And Prevention

You must have seen spineless people throughout your life, but neurosurgeons are the only people who have to deal with patients with spinal problems. You cannot perform your day-to-day activities without your spine in the right health.

There are several ways for you to follow to prevent a spinal cord impact.

Recognizing indications of spinal injury is crucial, as it can be life-changing. While every case is unique, some common signs and symptoms demand attention. Heightened awareness is necessary, as early intervention can make a significant difference. Some critical indicators of spinal cord injury include:

- Severe pain or pressure on the neck and head back at the site of the injury.
- Loss of sensation, itching, or numbness in the extremities (arms/feet).
- Lack of control over bladder or bowel movements.
- Difficulty walking or maintaining balance
- Impaired coordination or weakness in the limbs.
- Difficulties in breathing or shortness of breath.
- Twisted or oddly positioned neck or back.
- Inability to move the arm or leg.
- Unconsciousness or altered levels of consciousness.

Story of Christopher Reeve- The First Superman actor.

The story of Christopher Reeve, the famous protagonist who portrayed Superman and tragically became quadriplegic after a horse-riding accident, is a poignant illustration of the devastating effects of spinal cord injury. He tried all the treatments, conventional, experimental, alternate medicine, and the works. Still, for the 7-8 years that he lived after the accident, he was wheelchair-bound and had a tracheostomy and a portable ventilator to help him breathe. You can also relate to Hrithik Roshan's character in Guzaarish, a movie dedicated to a life of high cervical spine injury leading to quadriplegia with an Indian twist!

Initial Injury and Assessment: Neurosurgeons recognized Reeve's injury's immediate urgency and severity. The trauma likely resulted in a cervical spinal cord injury, given the paralysis of both his arms and legs. Initial assessments focused on stabilizing his spine to prevent further damage and assessing the extent of neurological impairment.

Surgical Intervention: Depending on the specific nature of the injury, neurosurgeons perform emergency surgery to decompress the spinal cord and stabilize the injured vertebrae. This could involve procedures such as spinal fusion or the placement of hardware to support the spine.

Rehabilitation and Long-Term Care: Neurosurgeons understand that spinal cord injuries require comprehensive rehabilitation efforts to optimize recovery and function. This involves a multidisciplinary team of healthcare workers, including physiotherapists, occupational therapists, and rehabilitation specialists, addressing Reeve's mobility, strength, and daily living skills.

Challenges and Hope: Despite the best efforts of modern medicine, neurosurgeons would acknowledge the significant challenges faced by individuals with severe spinal cord injuries. Reeve's story highlights the physical, emotional, and financial burdens of paralysis. However, his advocacy for spinal cord injury research and his determination to overcome his disability serve as a ray of hope for patients and healthcare providers alike.

Research and Innovation: From a neurosurgeon's perspective, Reeve's case underscores the importance of ongoing research and new inventions in spinal cord injury. Advances in neuro-regeneration, stem cell therapy, and neural interface technology offer promising avenues for improving results and quality of life for people with spinal cord damage in the future.

Christopher Reeve's journey serves as a reminder of the profound impact of spinal cord injury and the ongoing quest for advancements in treatment and rehabilitation within the field of neurosurgery.

Preventive measures for spinal cord injuries encompass adherence to road safety guidelines, such as consistently wearing seatbelts in cars and helmets on bikes. Moreover, off-road equipment requires strict adherence to regulatory standards. Sports, notably American football, have a notorious history of causing life-altering injuries, particularly to the brain and spine. Therefore, prioritizing safety protocols within sports is imperative to mitigate the risk of such injuries. Sports have come a long way since then, but the world of sports, like many things, is slow to change, such as the regulation of gloves in boxing or the regulation of grappling gloves in mixed martial arts. In the aquatic field, since people enjoy splashing around in the summer, it is common for people to dive into pools, not realizing that they could be shallow. This also can cause severe injuries to the spine due to the impact of which the person falls, which, in many cases, is not being broken by less water.

Another cause can be unclean environments since slips and falls commonly cause back issues. This is exaggerated in the old cartoons where the character slips on a banana peel. However, it is a real-life risk, like in the case of Bobby Leach, who was a daredevil and the second person to survive the fall of Niagara Falls in a metal tube. Unfortunately, however, he slipped on an orange peel and injured himself. That injury got infected, and he passed away. Things like this are sometimes freak accidents, and it's a one-in-a-hundred chance, but we have to be very careful. As the odds keep adding up over the amount of probability of chances of accidents, we as people are to be careful because the likelihood of problems is a possibility. Thus, we must be vigilant and aware that this could happen to anyone. So, you have to know the proper precautions to maintain security.

General prevention

It is advised that you do not move a person suffering from spinal problems and wait until the medical professionals arrive at the scene. They would be well-equipped to assess the situation and take measures to minimize the damage. It is essential to perform first aid. However, only if you are certain that the measures you are pursuing will do net good, as in some cases, it could just aggravate the situation.

Treatment options are mainly based on the kind of damage that the spine has sustained since. The severity of the injury can limit treatment to medication for the symptoms and stabilize the spine.

Common causes

Road traffic accidents are the most common cause of spinal injuries in the world. With the rising rate of urbanization and failing infrastructure, the chances of meeting in an accident are high. Rapid urbanization that comes with increased motorization, especially in developing countries, has contributed to the rise of road traffic accidents.

According to the research conducted by the Indian Spinal Injuries Centres, despite the implementation of safety measures and the improvement of the road infrastructure, there is a significant high point in the victims of spinal cord injuries among the demographic of lower mean age, males on two-wheelers. Road traffic accidents were 45 percent of spinal cord injuries compared to 39 percent of falls from heights. A comparative study in Birmingham's National Spinal Cord Injury Statistical Centre made a finding that made it apparent that the ratio of accidents was as follows. Vehicular accidents were 38.52 percent, falls from heights were 31.13 percent, acts of violence were 13.55, and sports and recreational activities were 8.57 percent.

However, the case with road traffic accidents is not only through collisions or incurred by the driver. There are cases where freak judgments could cost the mobility of the passenger. There was a case in Goa where two boys returning from a football game, caught in a moment, sped on a speed breaker. This launched the passenger pretty high, making him land on the metal bar on the back of the scooter seat. This caused him severe pain in the back; shrugging it off, he stumbled out of the scooter and went straight to sleep. The situation worsened to the point where he couldn't move his legs. This happened a few years ago, and now he has passed away. It shows that just because you aren't the driver doesn't mean you're safe.

Falls from heights like trees, scaffoldings, construction sites, and buildings play a significant role in the causes of Spinal cord injuries, specifically in developing countries. Some factors contribute to this issue, one of which is workplace safety. In many developing countries, safety measures are inadequate on construction sites. This leaves the workplace with a high risk of fall damage and life-threatening outcomes. In many cases, the equipment required to ensure the safety of the worker is scarce, which increases the likelihood of spinal injuries.

Whiplash injuries are a type of SCI that occurs when the neck is forcefully jerked back and forth, commonly during rear-end car collisions. This sudden movement can cause neck pain, stiffness, and headaches. Central cord syndrome, a form of spinal cord injury, may also occur in severe cases. It involves damage to the central part of the spinal cord, affecting functions in the arms more significantly than in the legs and potentially leading to varying degrees of sensory loss and motor dysfunction. Prompt medical assessment is crucial for managing symptoms and preventing long-term complications. Both conditions highlight the importance of using seat belts and proper head restraints in vehicles.

In rural areas, the risk of fall-caused injuries comes from falling from trees for multiple reasons, stemming from gathering fruit, honey, or coconuts. Since natural wild honey found on trees is a heavily sought-after commodity, there is a demand for golden nectar. However, to attain this, liquid gold comes at a price. With a poison-tipped yellow swarm and the high altitude, this endeavor is an easy recipe for a severe injury.

Also, occupations like the electricity department in rural areas are risky. This is because, due to the high concentration of flora in rural areas, the powerlines constantly get tangled into the trees, which is why the electricity department is meant to trim the trees, causing them to have the risk of falling. Lack of medical facilities is a major cause of prolonged spinal issues and even the demise of the affected person. The situation in rural India is bleak since barely any facilities can provide life-preserving aid to the affected persons.

War Zone Injuries

During the Indo-Pak War of 1971, a significant number of spinal injuries were recorded by the Indian Spinal Injuries Centre. This included 45 spinal cord injuries from war, including 11 Mukti Bahni volunteers of Bangladesh.

The military hospital in Kirkee, Pune, established an 80-bed spinal cord injury center in 1971, which was instrumental in aiding and supporting the soldiers in conflict to recovery. However, during the high point of the conflict, the center had an occupancy of 46 cases of spinal cord injuries in 30 days due to the war. These injuries were caused because of direct bullet injuries or indirect shrapnel and the lack of adequate medical measures. This caused the situation to worsen to a point where the injury was either irreparable or fatal.

The Indian army was the first to understand the gross effects of the war on a person's mobility capacity. Thus, due to this realization, the Indian army set up the paraplegic center following the Indo-Pak War, which happened from 1962-1965. In the last decade, the center has caught the appreciation of the armed forces, which has led to the initiation of centers to improve a better sense of rehabilitation for the soldiers who suffered in the war.

Improving soldiers' safety in war zones can be achieved through various means, including upgrading infrastructure and providing cutting-edge equipment to operatives in the field. Additionally, training personnel with the necessary skills to effectively care for soldiers in life-threatening situations and recognize the symptoms of spinal injuries is essential. This training ensures that informed decisions are made, avoiding hasty judgments that could jeopardize the life or mobility of a fellow soldier.

Provide adequate protective gear to soldiers since, with the proper equipment, the soldier will likely walk out of this alive rather than be severely injured. The equipment should include the basics, like armor, which is the newest version since a lot of armor has a likelihood of failing with certain types of ammunition; also, equipment that can save the joints in the armor so that the soldier is not put at risk of the possibility of shrapnel causing harm. However, this technology is a way away since there have been delays in producing quality and effectiveness.

Implementing conflict resolution strategies means that the country that can evade the chance of conflict entirely has a good chance of not suffering many casualties. This is why the country is involved in setting up a lot of peace talks and treaties, as it is a sad sight to see a soldier in pain, let alone losing his ability to walk in this respect. India is constantly making efforts in the jurisdiction of the country and away and is involved in peacekeeping efforts.

The Indian armed forces have taken a lot of measures to make sure their soldiers affected by the tragic injury of spinal damage are well taken care of. India has set up a lot of centers for these injuries.

Soldiers Independent Rehabilitation Foundation (SIRF) is a leading NGO whose welfare organization spearheads the movement to ensure that soldiers can avail themselves of as much welfare as required to sustain themselves and their families.

The perpetual conflict in the Middle East has left deep scars on the region and its people. Long-standing geopolitical struggles, resource access, and ideological clashes have fueled wars and unrest. Civilians often bear the brunt of these conflicts, facing displacement, loss, and the shattering of communities. The aftermath is not just physical but psychological, with generations growing up amidst violence, which disrupts the foundation of society and hampers development and peace. Efforts for resolution and rehabilitation continue amid these challenges as the international community seeks pathways to stability and healing for the war-torn areas and their inhabitants. The number of patients from this region who have suffered brain and spinal cord injuries and who have come to us for help and possible respite is HUGE and SAD. They are all victims of the power games being played by someone else. There are no winners EVER in such wars! The civilians lose their normalcy, the families of the soldiers lose their loved ones, and the nation loses its independence, all just to sustain more injuries.

Here's a rare success story of one such victim from Yemen.

Saddam Hussein, a healthy Yemeni, had sustained a severe bomb blast, and shrapnel got lodged in the back portion of his brain. He also had sustained a whiplash cervical spinal cord injury. For seven long years before he was brought to me, Saddam was bedridden and could only use his left upper limb productively. The right upper and both lower limbs were not only paralyzed, but they also had a peculiar problem – the moment anyone touched one of these three limbs and attempted to move them, they would start shaking violently, causing so much pain and discomfort to him that he would try to sit up and hit both his legs with his left hand in a way to stop this shaking! Life's simplest tasks became an unbeatable battle for the middle-aged man, and hope seemed like a far-fetched wish. Accessing treatment for his condition remained nearly impossible since Yemen isn't a developed country, leaving him trapped in a cycle of despair. He did not know where to go; all he had for this long period was stress.

But then, a glimmer of hope rose when he discovered his road to me at PRS Neurosciences. After taking a detailed history and evaluating his neurological condition, I felt that the only solution for him was the implantation of the baclofen pump. They agreed out of desperation, and the implantation happened. Chapter 7 gives details of this surgical procedure.

Magically, the moment he was out of general anesthesia and wheeled into the recovery, he called me excitedly! He showed me that the toes of his left foot showed some flicker of movement. And when I examined him, the touch or movement-induced shaking of his lower limbs had already come down drastically! Seemed like a 'miracle', even for me... cos I hadn't anticipated such a drastic result so quickly after the surgery. He was ecstatic and gave him a BIG HUG (you can see the video of Saddam on our YouTube channel)

Here, amidst the compassionate care of dedicated professionals, Saddam's journey took a beautiful transformative turn. With each day of treatment, he felt the tendrils of possibility wrapping around him, promising a life beyond his limitations. Since he was a Yemeni, he spoke Arabic, and none of us knew his language. That is when technology came as a savior. We used Google Translator to communicate.

As he reflects on his journey, Saddam's eyes shine with gratitude and newfound determination. He speaks of the changes with a tremble of emotion, his voice echoing the depths of his journey. Despite his challenges, he finds solace in the support of those around him and the progress he continues to make. With each step forward, Saddam inches closer to his dream of returning home to Yemen. His heart is filled with anticipation for the embrace of loved ones and the familiarity of his homeland.

As he gazes towards the horizon, he knows that with the unwavering support of PRS Neurosciences, he will soon reclaim his life and stride confidently towards a brighter future. Disability resulting from a spinal injury is heavily influenced by two main factors: the level of the injury along the spinal cord and the completeness or incompleteness of the injury.

After 6-8 months of intensive neuro rehabilitation and customized programming of the ITB pump for appropriate medication dosing, Saddam can now get up from bed and walk comfortably with a walker, even outside the house and in the community. This is a huge improvement for someone who, for seven long years, could not even turn in bed without support! He is now back in his home country, happy to be with his three daughters, who anxiously awaited his arrival.

Level of the Spinal Injury: The spinal cord is divided into different segments, each corresponding to specific body areas. The higher the level of the injury along the spinal cord, the more extensive the potential impact on bodily functions. For instance, injuries higher up on the spinal cord, such as in the cervical (neck) region, can result in more profound impairment because they may affect the functioning of the limbs, trunk, and even respiratory muscles. In contrast, injuries lower down on the spinal cord, such as in the lumbar (lower back) or sacral region, may primarily affect functions related to the legs and lower body.

Completeness of the Injury: Spinal cord injuries can be categorized as complete or incomplete based on the magnitude of damage to the spinal cord.

Complete Injury: In a complete injury, there is a complete loss of feelings and voluntary movement below the level of the injury. This means the individual has no motor or sensory function in the affected areas.

Incomplete Injury: In an incomplete injury, there is some retention of motor or sensory function below the level of the injury. The degree of disability can vary widely depending on the intensity of damage to the spinal cord. Individuals with incomplete injuries may sometimes retain partial sensation and movement in affected areas.

The combination of the level and completeness of the injury determines the extent of disability experienced by the individual. Severe injuries at higher levels of the spinal cord that result in complete loss of function often lead to profound disabilities, including paralysis and loss of sensation below the injury site. In contrast, individuals with incomplete injuries may retain some degree of function and sensation, allowing for varying levels of mobility and independence. Treatment and rehabilitation efforts focus on maximizing functional abilities and improving quality of life based on the specific characteristics of the spinal injury.

14

FROM STRUGGLE TO STRENGTH

THE REHABILITATION JOURNEY WITH SPINAL CORD INJURIES

"Successful rehabilitation from SCI isn't just physical; it involves re-engineering the entire thought process to adapt to a new way of living."

Dr. Stephanie Kolakowsky-Hayner

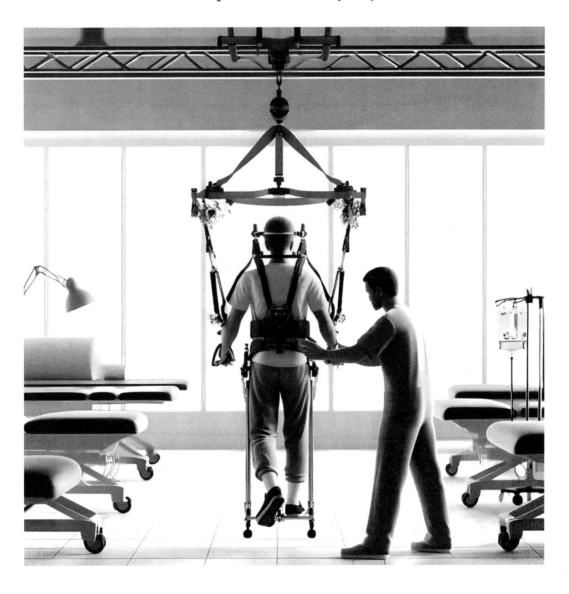

Kodandaram's story revisited

Only a handful, which is about four or five, of the hundred SCI patients tread the path to recovery with the vigor and tenacity of a warrior. No one dares make promises of complete restoration, for the journey is fraught with uncertainties.

Here is the story of Kodandaram, a vibrant 32-year-old whose life took an unexpected turn on the bustling streets of Bangalore. Once a dynamic bank employee, his world was suddenly interrupted by the screech of tires and the loud impact of a two-wheeler collision against an immovable pillar. The aftermath left him grappling with a shattered spine, confined to the sterile walls of a hospital.

But Kodandaram's story doesn't end there. Enter yours truly and PRS Neurosciences, where miracles are not just a distant dream but a tangible reality. Under the skilled hands of the therapists at PRS, Kodandaram embarked on a journey of restoration that defied all odds.

With each surgical procedure, ITB pump programming, and therapy session, Kodandaram's spirit soared higher, fueled by his family's unwavering support and his medical team's relentless determination. He emerged as a true fighter from the depths of despair, pulsating with newfound strength.

Today, Kodandaram stands tall, a testament to the miracles that unfold within the walls of PRS Neurosciences. His journey is all about the fact that even in the darkest times, there's always a glimmer of hope waiting to illuminate the path forward. And for Kodandaram, that path leads back to the vibrant streets of Bangalore, where he has re-embraced life with a newfound appreciation for every step he takes.

As Kodandaram recounts the harrowing details of his accident, the gravity of his ordeal becomes palpable. It was a seemingly ordinary morning, the sun just beginning the ascent, when chaos erupted on the streets. Three intoxicated individuals careened towards him on a collision course, their recklessness shattering the tranquillity of the day. Kodandaram's life hung in the balance in a split second as he desperately tried to evade the impending disaster. But fate had other plans. The borrowed bike he rode, an innocent bystander in the chaos, became a vessel of destruction as it skidded out of control, hurtling him toward the unforgiving pavement. The impact was brutal, the weight of three bodies and a metal machine pressing down on his fragile frame. At that moment, his spine bore the brunt of the force, leaving him paralyzed and robbed of sensation from T5 to T6.

From that fateful April 2019, Kodandaram's world turned upside down. Every facet of his existence, once filled with vitality and motion, ground to a halt. His legs, once the pillars of his mobility, lay dormant, devoid of sensation or strength. It was as if a vital part of him had been stolen away, leaving only fragments of his former self intact.

With each passing day and the unwavering support of a dedicated team and bystanders, Kodandaram began to reclaim fragments of his former life. Two months of relentless effort yielded small victories - the faint stirrings of movement in his legs, a flicker of sensation returning to his once numb limbs.

Once confined to his bed, unable to move a muscle, Kodandaram now strides confidently, covering distances of up to 100 to 200 meters with the aid of a walker. Once daunting, his daily routine has become manageable as he navigates tasks like getting ready, using the restroom, and even taking a bath with newfound autonomy. He even drives a car around independently, with his wheelchair in tow!

Despite initial prognoses that painted a bleak picture of his future, Kodandaram refused to succumb to despair. Driven by faith and an unwavering resolve, he embarked on a journey of rehabilitation that defied all odds. Though the road was fraught with challenges and setbacks, Kodandaram pressed on, inching closer to his goal each day.

Let's now take a look at the story of Shrijith Ram-

In July 2019, Shrijith encountered a challenging case that would have a lasting impact on his career and life. Shrijith, a young man who had recently completed his tenth standard and embarked on a diploma course, suddenly grappled with alarming symptoms. It began with persistent vomiting and a neck sprain, which initially seemed like minor issues. However, as his condition worsened and his symptoms intensified, it became clear that something far more serious was at play. Within about 6 hours, he had lost control of all his four limbs, and he was completely paralyzed from the neck down!

Upon his arrival at Mahaveer Jain Hospital, my team and I wasted no time conducting a thorough examination and ordering the necessary tests. The results were concerning—the MRI of his neck showed a non-cancerous intramedullary tumor called Cavernoma, occupying the center of his cervical spinal cord, from C2-C6, and it had bled! This discovery shed light on the root cause of his symptoms, including mobility issues, breathing difficulties, and compromised hand function.

In moments like these, when a patient's life hangs in the balance, every decision carries immense weight. Drawing upon my years of experience and expertise in neurosurgery, I carefully assessed Shrijith's case and presented his family with a detailed explanation of the proposed surgery. Despite the risks involved, including death, we approached the situation with determination and a commitment to ensuring Shrijith's safety above all else. Throughout the pre-operative consultations and discussions, I made it a point to provide Shrijith's family with the support and reassurance they needed during this challenging time. My goal was not only to save Shrijith's life but also to instill hope and confidence in his loved ones as we go forward.

As I prepared for the surgery, I couldn't help but feel the weight of responsibility resting on my shoulders. However, I was driven by a sense of purpose and a deep-seated commitment to my patient's well-being. The operation itself was a complex process, but I approached it with the same precision and dedication that defined my career as a neurosurgeon.

In the end, the surgery was a success, and I was able to delicately remove the entire tumor from his spinal cord. Shrijith's life was spared thanks to the collective efforts of the medical team. Witnessing his recovery and the gratitude in his family's eyes served as a poignant reminder of why I chose this profession—to make a difference in the lives of others, one patient at a time.

As a neurosurgeon, witnessing Shrijith's journey from the initial diagnosis to his remarkable recovery has been profoundly rewarding. Collaborating with the neuro rehabilitation team, led by Dr. Prathiba, to guide Shrijith through the post-operative phase was challenging and fulfilling. When Shrijith first arrived at Mahaveer Jain Hospital, his condition was dire—his mobility was non-existent, and he struggled with basic functions like speaking and breathing.

Working closely with the dedicated team of physical therapists, occupational therapists, and speech therapists, we devised a comprehensive rehabilitation plan tailored to Shrijith's unique needs. Each team member brought expertise in their respective areas, allowing us to address every aspect of Shrijith's recovery with precision and care. Our biggest challenge with his rehabilitation plan was a complete loss of joint sensation because of the loss of dorsal column sensations. It's like you see you are standing but do not feel any standing sensation. If the light is turned off, he will fall immediately because he uses his vision to balance. Do you think you only use your feet to walk?

Over time, Shrijith's progress was nothing short of remarkable. With the dedication of the neuro rehabilitation team, he gradually began breathing by himself and, after over 50 days, came off the ventilator, regained his speech, improved his breathing, and relearned essential skills like sitting and standing. He can now walk about ½ a kilometer with one-person support, albeit slowly. Witnessing his transformation from a patient in distress to a resilient individual thriving in his studies fills me with immense pride and gratitude.

I am deeply thankful for the opportunity to play a role in Shrijith's journey to recovery and for the trust placed in me by his family. Their gratitude is a testament to the collaborative efforts of the medical team involved in Shrijith's care. Moving forward, we are committed to continuing to provide exceptional care to our patients, guided by compassion, expertise, and dedication principles.

Bladder and Bowel Related Problems after SCI

In the unfortunate occurrence of a spinal cord injury (SCI), the bowel and bladder functions can get affected and go haywire. This happens because the neurological signals controlling the pelvis organs' functions get interrupted, like how our phones stop working when there's a bad network or no signal.

This leads to conditions such as neurogenic bladder or neurogenic bowel.

Signs and symptoms of neurogenic bladder can range from inability to empty the bladder, loss of bladder control, urinary frequency, and urinary tract infections.

Similarly, signs and symptoms of neurogenic bowel can range from loss of bowel control, constipation, bowel frequency, and lack of bowel movements.

The methods to control and alleviate neurogenic bladder include:

- **Lifestyle Changes** - Some measures include regular bathroom breaks, diet changes to non-irritant foods, and exercises that help control and strengthen the bladder muscles.

- **Medications** - Doctors can prescribe medications that can help reduce the frequency of bladder contractions, improve bladder control, increase bladder storage, or empty the bladder completely.

- **Botulinum Toxin (Botox) Injections** - These injections can help reduce the frequency of bladder contractions, but they may need to be repeated every six months.

- **Clean Intermittent Catheterization (CIC)** involves inserting a catheter through the urethra or abdominal wall into the bladder to empty it.

- **Stimulation Therapy** is employed when lifestyle changes and medications cannot alleviate the neurogenic bladder symptoms. It includes sacral nerve stimulation (SNS) therapy and percutaneous tibial nerve stimulation (PTNS). These techniques involve connecting a device to nerves in the bladder and sending electrical impulses to control the bladder.

- **Surgery** - Qualified doctors can perform bladder reconstructive surgery, which may help resolve the issue or improve the patient's condition. The surgery can include creating an artificial sphincter, bypassing the bladder, increasing bladder size, and removing the weakened section of the sphincter.

Sexual Function Related

Sexual function and fertility are prone to changes when a spinal cord injury (SCI) occurs.

Men and women with SCI both experience sexual dysfunction; there are changes in sexual desire, genital arousal, orgasm, menstrual cycle, and pain during sexual intercourse. For men, a major area of concern after SCI is the ability to get and maintain an erection. The solution to this problem includes -Using Specially Designed Devices and Tools - Constriction bands and vacuum erection devices are two such apparatus that increase the blood flow into the penis and maintain an erection.

1. Medication - Drugs like Viagra (sildenafil), Cialis (tadalafil), Levitra (vardenafil), Staxyn (vardenafil), and Stendra (avanafil) can help in maintaining an erection.

2. Urethral Suppositories - A suppository with Alprostadil is used as a penis blood vessel relaxant.

3. Penile Injection Therapy - A combined injection of one to four medications is administered directly to the penis to relax the blood vessels and increase the flow of blood.

4. Surgically Implanted Prosthesis - A three-piece penile prosthesis is placed in the muscle of the penis. This can cause structural damage and may affect the ability to get erections.

Ejaculation is also an area that is affected by SCI. A large demographic of men with SCI are unable to achieve ejaculation. This is because the spinal cord injury can prevent the bladder neck from closing, which can make the semen go into the bladder instead of going out the penis. This is called retrograde ejaculation.

For women, menstrual periods can stop after SCI because of the shock received from injury. It usually starts again after between three to six months.

Pregnancy is possible for people with spinal cord injury, and the pregnancy rates are close to the non-injured population. To avoid pregnancy, birth control is an option. Many different types of birth control measures can be explored after talking with a gynecologist.

- Condoms - Condoms are safe to use for people with SCI, and they are 98% effective in pregnancy prevention.

- Birth Control Pills - People with SCI can use birth control pills, and a lot of women do use them. They are 91% to 99% effective in preventing pregnancy, but an important observation is that people with new onset SCI who take birth control pills have a risk of developing blood clots. However, this risk decreases after three months from the injury.

- NuvaRing - It is a ring that is vaginally inserted and changed once a month.

- IUDs - Intrauterine devices (IUDs) are 99% effective in pregnancy prevention. For people with SCI, there is a chance that they may not be able to detect pain, and this can make it harder to feel when the device has become dislodged or if there is an infection.

- Implanted Hormonal Devices - They are 99% effective in preventing pregnancy, and the risk of blood clots is lower than using birth control pills.

- Depo-Provera Injection - The injected hormonal birth control option is administered every 12 weeks. With a 99% effectiveness in preventing pregnancy, it has a lower risk than birth control pills, but it can increase blood clot risk. However, women using Depo-Provera can experience a loss of bone mineral density, which can further lead to osteoporosis, which is already prevalent in SCI.

People with SCI can orgasm after their injury. This can be attained differently for every person, and it is up to them to explore how their body reacts to different stimulations.

Some stimulants that can be experimented with are audio stimulation through verbal expressions, sounds or music, visual stimulation, candles, incense, sexual devices, etc. Lubrication is also important for women as the body's ability to self-lubricate reduces after spinal injury. Autonomic dysreflexia (AD) can occur during sexual activity for people with SCI. AD refers to increased blood pressure due to a stimulus below the area of injury.

It can be triggered due to the following reasons -

- Rough stimulation of the genital area
- Stimulation through a vibrator
- Orgasm
- Menstruation
- Vaginal infection and inflammation

Some things to keep in mind for people with spinal cord injury while engaging in sexual activity with regards to bladder, bowel, and skin care are as follows -

- Empty the bladder before any sexual activity.
- A suprapubic catheter can be taped to the lower abdomen to keep it out of the way and prevent pulling.
- The regular bowel program should be followed to empty them before any sexual activity.
- A pillow or wedge can be used to ease pressure off the bladder and lower bowel during the activity.
- Skin damage can occur from shearing, pressure, or rubbing during the activity.
- Padding and positioning can help prevent injuries.
- The skin should be monitored for redness and injury.
- Lubrication should be used in ample amounts.
- Wash and dry the genital area with soap and water after sexual activity.

Seating, Mobility, and Pressure Sore Related

The management and rehabilitation of SCI depend on the level and type of injury. People with SCI require initial treatment in an ICU (intensive care unit), with the rehabilitation process starting in the acute care setting, which is followed by extended treatment in a specialized Spinal Injury Unit. Managing an individual with SCI is complex and lifelong, requiring a multidisciplinary approach.

A functional, goal-oriented, interdisciplinary rehabilitation program is needed to allow the individual with spinal cord injury to live a fulfilling and independent life.

Reduction in Range of Movement (ROM) may lead to contractures due to immobility, poor positioning, increased tone, and spasticity. Treatment methods include passive stretches, lengthened positioning, and other common exercises like active assisted ROM exercises, PNF, PRE, RRE, and tone inhibitory techniques in cases of spasticity. The occiput, elbow, back side of the shoulder, sacrum, and heels are prone to pressure sores or ulcers when lying in the supine position. The ear lobes, the outer side of the shoulder, the greater trochanter, and the malleoli are more prone to ulcers in a side-lying position. Preventive measures include passive pressure care, like frequent rolling exercises and mobilizing, adequately moisturizing the skin, nutrition and monitoring, and two hourly turning schedules. Individuals can also be taught how to perform frequent self-lifting exercises to relieve pressure.

Progressive resistance and functional strength training are clinically identified as achieving good results in maintaining and improving innervated muscle groups. Those with C6 and lower-level SCI can attain five motor skills: rolling, mobilizing from supine to long-sitting, unsupported sitting (short and long sitting), lifting vertically, and transfers.

Individuals with C1-4 tetraplegia require powered wheelchairs. These wheelchairs may be controlled by chin, sip, and puff or head movement. Those with C5 tetraplegia mostly use hand-movement-controlled powered wheelchairs. Most individuals with C6-8 tetraplegia can navigate independently with a manual wheelchair, but they may use a hand-controlled one as an alternative. Individuals with SCI below C8 can independently mobilize with a manual wheelchair. Since these people spend a significant amount of time in a wheelchair, it is crucial to have a well-designed and appropriately selected wheelchair cushion to prevent any further spinal deformity or pain owing to improper sitting position. These days, standing wheelchairs are available. There are manual wheelchairs that enable the person to stand while still in the wheelchair! The advantage is that it makes it easy to reach higher shelves, which is common in Indian households and workplaces.

Individuals with spinal cord injuries should be familiarized with their new way of mobilizing. Turning, opening, and closing doors, going up and down inclines, going around and over obstacles, and mobilizing indoors and outdoors are important activities to practice to ensure safe and independent movement.

Strengthening is the most common group activity across all types and levels of spinal cord injury. While the ability to stand or walk relies on several factors, the activity of standing has many benefits, even if standing independently may not be possible. These benefits include emotional well-being, orthostatic hypotension, bone mineral density, spasticity, and bladder and bowel function. Assistive devices such as tilt tables, standing wheelchairs, and standing frames can achieve standing. Individuals with paraplegia may stand in parallel bars with the help of knee extension splints or orthoses. Gait training is possible among individuals with complete paraplegia to partially paralyzed lower extremities using orthoses and walking aids such as knee-ankle-foot and hip-knee-foot orthoses.

Depending upon their level and type of lesion, individuals with SCI may have many complex needs and face a range of long-term restrictions in their ability to live independently, commute, work or complete their education, and take part in social gatherings. Coordinated community rehabilitation services and long-term support are required to ensure the long-term needs of individuals with SCI. Active case management with managers with appropriate training and skills is considered the leading practice to ensure coordinated care post-initial rehabilitation and personalized case management for patients with complex requirements.

Caregiver Burden in India and Developing Countries

Experts have expressed the need for Family Caregivers (FCGs) to be knowledgeable about the neurological condition, such as the nature of the injury, type, causes, symptoms, management, prognosis, and recovery. We should inform caregivers about techniques for managing symptoms such as bowel incontinence, bladder incontinence, and pressure ulcers; otherwise, in the long run, these complications will impact the recovery and rehabilitation outcomes, thereby increasing the caregiver burden.

The first question the CGs propose is, 'When will my loved one start walking?' Educating the family and caregivers about their loved ones' neurological conditions, especially the prognosis and recovery phase, is important to help them have realistic expectations and plan accordingly.

Experts have stated that in an attempt to cater to the needs of Persons with Spinal Cord Injury (PwSCI), FCGs tend to ignore their own mental health needs. Experts have identified numerous psychological needs for FCGs, such as acknowledging their feelings, problem-solving abilities, stress management, positive coping skills, and emotional regulation. The CGs of PwSCI often lack time to process their own emotions with others, as they must always be with the PwSCI. Thus, they are unable to even think about their needs and unknowingly put their mental health at risk.

Different from other illnesses, FGCs tend to be more attached to their PwSCI. This leads to FGCs having no time to perform their daily activities. Some experts have stressed the importance for FCGs to take care of their personal needs, such as a normal daily routine (including diet, sleep, hygiene, and leisure), sharing responsibilities, managing marital, sexual, and interpersonal issues, and asking for help to make time to engage in recreational and spiritual activities.

The CGs of PwSCI must think about their care and focus on normalizing their daily routines. They must also manage their physical and mental health to care for the PwSCI. Otherwise, the PwSCI will bounce back to the CGs, increasing their burden.

In a country like India, many PwSCI are from low socioeconomic backgrounds, because of which they are unable to afford the costs of treatment and other associated expenses. Experts have pointed out several financial requirements for buying medicines, meeting household expenditures, and providing education. At PRS, we understand your situation very well and don't mind providing free treatment so you can spend your hard-earned money on other basic necessities.

Experts have expressed the need to establish rehabilitation centers, peer support groups, respite care centers, social participation, and secondary family support to intensify the FCGs' support role.

We must empower CGs with respite care services and the ability to seek support from extended family members and society to reduce their burden. Many CGs have inadequate time to participate in various social gatherings; thus, we must educate them and others about the importance of community participation.

Experts have identified the need for welfare, such as unique disability identity (UDID) registration and certification, disability welfare benefits, rights of persons with disabilities, and government schemes.

All persons with a disability (PwD) and their CGs should know about the rights of the PwD, particularly supported education, supported employment, and concepts of the Rights of PwD Act.

Experts have expressed concern about FCGs' vocational needs. They have stated how the injury would affect the vocational components of PwSCI and FCGs. It has been pointed out that FCGs would need assistance obtaining jobs, starting self-employment, and pursuing their education.

As many of the PwSCI are young males and their spouses must remain with them at home, we must educate them on the self-employment options available. This can enable the CGs to earn money to run the family and care for the PwSCI.

Experts have presented the significance of telemedicine needs for PwSCI and their FCGs, such as regular check-ups, prescription orders, and exercise over video calls.

Traveling from far distances for follow-ups is very difficult for the PwSCI and their CGs. We should initiate telemedicine services to reduce their travel difficulties and treatment costs.

Experts have highlighted the importance of referral needs for FCGs, who play a huge role in the recovery process of PwSCI. Regular exercise and following treatment are important factors for better recovery from SCI. Therefore, FCGs should be knowledgeable about nearby therapy centers and hospitals. They must find out about trauma care centers, occupational and physiotherapy centers, and local NGOs.

We must inform CGs about the local NGOs and their services so they can seek community support whenever needed. This will enhance their social support, which is important.

15

THE SECRET SAUCE OF PRS NEUROSCIENCES...

NEWRO'S LOGICS = newro LOGICS!

"The only thing worse than being blind is having sight but no vision."

Helen Keller

What the brain does not know... The eyes cannot see...

Dr. Sharan Srinivasan

What does that mean to you?

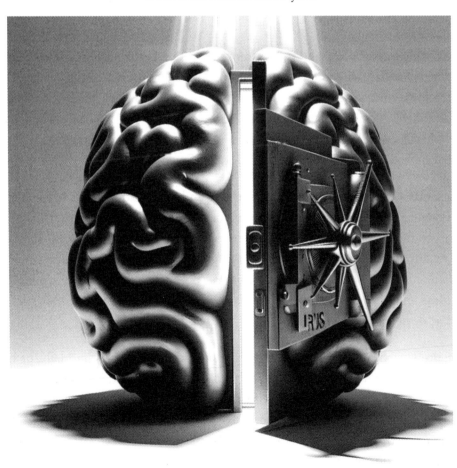

The software of the human brain - CVC – Cog-V-Com

Now, let me hand over the baton again to Dr. Prathiba, who will talk about the software of the human brain, especially when it gets disrupted.

Dr. Prathiba, CEO of PRS Neurosciences, a medical doctor and trained neuropsychologist, and Director of the clinical and rehab services, says that Mr. Rao was a retired banker by profession. Mr. Rao's journey from a dire situation to near-normalcy is a testament to resilience and the marvels of neuro rehabilitation. He experienced a sudden cardiac arrest that led to a hypoxic brain injury. As a retired banker, his life was numbers and precision, but post-arrest, he couldn't even recall his name or identify his wife and son, let alone the numbers he once managed with ease.

Initially, he mistook the hospital for a resort, oblivious to his surroundings and condition. When I first assessed him, his confusion was palpable and profound. Despite this, physically, his body responded nearly as well as it ever had—his sensory-motor control (SMC) remained almost untouched. If you saw him walking around in the ward, you would say he looked 'normal.' But cognitively, the damage was significant.

The software of his brain – the intricate network of cognition, vision, and communication, Cog-V-Com or CVC as we call it – was impaired. I enrolled him in an intense cognitive and visual retraining program, and despite his initial struggles with basic arithmetic, object identification, and color recognition, he persevered. When I asked him how much 2 + 2 was in the initial stages, He said 14! And then he pointed to the '+' mark on the paper and asked me, "What is this?"

Can you imagine such a question coming from a retired banker? Unbelievable! He couldn't tell me the color of his hair, the sky, etc. One day, when he was having breakfast at home, he got up to get a glass of water and disappeared for much longer than usual. When his wife went looking for him, she found him in the toilet, glass in hand, trying to get water from the western closet!!! He wrote neatly and perfectly when I asked him to write '1 to 10'! And then when I asked him to read what he had written... he read perfectly till '9' and then when he looked at the '10' that he had written... he paused and looked foxed.

He said – I have written wrong here – pointing to the '1 and 0' he had written. I have written 1 and 0. This is wrong! Can you imagine! I have many such instances that I can share with you, but I won't be able to do so right now. But you get the point. And such problems of any patient can never be seen, even in the most sophisticated MRI or any other machine today! But things like these are what make my apparently 'normal' looking patients dysfunctional. Are you getting my point? You are trying to attach a picture or video to your WhatsApp chat. Unless and until you try to do that task, you DO NOT know if that part of the software is working properly. The devil is in the details.

Through daily sessions, each lasting hours, we noticed a slow improvement. Gradually, he began to remember his loved ones and his past life as a banker. Although full recovery eluded him initially, he made substantial progress. Eventually, he could manage daily life with minimal assistance, thanks to the rigorous rehabilitation process. This journey of recovery highlights the incredible ability of the human brain to heal and adapt, as well as the importance of tailored, persistent rehabilitation efforts. It's a powerful reminder that even when the 'hardware' of our bodies remains intact, the 'software' – our mental functions – is equally crucial for a full and vibrant life.

Software in our 'digital' lives is merging with the software of our 'real' lives!

Imagine software as the unsung hero of our digital lives, the silent puppeteer orchestrating every click, tap, and swipe we take for granted. From the moment you scroll through your morning news feed to the last 'Goodnight' you say to your smart home device, software is the invisible thread weaving through the tapestry of our daily routines. Whenever you check the weather on your phone, you use the software. You use the software whenever you open a message on Facebook, create a budget spreadsheet, or join a Zoom call. Do you know and even realize that each of our brains has such a puppeteer that we have trained?? And successfully?

This magical essence of the digital realm comes in five primary avatars or types of software, each with its realm of influence:

The first step is system software, the backbone of our devices, which ensures that the hardware and software speak the same language. It's like an orchestra conductor, ensuring every section comes in at the right time. Contrast this with system software: the behind-the-scenes maestro orchestrating the symphony of hardware and applications. It's the foundation upon which your applications perform, quietly ensuring that your device functions smoothly, almost like a reflexive action of the digital body. It's embodied by operating systems like Windows or iOS, which, much like a diligent butler, quietly keeps the household running without your direct interaction. It often announces its presence only when it's time to enhance its capabilities through an update, maintaining the digital equilibrium we rely on daily.

Secondly, we have the application software, tools, and gadgets of the digital world. These apps help you hail a ride, the programs that transform your keystrokes into visual masterpieces, and the platforms where virtual meetings occur across continents. In digital tools, application software is akin to a Swiss Army knife, offering various features tailored to fulfill our tasks. These programs you enlist to get the job done, whether drafting a document on Microsoft Word, editing a photograph in Adobe Photoshop, or exploring the vast digital world through internet browsers like Chrome or Firefox. Each application is a specialist honed to deliver results for the end-user – that's you, leveraging the tool for your personal or professional objectives.

Thirdly, there's also the developmental or programming software, a playground for the creators, where lines of code are spun into complex applications and systems. This is where magic happens, ideas becoming tangible tools to solve problems or create new possibilities. Programming software is the craftsperson's toolkit for the digital world, vital for those who weave the intricate tapestry of code. These tools bridge human ingenuity and machine execution, translating languages like Python or C++ into commands a computer can execute. It's not just about creation; it's also about refinement—ensuring the code is sharp, effective, and error-free.

Fourth is the driver software, often grouped with system software, which is like the universal adapter for your computer. It speaks to the peripherals—the printer, the mouse, the keyboard—and ensures they all play nicely with the computer. When you plug in a new device, like a printer, driver software is like the interpreter that helps your computer understand the printer's language, enabling a seamless conversation that culminates in the physical expression of your digital documents.

Lastly, we have utility software, the unsung heroes working behind the curtain. They keep your devices clean from digital clutter, defend against viruses, and ensure your machine runs as smoothly as a freshly serviced race car.

Software is the guiding force behind our digital interactions, a complex yet essential element in both personal and business realms. Each type of software has a role to play, and understanding them is like getting a peek behind the curtain of the great digital show that plays out in our lives each day.

Similarly, our brain's software is the guiding force behind all our 'real-life' interactions with the world around us—other humans, animals, devices, etc. @PRS Neurosciences. Our brain also has all this software, and we are trying to understand how our brain processes all these things in a second without us even realizing the computations of the brain. We call this software Cog-V-Com.

Let's start the chapter with one of my co-drivers, Ganapathy Arumugham.

In Mr. Ganapathy Arumugham's words:

"My background lies primarily in occupational therapy. I completed my undergraduate studies with a Bachelor of Occupational Therapy and a postgraduate specialization in Paediatrics. I hold a dual interest, focusing on child development and neurological disabilities in both children and adults. My central fascination lies in examining brain and spinal functions across these two demographics, particularly how various brain conditions manifest in symptoms among these populations. My interest extends beyond merely understanding the structure and function of the brain; I'm equally intrigued by its practical application in daily life. It's essential to grasp how the brain functions daily and what cues we observe to gain insights into its operation. If you love neuroscience and want to understand the human brain, see the brain through the eye and its circuits!

Let me share a story: "A NOT SO USUAL DAY IN MY ROUTINE."

On a usual day in the OPD, my professional brain was perked up by this young, smart, 46-year-old man, Girish, who enthusiastically interacted with me as if he had known me closely. A sample of our everyday conversation would be: "Hi Girish, how are you?" … *"I am fine. Who are you?"*

"I am Ganapathy."

"Hi Ganapathy, I love you." This kind of interaction would make any clinician ready to intervene.

Seeing the amazing results of one of our other neurologically disabled patients and Girish 'looked okay' but was 'not okay,' the family had come for a consultation with Dr. Sharan, hoping that some 'Jadoo' could be done by him and his team. Dr. Sharan quickly realized that Girish had significant disabilities due to the damage to his 'visual processing system,' which gets missed by most rehab professionals. He then immediately referred the patient to me for a detailed evaluation. I learned from the previous reports that Girish had suffered a cardiac arrest two years ago and was being treated with a diagnosis of Hypoxic Ischemic Encephalopathy (HIE) with spastic quadriparesis and Ischemic Heart Disease (IHD). He was treated in popular residential rehabilitation care for seven months with the goals of improving his sensorium, speech, swallowing, hand function, ADL, and mobility. The approaches adopted were neuromuscular, biomechanical, functional ability training, and even robotics.

When the family approached me, they were visibly bothered, and I felt an element of overprotection and overinvolvement as the caretakers tended to advise and guide my evaluation and intervention. This created a momentary reluctance in me to intervene further. However, I gathered all my professional experience and expertise and geared up to deliver to the best of my abilities.

My first step was to understand Girish from a different perspective, as the presenting complaints were more focused on the inability to see and recognize people and objects. However, when I went into the depths of the concerns and observations of the family, I could figure out that the difficulties were more precise, in the sense that Girish could understand what was happening in front of him but couldn't understand what and who they were. This was when my professional self lit up, and I decided on a detailed functional analysis of Mr. Girish's vision. Subsequently, I could deduce that Girish might be dealing with a condition known as 'Aperceptual Agnosia' wherein a person finds it difficult to perceive or visually understand the characteristics of an object or person in terms of their color and form, which in turn renders them unable to identify or name a particular object or person who was already in their repertoire and memory before the catastrophic medical event (here HIE). For instance, when a cup was presented before him, he couldn't identify it. However, when I tried using the cup as if for drinking, Girish could instantly tell that I was drinking water.

Now let me try to explain this further, in layman's words.

Our brain works like a system, processing inputs (like sensory data), internal activities, outputs, and feedback loops. The information we get from seeing, hearing, smelling, tasting, and touching helps shape our reality. Humans, with sophisticated brains, experience the world in complex ways, thanks to our advanced language skills and frontal lobe functions. Unlike animals that mainly act on instinct, we can quickly adjust to new situations using complex thinking. Our brain turns sensory data into meaningful experiences and language, helping us navigate life. Sensory information goes through a process in the brain involving enhancement, calculation, and communication between brain areas to become part of our experiences. These experiences become part of our brain's storage system, affecting our future actions. Language is key to sharing and understanding these experiences. Our brain combines sensory information in a special area; if this process is disturbed, it can change how we perceive and react to the world.

Imagine a child experiencing the world for the first time. They don't have memories to guide them, so they use basic reflexes to understand their environment. When something touches their cheek, they turn their head toward it, or if their palm touches an object, they might grab it. These reactions are automatic, not learned.

As children grow, they start to make sense of what they sense. Touch, sound, and sight start forming patterns in their brains. They might smile at familiar faces or follow moving objects with their eyes, even if they don't understand what they're seeing yet. Parents and family help guide them, teaching them words and concepts. Over time, the child starts recognizing and learning from new and known things, developing their thinking and perceiving abilities.

Think about an adult's brain working like a busy office. It has five main tasks. Paying attention is like the security guard making sure important stuff gets through. Perception is the worker who unpacks the information. Then comes registration, like filing away what we've just understood. Memory is the storage room where all this information is kept for later use. And language is our messenger, helping us share and explain what we've learned.

Take talking in a second language as an example. It's like using a translation app; we might speak one language but often think in our first language. This shows how deep our mother tongue is rooted in our thinking. It's our home base for making sense of the world.

Sight is like the biggest window in our office, showing us around 80% of what we learn. It's linked up with many different departments in our brain, ensuring we understand what we see. We've got focused vision, like looking through binoculars, and peripheral vision, like a wide-angle lens. Together, they help us get around and figure things out. This operation is our brain's way of building a picture of the world.

Mr. Ganapathy Arumugham highlights the visual system of human beings as follows.

Mr. Ganapathy Arumugham makes an interesting point about how we see. Our eyes work together to show us a single picture, even though we have two eyes. Think of it like a camera. The retina is the screen inside, and the pupil is the tiny hole that light passes through, just like the lens of a camera. When we look at something, the light from it comes into our eyes, flips upside down, and turns around on the retina. The retina's center has a spot packed with cells for seeing color, while the edges are more for seeing when it's dark.

The optic nerve is like a big cable sending all this information to the brain, where special cells sort out things like how bright it is, the colors, and seeing in dim light. The pupil also changes size depending on how much light there is, like auto-adjust on a camera. But that's not all. How our eyes see also helps set our body clock and even affects how we feel awake or sleepy. The brain uses the information from our eyes for more than just seeing. It helps us recognize faces and understand the world, which is important for learning and hanging out with people. So, seeing is a big deal, more than just looking at stuff. It's a whole system that affects much of what we do daily.

Visual perception is a complex process, and our brains use three main elements to interpret what we see: shape, color, and movement. Imagine our brain as a detective, always looking for patterns. When we see the moon, our brain notes its round shape and white color against the night sky. Recognizing a mango on a tree, our brain picks out its unique form and vibrant color among the leaves.

We have two main brain pathways for processing vision. The 'where' pathway is like our body's GPS, helping us figure out where things are and how they're moving so we can reach for something or walk around without bumping into things. The 'what' pathway is like an ID scanner, focusing on identifying things, faces, and words.

When we wonder what we're looking at, our brain's language centers jump in to help us name and understand these objects. So, our ability to see isn't just about getting from point A to point B; it's also about recognizing, responding, and connecting what we see to language.

Experiments have shown that when our visual perception is off, it can mess with our ability to recognize objects or do tasks correctly. This can affect everything from how we do our jobs to driving safely. Understanding how we see can help us understand and act in the world. Even the part of our brain that helps us with directions and figuring out where we are in space, the parietal cortex, is involved in visual processing.

Lastly, our eyes play a crucial role, with their movements fine-tuning our vision and awareness of space. All these parts work together, making our visual system not just about seeing but also about understanding and interacting with our surroundings. It's fascinating how this complex system influences our daily lives, behavior, and even how we think.

Understanding the Oculomotor System: Function, Coordination, and Dysfunction

The oculomotor system is like the control center for our eyes' movements, allowing us to look up, down, and side to side. It comprises muscles and nerves that work together to move our eyes and help us focus on different things. Think of it as a team of tiny pilots moving your eyeballs precisely where they need to go.

Our eyes can make quick jumps from one point to another, called saccades. They can also smoothly follow a moving object called pursuit. This coordination is super important because it helps us see one clear image even though our eyes move.

Sometimes, this system can have issues. If the brain, which is the command center, or the nerves, like the communication lines, get damaged, we might be unable to move our eyes properly. This can lead to problems like gaze palsy, where you can't move your eyes to one side, or neglect, where you don't notice things on one side of your space.

Understanding what's going wrong can be tricky. Neglect, for example, usually happens after a stroke in the right part of the brain, making someone ignore the left side of their world. That side becomes invisible to them because that part of the brain oversees paying attention to it.

Then there's hemianopia, where you lose half of your field of vision. It's like looking through binoculars with either the right or left half of both lenses covered. Depending on the brain or eye nerve damage, the missing part of vision can be different.

Saccade issues, gaze palsy, and neglect involve how our brains and eyes communicate. When things go wrong, they can affect daily life, making simple things like walking or reading tough. Understanding these problems helps doctors and therapists determine how to help someone recover or adapt.

The real-world impact of visual deficits is illustrated poignantly by a woman experiencing visual disturbances while navigating her surroundings while teaching. She should be aware of the students' seating arrangement and from where they are calling so that she can promptly respond to them. Auditory cues can compensate for visual deficits, prompting us to elaborate on the brain's sensory processing complexity. While acknowledging the potential for reflexive eye movements based on sound, you can emphasize the intricate interplay between sensory modalities in complex scenarios.

What is cognitive fatigue?

Cognitive fatigue is like mental exhaustion. It happens when your brain must work too hard, for too long, or under tough conditions—like how your body feels tired after a long run. Imagine your brain as a phone; when you use it a lot, the battery drains faster, especially if many apps open simultaneously. If you're studying a lot, dealing with stress, and not eating or sleeping well, your brain's "battery" can run low. This can make you feel dizzy, forgetful, or shaky.

Now, about neglect and visual field deficits: neglect is when someone doesn't notice things on one side of their space—it's like half of the world just doesn't register with them, even though they can technically see it. Hemianopia is different; it's losing sight of half of your visual field like a curtain is drawn over one side.

Neglect has a bit of an advantage for recovery because it's about attention—not actual vision loss. The brain can sometimes learn to pay attention again to the side it ignores. Hemianopia is tougher because it usually involves damage to the parts of the brain or eyes that process vision, and that's not as easy to fix.

How will you explain vision problems to the caregiver?

Explaining vision problems can be tricky because they're less obvious than other physical disabilities. There's sometimes an unfair judgment around blindness because it's not easy for others to see the problem. It's important to realize that vision issues are complex—they're not just about the eyes but involve different parts of the brain and the visual system.

Take, for example, someone who has had a stroke and starts bumping into things on one side. Their family might think they're just weak, but the real issue could be with how they see and understand space, which is what happened in a stroke survivor's case. After the stroke, the person had trouble with balance and knowing where things were around them. But once they got help for their vision, they got much better quickly.

Getting families to see how important it is to work on vision, even when the problems aren't obvious, can be a big part of recovery. Healing the brain, especially for seeing and moving, differs from fixing a broken bone. It takes time, and you must understand how the brain connects seeing with doing. It's not just about the physical act of seeing; it's about how the brain uses what we see to help us move and interact with the world.

FIL: FUNCTIONAL INDEPENDENCE LEVELS
THE CONCEPT OF FIL

What is FIL?
Functional Independence Levels (FIL) describe how well someone can look after themselves and participate in social life. They're a way to check what a person can do day-to-day and see where they might need help to improve their independence. This can make life more satisfying and ease the load on caregivers. Getting a good FIL is crucial for returning to community life, which is enjoyable and can ease the pressure on caregivers.

Where is FIL used?
Rehab professionals use FIL to set goals and measure a patient's progress. It's a big-picture look at a patient's ability to interact with their environment. Cognitive therapists, speech-language pathologists, physical therapists, and occupational therapists all use it to get a broad understanding of a patient's abilities. It's like zooming out to see the whole picture of how they're doing.

Why do we need FIL?
FIL helps the rehab team kick-start the recovery process with a clear goal in mind. It's like dropping a pin to begin the process. They plan backward from the ideal FIL to specific evaluations, figure out the final steps needed for the patient, and work from there toward the goal. It keeps hopes realistic.

What does FIL include?
Occupational therapists mainly run FIL and give useful information to:

1. Occupational therapists themselves
2. Physical therapists to understand physical baseline levels

3. The cognitive-visual-communication team to gauge cognitive and communication needs
4. Caregivers to know what to expect and prepare for the recovery process

FIL helps patients reach their best levels of recovery.

What are the FIL factors?

FIL looks at whether someone can:

1. Understand and plan daily routines, remembering important past events to make quick decisions
2. Socialize with family and strangers when needed
3. Move safely around their home
4. Use what they've learned before in new places to complete tasks

The five signs of successfully reaching FIL are:

1. Skilled task performance
2. Being appropriate for the environment
3. Energy efficiency
4. Social acceptability
5. Confidence

How are FIL levels defined?

Each FIL level has specific daily routines that patients should do to reach their rehab goals and move to the next level if that's what they and their families want. FIL connects what the patient wants and expects to the next steps in recovery, using a common language for both the patient and clinical teams. It includes physical levels, upper limb function, swallowing, cognition for understanding and planning, visual perception, and communication. Each area has different sub-levels, but going into more detail is beyond FIL's scope because it gets very complex.

Example:

A caregiver might say they want their father to go to the bathroom by himself at night. In clinical terms, this means he needs to:

1. Get out of bed and walk to the bathroom without falling.
2. Use the bathroom without help.
3. Manage the whole toileting process with his hands.
4. Return to bed safely.
5. Move around with low light.

This goal is what we aim for at FIL level 3.

FULL: FUNCTIONAL UPPER LIMB LEVELS
THE CONCEPT OF FULL

What is FULL?

Functional Upper Limb Levels (FULL) assess the ability of both arms to perform everyday tasks. It's crucial for interacting with the world around us and for living independently.

Where is FULL used?

Rehab professionals need to understand and improve a person's ability to use their arms and hands in goal-directed activities. It helps track the progress of a patient's arm function in both non-conscious movements and conscious skills.

Why do we need FULL?

FULL provides a detailed look at the functional abilities of a person's arms after recovery from an injury or illness. It's important because even if arm movement and strength are restored, it doesn't mean a person can automatically do everyday tasks efficiently and safely. FULL is used to guide specific training for these tasks.

What does FULL measure?

FULL is mainly for occupational therapists but also gives important information to:

1. Physical therapists
2. Cognitive-visual-communication teams
3. Caregivers

This information helps the patient achieve the highest possible recovery level.

When do we need FULL data?

FULL is needed to assess how well a person can:

a. Move in bed
b. Sit and balance
 c. Use their arms for various tasks in different positions, ensuring activities are done properly and safely.

What is the concept of SAREES?

SAREES stands for

S - Speed
A - Accuracy
R - Rhythm
E – Endurance
E - Error corrections/minimization
E- Environment
S – Safety

It's a set of criteria to ensure tasks are performed well.

How does FULL help occupational therapists?

FULL helps occupational therapists gauge a patient's current arm function, from movement to skill level, and decide on the training needed for efficient, safe task performance.

How does FULL assist other rehab professionals?

FULL informs the rest of the rehab team about a patient's arm abilities. They must plan their part in the rehabilitation process and ensure a smooth and effective recovery.

How is FULL structured and measured?

FULL is set up so that once one arm (usually the less affected one) can do basic actions, therapy can begin to include both arms. The goal is to teach the patient to perform tasks with the right speed, accuracy, rhythm, endurance, error correction, environmental adaptation, and safety at each level of recovery.

FBL: FUNCTIONAL BODY LEVELS
THE CONCEPT OF FBL

What is FBL?

Functional Body Levels (FBL) measure how well the body—specifically the head, neck, trunk, and lower limbs—can perform day-to-day actions, either with or without using the upper limbs. It's crucial for starting voluntary interaction with the environment.

Where is FBL used?

Rehab professionals use FBL to determine if a patient is ready for functional retraining. It organizes functions from simple movements like bed mobility to more complex ones like moving outside the home for various purposes.

Why do we need FBL?

FBL helps track patient progress and outlines the steps needed for continued recovery. It ensures that patients are trained safely and effectively without risking injury or delays in recovery.

What does FBL measure?

Physical therapists mainly use times occupational therapists for lower limb retraining. It provides functional data for:

1. Physical therapists
2. Occupational therapists assessing upper limb rehab potential
3. Cognitive-visual-communication teams evaluating physical body function understanding
4. Caregivers planning logistics for patient mobility

FBL aims to help patients reach their highest potential for recovery.

When do we need FBL data?

FBL data helps clinicians understand a patient's current ability to interact with their surroundings and determine the level of assistance needed for self-care. Caregivers use this information to decide on assistive devices and home modifications for safer patient interaction.

How does FBL help physical therapists?

FBL allows PTs to distinguish between compensation and true restoration of motor control. It assesses the training needed for a patient to perform activities safely and effectively and helps PTs understand a patient's potential versus their current performance.

How does FBL assist other rehab team members?

FBL informs the rehab team about the patient's functional abilities, ensuring that everyone's efforts are coordinated and contribute to quality outcomes.

How is FBL structured and measured?

FBL is designed so that as soon as a patient achieves a certain functional level, they begin training for the next level. Patients must demonstrate a basic ability to maintain safety in one position before moving on to more challenging tasks. As skills improve, FBL tasks become more automatic, allowing for more complex participation in activities.

CVC = Cognition Vision Communication or Cog-V-Com

The Cog-V-com module, the USP of PRS neurosciences, represents a ground-breaking advancement in neurocognitive assessment and rehabilitation. Developed as a proprietary, multidimensional tool, its primary function is to comprehensively evaluate and analyze the 'software dysfunctions' of the human brain—the combined functions of cognition, vision, and communication in individuals affected by brain-related disorders or injuries. At its core, the *Cog-V-com module* is a sophisticated assessment system, leveraging state-of-the-art technologies and methodologies to provide detailed insights into an individual's cognitive, visual, and communicative abilities. Integrating data from various sources and employing advanced algorithms offers a holistic understanding of the individual's brain function, enabling healthcare professionals to make informed decisions about their level of functionality and tailor treatment plans accordingly.

One of the key features of the *Cog-V-com module* is its ability to assess cognition, vision, and communication simultaneously, yet distinctly, recognizing the intricate interplay between these domains in everyday activities. Through a series of carefully designed tasks, tests, and simulations, it captures a comprehensive picture of the individual's cognitive processes, visual perception, and linguistic abilities, allowing for a nuanced assessment of their strengths, weaknesses, and areas for improvement.

Moreover, the *Cog-V-com module* is designed to be adaptable and customizable, catering to a wide range of neurological conditions and patient profiles. Whether it's assessing cognitive function in individuals with Alzheimer's disease, evaluating visual processing in patients with traumatic brain injuries, or analyzing language comprehension in stroke survivors or any other brain-related disorder, the module can be tailored to meet specific clinical needs and objectives.

In addition to its assessment capabilities, the *Cog-V-com module* also serves as a valuable tool for rehabilitation and intervention. Identifying areas of impairment and potential avenues for improvement empowers healthcare professionals to develop targeted rehabilitation programs to enhance cognitive, visual, and communicative abilities, ultimately promoting better functional outcomes and quality of life for individuals with brain-related disorders.

In summary, the *Cog-V-com module* represents a paradigm shift in assessing and managing neurological conditions, offering a comprehensive and integrated approach to understanding and addressing the complex interplay between cognition, vision, and communication in individuals with brain-related disorders. Its advanced capabilities hold immense promise for improving clinical decision-making, optimizing rehabilitation strategies, and, ultimately, enhancing the well-being of patients worldwide.

CVC for Software (CVC4S) or Cog-V-Com4S

The *Cog-V-Com4S* aspect of the module is dedicated to assessing and addressing problems related to internal cognitive processes. These processes encompass a wide range of mental activities involved in perception, memory, attention, language, reasoning, and decision-making. Here's how the CVC4S module functions:

Cognitive Assessment: Utilizing a variety of standardized tests, cognitive tasks, and psychological assessments, the *CVC4S* module evaluates the individual's cognitive abilities across different domains. This may include tests for memory retention, attention span, executive function, problem-solving skills, and abstract reasoning.

Neurocognitive Profiling: The CVC4S module generates a detailed neurocognitive profile for each individual by analyzing cognitive strengths and weaknesses patterns. This profile helps clinicians understand the underlying cognitive processes affected by brain-related disorders or injuries, such as Alzheimer's disease, traumatic brain injury, or even neurodevelopmental disorders.

Cognitive Rehabilitation: Based on the neurocognitive profile, the CVC4S module recommends personalized cognitive rehabilitation strategies aimed at improving specific cognitive functions, the pinnacle of our 'precision and personalized medicine.' These strategies may involve cognitive training exercises, compensatory strategies, behavioral interventions, and psychoeducation to enhance cognitive skills and promote functional independence.

Monitoring Progress: The CVC4S module tracks the individual's progress in cognitive rehabilitation programs through ongoing assessments and monitoring. It provides valuable feedback to clinicians, allowing them to adjust intervention strategies and optimize treatment outcomes over time.

CVC for Hardware (CVC4H) or Cog-V-Com4H

In contrast, the *CVC4H aspect* of the module focuses on problems related to producing motor outputs that are goal-oriented and skilled. This encompasses motor control, coordination, agility, and the execution of purposeful movements. Here's how the *CVC4H module* operates:

Motor Function Assessment: The CVC4H module evaluates the individual's motor function across different levels of complexity using a combination of standardized motor assessments, functional tasks, and kinematic analysis. This includes assessing basic motor skills (e.g., grasping, reaching) as well as higher-level motor tasks (e.g., fine motor coordination, tool use).

Task Tree analysis: The task tree analysis is a comprehensive analysis of a self-care, work, or leisure-related activity that an individual finds purposeful and identifies with self. This tree creates an organized and systematic breakdown of the selected task and helps the rehabilitation professional understand the connection between participation and limitation. Through this holistic understanding, all rehabilitation professionals can anchor their goals by focusing on what the patient wants to achieve and working 'together-together' with a clear plan!

Kinematic Analysis: Leveraging motion capture technology and biomechanical analysis, the CVC4H module quantifies the individual's movement patterns, joint angles, velocity, and accuracy during motor tasks. This objective data provides insights into motor control deficits, movement abnormalities, and compensatory strategies employed by the individual.

Motor Rehabilitation: The CVC4H module prescribes tailored motor rehabilitation interventions to restore or improve motor function based on the motor assessment findings. These interventions may include physical therapy exercises, occupational therapy techniques, assistive devices, and adaptive strategies to enhance motor performance and functional independence.

Cognitive-Motor Integration Analysis: Leveraging cognitive neuroscience principles, the CVC4H module examines the integration between cognitive and motor processes during task performance. It identifies areas of dysfunction or disconnection between cognitive planning and motor execution, providing insights into the underlying neurocognitive mechanisms affecting motor function.

Cognitive-Motor Rehabilitation Strategies: Based on the assessment findings, the CVC4H module designs tailored rehabilitation strategies aimed at improving cognitive-motor integration and functional motor performance. These strategies may include cognitive training exercises targeting motor planning, dual-task training to improve multitasking abilities, and motor imagery techniques to enhance motor preparation and execution.

Progress Tracking: Similar to *the CVC4S module, the CVC4H module* facilitates ongoing monitoring of motor rehabilitation progress. It enables clinicians to objectively measure changes in motor function, adapt rehabilitation protocols as needed, and optimize the individual's ability to perform activities of daily living and achieve personal goals.

By integrating *CVC4S and CVC4H functionalities, the Cog-V-com* module provides a comprehensive approach to assessing and addressing the complex interplay between cognitive processes and motor function in individuals with brain-related disorders or injuries. This dual-focus framework enables clinicians to develop personalized intervention plans that target both cognitive and motor aspects of rehabilitation, ultimately maximizing functional outcomes and improving patients' quality of life.

It is a story about a mother who underwent Cognitive Retraining for Hardware.

Jayamma, hailing from a small town near Tumkur, suffered a concussive head injury and received initial treatment at local hospitals before being referred to me for cognitive retraining. Given her illiteracy, I utilized an illiterate battery for assessment due to her comprehension challenges.

Although she could manage basic activities of daily living (ADL) to some extent, she required frequent instructions and close monitoring from her family, particularly her three cooperative sons.

Upon her arrival, it became evident that Jayamma faced difficulties even in simple tasks like dressing and grooming. Despite her physical capabilities, she struggled with tasks such as combing her hair and wearing a sari. Her sons' attempts to assist her, like tying a rubber band around her hair, underscored the extent of her challenges. However, her speech remained coherent, albeit lacking clarity. The focus of her rehabilitation was not only on regaining functional independence but also on restoring her culinary skills, which she had completely forgotten post-injury. Despite being renowned for her cooking prowess before the accident, Jayamma had no recollection of her culinary expertise. Over three to four months, using visual aids and guided instructions, she gradually reacquainted herself with cooking techniques and ingredients, with her sons attesting to the effectiveness of this approach.

With consistent effort and support, Jayamma regained her cooking proficiency and even resumed wearing a sari independently. Furthermore, she expressed a desire to contribute financially to her family's welfare, prompting her involvement in her husband's petty shop. Initially assisting with basic tasks like customer interactions and stock management, Jayamma gradually assumed more responsibilities, eventually managing the shop efficiently.

Her journey from struggling with basic tasks to successfully managing household chores and a petty shop exemplifies the transformative power of family support and dedicated retraining efforts. Despite her humble background and initial setbacks, Jayamma's determination and perseverance ultimately led to her remarkable recovery and newfound independence.

The ultimate goal is to help us interact with the external environment productively and meaningfully.

Cognitive Behavioral Therapies (CBT) Integration

The CVC model incorporates Cognitive Behavioral Therapies (CBT) elements to address maladaptive thought patterns, emotional regulation, and behavior modification. Through targeted interventions and structured sessions, individuals learn to identify and challenge negative thought patterns, develop coping strategies for managing stress and anxiety, and cultivate adaptive behaviors conducive to their functional goals. The integration of CBT techniques within the CVC model allows for a comprehensive approach to addressing cognitive, emotional, and behavioral aspects of rehabilitation.

Deep Relaxation Techniques (DRT)

Deep Relaxation Techniques (DRT), including mindfulness meditation, progressive muscle relaxation, and guided imagery, are integrated into the CVC model to promote stress reduction, emotional regulation, and overall well-being. By incorporating DRT sessions into rehabilitation programs, individuals learn to cultivate a state of deep relaxation, alleviate physical and emotional tension, and enhance their ability to cope with challenging situations. The integration of DRT within the CVC model complements cognitive and motor rehabilitation efforts by fostering a conducive internal environment for learning, adaptation, and recovery.

Yoga and Pranayama

The CVC model incorporates yoga and pranayama practices to promote physical health, mental well-being, and emotional balance. Through yoga postures (asanas) and breathing exercises (pranayama), individuals improve flexibility, strength, and body awareness while enhancing respiratory function and stress resilience. The integration of yoga and pranayama within the CVC model offers holistic benefits for cognitive, motor, and behavioral rehabilitation, supporting individuals in their journey toward improved functional outcomes and quality of life.

Tailored Rehabilitation Plans

Within the CVC model, behavioral rehabilitation strategies are tailored to every individual's unique needs, preferences, and goals. Rehabilitation plans are personalized based on comprehensive assessments of cognitive, motor, and behavioral functioning, ensuring that interventions are targeted and effective. By integrating behavioral rehabilitation strategies into the CVC model, clinicians can address the multidimensional needs of individuals with brain-related disorders or injuries, fostering holistic recovery and promoting optimal functioning across cognitive, emotional, and behavioral domains.

In summary, the integration of behavioral rehabilitation strategies within the Cog-V-com (CVC) model enhances its capacity to address the complex interplay between cognitive, motor, and behavioral functioning in individuals with brain-related disorders or injuries. By incorporating Cognitive Behavioral Therapies (CBT) strategies, Deep Relaxation Techniques (DRT), yoga, pranayama, and other evidence-based practices, the CVC model offers a comprehensive approach to rehabilitation, supporting individuals in their journey towards improved quality of life and functional independence.

The therapists have their own life. Apart from their professional lives, they also have their family life. They have their friend's circle. They have their own life to deal with. They might have health problems. They might have psychological issues. They might have physical issues. They might have logistic issues. They may have emotional issues. Now, all these things need to be dealt with, and only then do I think there is sanity in the whole process. When these people, as therapists, have dealt with their problems and have positivity inside them, they can produce magical results with the positivity they have created for themselves in the patients. Since I believe a lot in energy levels, I make sure I train all my people to create positive energy, destroy negative energy, or negate negative energy, and keep that charge going to support their patients, their caregivers, and themselves. I think they should support themselves and go forward with producing the results. As in every workspace, there can be ego issues, emotional clashes, and times when they are compared with somebody else, and they feel bad about it.

So, all these subtle things do affect the therapist's mental status. Now, as an organization head, it is my responsibility to make sure I show them and direct them how they can recognize this in the first place. Then, how do you handle that? How do you get over it and go forward, creating positive energy for themselves and their patients? This is most important.

Finally...

Suppose one part of the story is the problems the patient is having, either after a stroke or head injury or whatever neurological deficit they've developed. In that case, the other part of the story, the half, is of the caregivers or the patient's family members. Everything went smoothly until that dreadful day came like a 'bolt from the blue' in their lives. And suddenly, if the patient had a stroke or a head injury or some kind of spinal cord injury, some neurological issue, the whole life becomes a turmoil for them, starting from the rush to the emergency, ICU admission, surgery if required, arranging the money for all that, arranging logistic issues for all these things, family support, do they have it or not, or do they have to hire somebody to look after the family member, the patient? Everything. If they are working, do they get permission from the job? How long should they take off? All these things are starting to burden the caregivers. The patients are lying on the bed many times in a coma or maybe just out of the coma. They don't even realize what's happening to them. The caregivers are the ones who have been looking after them all the time, morning and night, 24/7.

They must be responsible for giving feedback to the doctors or the therapists who go to them and ask them how the patient has been doing. Has the patient slept well or not slept? Are there any challenges? If any other problems, medical or nonmedical, that the patient is having, all this feedback is to be given by the caregivers or the family members. Now, sometimes, they are so overwhelmed. They finish the emergency, they finish the ICU, and if there is surgery, they finish up with that. They must organize money from somewhere. Not everybody is sitting with a pot of money to be used in an emergency like this because the hospitalization, the ICU, the nursing, and the logistics all cost a lot of money, a couple of lakhs, probably, for a few days. Now, in this situation. They run helter-skelter. They try their best to check all the resources. They bring in all kinds of possible money from every possible place, probably affordable or not affordable, and all kinds of people have trouble. Initially, they have the energy. They probably have the money also. They have some people coming and supporting them in the initial stages over a month or two since the deficits are long-bearing especially the neurological ones. So, after three months, six months, all these supports start slowly coming down. The money starts coming down. The people running around to the hospital to be around with them start slowly coming down. There may be pressure from the workplace that they have been missing for a long time, or they're unable to focus on work if they are also trying to work. A lot of these issues start mounting on the caregivers. Sometimes, if they are the ones looking after the patient day in and day out, they probably don't get sleep at night because the patient is awake or disturbed for some reason. They can't sleep during the day because therapies are happening. People are going in and out, and there are doctor visits and investigations. All these things are happening during the day. So, days together, there are times that caregivers don't get to sleep properly. They don't get to eat properly. They don't even get to take care of themselves and have time for themselves. In fact, after some time, their health starts getting affected because they've been focusing only on the patient.

So, for us, it's very important to make sure the caregivers are taken care of, whether it is the husband, the wife, or even a hired caregiver. Do they sleep well? Do they eat well? How are they able to balance all these things? Do they have some time for themselves? Are they able to talk to their other family members? How are they managing to balance their work and other family needs? Maybe they have small kids that they must look after all these things. So, we have to counsel these caregivers very frequently to get them out of that overwhelming situation they get into many times.

Here's another story!

Ramesh experienced a two-wheeler accident near Kolar while traveling towards Bangalore. He was promptly taken to the local hospital for emergency treatment and eventually recovered. Despite being discharged, he grappled with significant cognitive issues.

While he regained mobility and manual dexterity, there were noticeable deficits in his cognitive functions. Although his speech remained unaffected, comprehension and memory posed challenges. He required frequent repetition to grasp information and often struggled to retain conversations. Additionally, he exhibited severe behavioral problems, displaying aggression and irritability, a stark contrast to his previously mild-mannered demeanor.

Upon assessment, it was revealed that Ramesh was a second-year BSc student who had missed his exams due to the accident. Over 4-8 weeks, a home-based retraining program supported by his dedicated brothers began to yield results. Through intensive sessions at home and in Bangalore, Ramesh gradually regained some semblance of memory and comprehension. Within six months, he had progressed sufficiently to consider returning to college, although challenges persisted in the classroom and during self-study.

Despite ongoing difficulties, the brothers continued to seek guidance and support, diligently implementing the retraining program. With time and perseverance, Ramesh's memory and cognitive abilities improved significantly. He successfully completed his BSc, pursued an MSc, and ultimately entered the workforce, demonstrating remarkable progress and resilience. This achievement underscores the invaluable role of family support in overcoming cognitive challenges and achieving personal and academic milestones.

@PRS Neurosciences, the therapists are the core strength of the organization's rehab vertical. The clinicians study a lot. They understand not only the subject but also, they must understand the patient, the patient's caregiver. They must have the patience to understand and wait and to support the patient and the caregiver.

Most of the time, these are youngsters who probably do not have the maturity that some of the patients and caregivers have because they would have just come out of college. They would have probably had two, three, four, or five years of experience on the work front, and they probably haven't been exposed to all the difficulties that the patient and the caregiver probably would have seen in their lives.

However, knowing that they are in this place, handling these patients and caregivers who are already overwhelmed and really under a lot of pressure, the therapist plays a huge role in making sure that these people are comforted. And it is my job to make sure that these people keep up their sanity. So they work on themselves so that they have peace of mind, they have their inner strength and inner capabilities built up so that they can handle the stress, work stress, along with the patient, supporting the caregivers and making sure the results are produced in a way that is impressive to them and very impressive to the patient and the caregivers.

Understanding the Importance of Medical Insurance in India

Health insurance plays a crucial role in providing financial protection and peace of mind during medical emergencies, such as strokes, head injuries, or spinal cord injuries, as discussed in the passage. Health insurance can significantly alleviate the financial burden of hospitalization, surgeries, and ongoing medical care. However, many people underestimate its importance or mistakenly believe it won't be useful to them. This misconception often stems from the belief that it wastes money if they don't utilize the insurance benefits within a given year. Yet, the true value of health insurance lies in its ability to safeguard against unexpected and potentially catastrophic healthcare costs. It offers a safety net, ensuring that individuals and their families can access necessary medical treatment without facing crippling financial hardship. Therefore, it's crucial to encourage everyone to prioritize obtaining health insurance coverage. It's an investment in one's health and financial well-being, providing invaluable support and protection when it's needed most.

This book cannot end without a small note on our charity - Swaasthya Aarogya Foundation (SAF)

Swaasthya Aarogya Foundation (SAF) is our NGO wing, established with a deeply personal commitment to addressing the healthcare disparities faced by many in our community.

Establishing the Swaasthya Aarogya Foundation has been a deeply personal journey for us. It began before we even founded our company, PRS Neurosciences. As doctors, we've encountered countless patients who simply couldn't afford the surgeries or treatments they desperately needed. It's heartbreaking to see hardworking individuals, like auto-rickshaw drivers or cab drivers, suddenly faced with a medical emergency and unable to cover the exorbitant costs of hospitalization and care.

In India, the reality is that many people don't prioritize health insurance and even those who do often find themselves financially drained when a medical crisis strikes. We've witnessed families exhaust their savings, sell off possessions, and take out loans to save a loved one's life. But what happens after the acute phase of treatment, when long-term rehabilitation is necessary?

Rehabilitation is often overlooked, yet it's a vital part of the healing process, especially for those who can't afford ongoing care. That's why we felt compelled to establish our NGO alongside our medical practice. The Swaasthya Aarogya Foundation aims to bridge the gap by providing funding for surgeries and rehabilitation services to those who would otherwise be unable to access them.

Raising funds is challenging, but we've been fortunate to receive support from our network of friends, family, and compassionate individuals who believe in our cause. Whether it's a small contribution or a larger donation, every bit helps us make a difference in someone's life.

Running the NGO alongside our company isn't easy but incredibly rewarding. Knowing that we're helping patients get back on their feet, regain their independence, and reintegrate into society fuels our determination to keep going. Our focus isn't just on those who can afford care; it's on those who need it the most – the ones who would otherwise be left behind.

Through the Swaasthya Aarogya Foundation, we're not just providing medical treatment but restoring hope and dignity to those who need it most. And as long as there are people in need, we'll continue to run this organization, knowing that every life we touch is a testament to the power of compassion and community.

CONCLUSION

"It does not matter how slowly you go as long as you do not stop."

- Confucius

The Journey Of 'HOPE'

You may have been asking yourself why you should learn about functional neuroscience. It's a question that may not seem relevant if you haven't encountered neurological diseases within your circle of friends or family. However, as I have reiterated, understanding neuroscience is crucial because the **brain** is the **most vital organ** for human survival. Even if the brain is functioning at 100%, challenges can arise.

Neurological diseases and dysfunctions come in various forms, often perplexing even specialists like neurosurgeons and neuro physicians, let alone general practitioners who lack expertise in neuroscience. Yet, having even a basic understanding can make a significant difference when you or a loved one begins experiencing symptoms. It's about being proactive without succumbing to the anxiety of relying solely on internet searches or self-diagnosis.

Consider the landscape of health awareness. There's ample information available on cancer, heart diseases, liver health issues, and more. People monitor their steps with smartwatches for cardiovascular health, but only a few pay attention to brain health. As we move forward, knowledge about the brain should become as common as awareness about other organs and diseases.

In India, it's estimated that around 100 million people suffer from neurological disorders, ranging from Epilepsy to Parkinson's disease. This highlights the urgent need for effective treatments and interventions. Despite the high prevalence of brain and other movement disorders, there's a significant lack of awareness and understanding among the general population. Many people living with these conditions often face stigma and discrimination, hindering their access to proper care and support.

We also have one of the highest incidences of spine injuries in the world, with an estimated 20,000 new cases reported annually. These injuries result from various causes, including road traffic accidents, falls, sports injuries, and violence. Despite the significant burden of spine injuries, access to specialized spine care services, including surgical interventions and rehabilitation, remains limited in many parts of the country. This underscores the urgent need for improved infrastructure, expertise, and resources to address the growing challenge of spine injuries and ensure optimal outcomes for affected individuals in India.

So, how and why did I develop newro LOGICS as an initiative? It's a question that's been posed to me countless times over the past 25 years, and it's worth addressing once more for our audience.

Since I was 14, I have harbored the dream of becoming a neurosurgeon, and I've relentlessly pursued that dream ever since. As I embarked on my journey to become a neurosurgeon in the mid and late 1990s, I encountered patients who had undergone surgeries for strokes, head injuries, and brain tumors.

While our surgical interventions saved their lives, many remained in a state of dysfunction—semi-conscious, bedridden, and dependent on acute care support for extended periods.

As these patients languished in hospitals, occupying precious beds needed for acute care, their families faced the heart-wrenching dilemma of finding appropriate care facilities. I found myself at a loss, torn between my professional duty and the stark reality of inadequate post-surgical care options. That was a pivotal moment of introspection. This wasn't what I had envisioned for myself when I embarked on my neurosurgery journey. I didn't want to be just another surgeon; I wanted to be a healer, restoring my patients' quality of life. The seed of an idea began to germinate—a realization that comprehensive post-surgical care, encompassing rehabilitation, was sorely lacking in our healthcare landscape.

In the late 1990s, rehabilitation was virtually nonexistent in India beyond essential physiotherapy. I grappled with the realization that someone needed to address the neglected field of rehabilitating damaged brain circuits to facilitate recovery. Though the idea simmered in the background, it wasn't until 2005 that the situation's urgency became glaringly apparent.

For too long, I had held the misconception that my role as a neurosurgeon ended once the surgery was completed—that rehabilitation was someone else's responsibility. However, it became evident that the existing system failed our patients. In 2006 and 2007, I decided to take personal responsibility for guiding my patients through the recovery journey. I successfully enrolled my best friend and life partner, Dr. Prathiba, in this crazy but exciting journey! I recognized the imperative to support them holistically and facilitate their transition to functional independence to the best of my abilities.

Thus, the concept of newro LOGICS emerged—an initiative born out of a deep-seated commitment to ensuring that every patient receives comprehensive care, from surgery to rehabilitation, from hopelessness to

I've reiterated this point countless times, even in the ICU, to intensivists: all the monitors, all the beeping, all those numbers flashing on the screens—none of them provide brain data. It's all about blood pressure, sugar levels, heart rate, saturation, breathing patterns, etc. Everyone seems fixated on everything else except the brain. I always tell the ICU staff – that it takes less time for you to measure a patient's coma score using the GCS than to check his BP! I've often asked my colleagues in the ICU why there's a neglectful attitude towards the brain.

It's often dismissed with remarks like, "It's just a stroke, they'll be fine," or "They only lost consciousness for a few minutes." But what people fail to grasp is that it's incredibly challenging for the brain to stop functioning even for a brief moment. Just one minute of lost consciousness indicates a significant problem.

I often use dialogue to drive this point home, 'if a patient walks into the hospital talking and coherent despite a brain problem, their chances of leaving the hospital in the same state are much higher. However, if they're brought in semi-conscious or unconscious, the odds of a full recovery are significantly lower because more brain damage has likely occurred and will also take much longer. And unfortunately, we don't have spare parts for the brain.'

The key message here is that earlier intervention leads to better outcomes. We're advocating this concept globally, not just in India—a concept of **"time is brain."** That's why we have made a shift from using the term "stroke" to using "brain attack" instead in our efforts to instill the same sense of urgency associated with heart attacks, where every second counts.

Understanding concepts like the lucid interval and the complexities of the brain is crucial because, quite simply, we don't have a backup brain. It's a delicate organ; we must treat it with utmost care and urgency.

So, what about people's common misconceptions or misinformation about my field? I'd like to highlight three key points.

Firstly, let's talk about memory problems as we age. It's a common belief that memory naturally deteriorates as we age, but that's not always true. Take, for example, renowned figures like Ram Jethmalani, who practiced law in the Supreme Court at 97 years old, or Manmohan Singh, who served as the Prime Minister at 84. Even Joe Biden, the President of America, is 81 years old. These individuals demonstrate that age doesn't necessarily equate to memory decline. If someone is experiencing memory problems, it's essential to investigate further. Memory issues could signal underlying conditions like Alzheimer's disease, low sodium levels, brain tumors, or fluid accumulation in the brain. Don't dismiss memory problems as a normal part of aging—seek medical attention from a neurologist or neurosurgeon for proper evaluation.

Secondly, let's address headaches. Not all headaches are migraines, contrary to popular belief. Many people attribute all headaches to migraines, but there are numerous other types of headaches. I recall a story of a radiation oncologist who suffered from headaches for 25 years, assuming they were migraines without undergoing a scan. Eventually, when a scan was performed out of frustration, an unruptured brain aneurysm was discovered. This underscores the importance of proper diagnosis and not assuming that all headaches are migraines without medical evaluation.

Lastly, let's debunk the misconception surrounding spondylosis or spondylitis. These terms often evoke fear but are common conditions of spine wear and tear, which occurs with age. I've encountered patients as young as 35 who express distress over being diagnosed with spondylitis. Providing reassurance and proper context to patients is crucial, explaining that these conditions are manageable and don't signify the end of life. The psychological impact of the disease may be sometimes more debilitating than the condition itself, leading individuals to feel like they are living dead. Educating patients about their condition and alleviating their fears is essential for a holistic approach to their well-being.

Access to neurosurgical care remains challenging in many parts of India, particularly in semi-urban and rural areas. Still, it has improved by leaps and bounds, especially in the past two decades. This leads to delays in diagnosis and treatment, resulting in poorer outcomes for patients with brain tumors, traumatic brain injuries, spinal cord injuries, and other neurosurgical conditions.

Stereotactic neurosurgery, a minimally invasive technique used for precisely targeting areas within the brain, has seen significant advancements recently. With the introduction of advanced imaging technologies and robotic-assisted systems, neurosurgeons can now perform complex brain surgeries with greater accuracy and safety.

Despite the growing recognition of the importance of neuro rehabilitation in improving outcomes for individuals with neurological disorders, there's a significant gap in access to rehabilitation services and qualified neuro rehabilitation professionals across the country. Many patients lack access to specialized neuro rehabilitation centers and trained therapists, limiting their recovery potential.

Neuromodulation techniques, such as deep brain stimulation (DBS) and transcranial magnetic stimulation (TMS), offer promising avenues for the treatment of various neurological conditions, including Parkinson's disease, depression, and chronic pain. However, these advanced therapies are still relatively inaccessible to many patients in India due to cost constraints and limited expertise.

Addressing the complex needs of individuals with neurological disorders requires a multidisciplinary approach involving neurosurgeons, neurologists, rehabilitation specialists, psychologists, and caregivers. However, such integrated care models still need to be widely established in India, leading to fragmented and suboptimal care for many patients.

Despite the challenges, there's a growing emphasis on research and innovation in the field of neurosciences in India. Collaborative efforts between academic institutions, healthcare organizations, and government agencies are driving advancements in understanding movement disorders and developing novel yet affordable treatment modalities tailored to the patients.

This underscores the urgent need for concerted efforts to improve access to neurosurgical care, rehabilitation services, and advanced treatment modalities for individuals living with neurological disorders in India. By raising awareness, investing in healthcare infrastructure, and fostering collaboration among stakeholders, we can work towards ensuring better outcomes and quality of life for all affected individuals.

So far, in **'Rebooting The Brain®,'** we have explored the rising incidence of neurological disability in India, delving into the transition from dependence to independence for patients and families. We highlighted the journey from hopelessness to hope, likening it to a marathon race with an indefinite finish line—my childhood dream of becoming a neurosurgeon and the relentless pursuit of that dream. We recounted encounters with patients during training and the pivotal moments that shaped my journey, including my transformative experiences, like the trip to Japan in 2015 that led to my stereotactic practice. We ventured into the world of misbehaving brain and spinal cord circuits, discussing movement disorders and the role of neuromodulation in their treatment. We also explored neuromodulation surgeries and their benefits for different patient populations.

The "Guitar Surgeon" took center stage in Chapter 4, where we recounted a viral live surgery and the intricacies of treating Task-Specific Focal Hand Dystonia (TSFHD). We tried our best to provide in-depth explorations of Parkinson's Disease, dystonia, spasticity, and neuromodulation procedures, shedding light on these often misunderstood conditions and their treatment options. We even addressed chronic pain as the fifth vital sign, discussing its significance in treatment approaches and sharing stories of individuals grappling with chronic pain conditions like trigeminal neuralgia and musculoskeletal pains.

Gradually, we shifted our focus to strokes, emphasizing the urgency of time spent on stroke management and prevention strategies. We followed the journey of stroke survivors, highlighting their resilience in the face of adversity.

We also tackled traumatic brain injury and its staggering global impact, underscoring the importance of prevention and timely intervention. We delved into spinal cord injury, its causes, rehabilitation, and the experiences of survivors.

As we end our journey **exploring the emerging field of Functional Neurosciences – comprising neuromodulation with advanced neuro rehabilitation,** it's clear that understanding and treating neurological conditions is both complex and hopeful. We've seen how teamwork, new technologies, and caring attitudes have made a big difference in helping people with brain problems. In wrapping up this part, let's keep the spirit of teamwork and hope alive. Together, we can create a future where everyone can live their best life, regardless of their brain condition.

Within healthcare, neuro rehabilitation encompasses far more than restoring physical functions; it embodies a profound commitment to enhancing the quality of life and providing compassionate palliative care.

Let me leave you with a last story on how technology has allowed a fully paralyzed, terminally ill MND patient on a ventilator to communicate with the outside world and remain connected.

Unyielding Spirit: The Indomitable Entrepreneur with terminal MND, navigating Business and Life with a Gaze.

Set against the backdrop of a family's unwavering resolve and a community's steadfast support, the narrative of Shivakumar and his courageous battle against Motor Neuron Disease (MND) serves as a poignant testament to the transformative power of perseverance, technological innovation, and the enduring human spirit.

The New Year 2019 began a tumultuous journey for Shivakumar and his family. As they joyously celebrated the onset of a new year, little did they know that an invisible storm was brewing within Shivakumar's body. As his wife narrates, it is apparent that that particular night has been ingrained in their minds.

That night, five years ago, he began to stumble while walking, sometimes resulting in him falling. Initially attributing it to fatigue or a passing discomfort, Shivakumar and his family brushed aside the ominous signs.

Shivakumar, a resilient man who came to Bengaluru over three decades ago from his village to pursue a better life, had built a thriving business empire – SNAB GRAPHIX (INDIA) PVT. LTD. His journey from struggling for a job in 1991 to establishing an imports trading company in 1996 was a testament to his determination and entrepreneurial spirit.

Over the years, he has expanded his successful business to multiple cities, providing many jobs and opportunities, which he lacked when he began his journey in Bengaluru. His success was a personal triumph and a beacon of hope for those who knew him and depended on him.

The first day of 2019 unfolded with Shivakumar's leg discomfort persisting, gradually becoming more than a passing inconvenience. By November of the same year, the pain had intensified to a point where it couldn't be ignored any longer—not just the increase in discomfort but an ache coursing across his body to his arms. Alarmed by the escalating discomfort and the realization that this was more than a temporary ailment, Shivakumar and his family sought medical attention.

The progression of the discomfort from January to November 2019 manifested in a slowing gait. What was once a routine walk with his wife, where she struggled to keep up with this tall man's gait and pace, transformed into a struggle for him to maintain his wife's pace? Initially dismissed as inexplicable, the discomfort intensified, extending its grip from his legs to his arms. As the mysterious condition unfolded, Shivakumar relied on a wheelchair to navigate his surroundings.

The diagnosis was devastating – early stages of Motor Neuron Disease (MND). What began as an innocent discomfort in his legs had insidiously spread to his hands, causing them to curl involuntarily. The medical team provided a grim outlook, expressing the challenges of MND's unpredictable progression. Expectations were limited to short intervals of three to six months as the disorder relentlessly advanced, leaving uncertainty about the future. However, even as Shivakumar demonstrated resilience in the business realm and compassion on the personal front, a silent battle raged within him. This mysterious leg issue that had surfaced on New Year's night in 2019 and had evolved into a relentless adversary now had an identity. Despite his disciplined and healthy lifestyle, marked by regular walks and an absence of accidents or injuries, the issue persisted, gradually encroaching upon his ability to walk. Slowly creeping up, it made its way to his arms.

As the world grappled with the emergence of the COVID-19 pandemic in late 2019-early 2020, Shivakumar, the visionary entrepreneur, found himself navigating uncharted waters. Little did he know that his foresight, honed by years of business acumen, would aid him in extending a helping hand to those around him.

Shivakumar had unknowingly anticipated the global disruption caused by the pandemic. Observing the shutdown of Chinese markets, his primary supplier hub, he foresaw the possibility of similar closures in other parts of the world, especially India. Sensing the impending storm, he strategically relocated his family to Chikkamagaluru just before the widespread lockdowns commenced.

His proactive measures proved crucial as markets worldwide shuttered due to the unforeseen impact of the COVID-19 epidemic. Meanwhile, in the confines of his home, Shivakumar and his family found themselves amid the pandemic's early stages. A house help stayed with them, and with the scarcity of masks and sanitizers, Shivakumar and Kavitha decided to avoid capitalizing on the situation. Instead, they distributed the essential protective gear to family, friends, and well-wishers, embodying a spirit of generosity in adversity.

Shivakumar confronted a new challenge on March 26, 2022, at the height of India's third wave of the COVID-19 pandemic. Breathing issues emerged, adding another layer of complexity to his already formidable health struggles. By this period, the discomfort creeping into his hands had almost taken over, causing increased weakness. The physical toll became increasingly evident as he found himself 50% weaker, grappling not only with the debilitating effects of MND but also with the concurrent challenges posed by the global health crisis. As the MND progressed, he could not walk on his own due to the intense discomfort he felt. He decided to mount on a wheelchair for ease of movement.

Yet, Shivakumar faced these trials and tribulations with characteristic determination. His ability to foresee challenges in the business world proved paralleled by his resilience in the face of personal adversity. Guiding SNAB GRAPHIX through the ever-evolving global landscape, Shivakumar's son found inspiration in his father's strength. Though physically weakened, Shivakumar continued to inspire everyone with his unwavering spirit, symbolizing strength for his family, employees, and all who knew him.

As Shivakumar's battle with Motor Neuron Disease (MND) intensified, his cognitive abilities remained a beacon of resilience amid physical deterioration. The medical team, while unable to provide long-term prognoses due to the unpredictable nature of MND, marveled at Shivakumar's high-functioning cognitive skills. Even as his hands curled and speech slurred, his mind remained sharp.

Despite this daunting prognosis, Shivakumar's cognitive abilities remained remarkably intact. His sharp mind, honed through years of managing his business, continued to function at a high level. For the past five years, he has been guiding his wife, Kavitha, and, more recently, his son in steering the ship of SNAB GRAPHIX, while his daughter, inspired by her father's resilience in the face of medical challenges, has embarked on her journey in the healthcare field.

Currently, in her first year of medical school, she has been motivated to contribute to the field and make a meaningful impact on the lives of those facing similar health struggles.

As the years rolled on, the progression of MND took its toll. The weakness of hands and slurring of speech became more pronounced. Amid the third wave of the COVID-19 pandemic in March 2022, breathing issues surfaced, adding another layer of complexity to Shivakumar's health challenges. The physical weakness reached a point where he was 50% incapacitated.

Amidst these trials, a glimmer of hope emerged in the form of Mr. Vasanth Rao from the MND Association. Mr. Rao, who had experienced a similar ordeal through his late wife, Dr. Shyama Narang, contacted Shivakumar's family. Understanding the challenges they faced, he recommended the Tobii Dynavox Blink-tech software. This advanced communication tool would prove invaluable as Shivakumar's speech faltered.

Remarkably, with medical guidance, Shivakumar could anticipate the progressive nature of his MND. Even before the software became necessary, he had ordered it, ensuring that communication would not become a barrier in his journey. His foresight and meticulous planning became evident – a testament to his ability to stay three steps ahead of the disorder.

The MND Association has a broader mission beyond individual support. Its vision extends to advancing excellence in care and support for people with MND and promoting coordinated research communities dedicated to finding a cure. Mr. Rao's involvement, driven by the legacy of his late wife, reflected a shared commitment to fighting MND.

As he lost all mobility, Shivakumar was shifted to Bhagawan Mahaveer Jain Hospital about 2.5 years ago (2022). That is when I met this enigmatic and inspiring man. As a dedicated neurosurgeon, I could not help the family much medically. Still, I have since then become a regular presence in Shivakumar's life, boosting his energy during my bi-weekly visits, as his wife says. Even though it is a lifeline for communication, the Blink-tech software has become Shivakumar's window to the world. Despite being bedridden for two years, he watches the news, talk shows, and his favorite shows on almost all OTT/streaming platforms, maintaining a connection with the external world.

As the medical mystery unfolded, various professionals sought to understand Shivakumar's condition. Dr. Venkat Raman, a lead expert in India, explored the possibility of lead poisoning as being the cause of the MND. At the same time, a group of researchers from Delhi investigated the genetic aspect as a trigger. Both avenues proved to be dead ends, leaving the medical community perplexed.

His wife, Kavitha, and I are amazed at the seemingly contradictory medical reports. On medical reports, Shivakumar appears to be a healthy adult man, defying the reality of his condition. Even in the face of adversity, Shivakumar's disciplined hygiene stands out. Despite being bedridden, he has not developed a single bed infection or bedsore and has maintained his nutritional status without any coercion from his caregivers!

The Tobii Dynavox Blink-tech software continues to be a vital tool, allowing Shivakumar to communicate with his family and caregivers and engage with the world through news and entertainment. The software, produced by the Sweden-based organization Tobii Dynavox, is a testament to the power of technology in empowering individuals facing complex communication and mobility challenges.

As the Tobii Dynavox Blink-tech software integrates into Shivakumar's life with a cost nearing 17 lacs, he acknowledges the privilege of financial means facilitating access to such advanced technology. Given his background in the import business, acquiring this technology was more accessible to him. In his immobile state, relying on the screen that serves as his lifeline, Shivakumar consistently emphasizes to visiting doctors that he is not only concerned about his fate but also about the rarity of this condition, which limits awareness.

Many individuals only discover it when they become caregivers for MND patients. The scarcity of resources and their high costs compound the challenges. He endeavors to bring MND-accessible technology and resources to India, ensuring future generations and those unaware of the condition have better support.

While his family understandably worries primarily about his well-being, Shivakumar's humble vision extends to the well-being of others facing similar struggles.

Despite ongoing neuro rehabilitation at Bhagwan Mahaveer Jain Hospital, Girinagar, Shivakumar's commitment to giving back remains unwavering. Even in a seemingly vegetative state, he and his family continue to provide for various not-for-profit organizations, exemplifying a spirit of generosity that transcends his physical limitations.

Shivakumar's story will become a mosaic of resilience, foresight, and adaptability as the years progress. Through the highs and lows, he faces the challenges of MND head-on, leaving an indelible mark on those who know him. His family's unwavering support, the dedication of his caregivers and healthcare professionals, and technological aids have become the pillars supporting Shivakumar in his courageous journey.

"It is a waste of time to be angry about my disability. One has to get on with life, and I haven't done badly. People won't have time for you if you are always angry or complaining."

— Stephen Hawking

But fret not yet because we've got more to come!

In our upcoming book, **Rebooting The Brain® – Part-2**, we invite readers to embark on a journey into the realm of **"Neuro Justice,"** offering a comprehensive exploration of the intersection between neurology, law, policy, and rehabilitation and **"Functional Neurosciences – the newro LOGICS® way,"** offering a comprehensive exploration of the intersection between clinical neurology, IoMT-based technology, and cutting-edge clinical research. Here's a glimpse of what to expect:

1. **Understanding the Global Burden of Neurological Disabilities:** Dive with us into the intricate web of neurological disabilities, including stroke, traumatic brain injury (TBI), spinal cord injury (SCI), and Parkinson's disease, as we explore the profound impact of these conditions on individuals, families, communities, and economies worldwide.

2. **Policy, Perception, and Advocacy:** Examine the role of policymakers, social influencers, and advocacy groups in shaping public policy and perception surrounding neurological disabilities with us as we delve into the legal frameworks, regulations, and ethical considerations involved in addressing these complex issues within the legal system.

3. **Navigating the Medico-Legal Landscape:** Gain insights into the challenges faced by individuals with neurological disabilities and their caregivers as they navigate healthcare and legal systems. Explore the nuances of assessing functional disabilities for just compensation, including the limitations of traditional diagnostic methods and the importance of multidisciplinary approaches.

4. **Revolutionizing Neuro rehabilitation:** Discover the transformative potential of functional neurosciences in revolutionizing rehabilitation for individuals with neurological disabilities. Explore concepts such as neuroplasticity, rewiring the brain, and the role of IoMT-based technology in enhancing rehabilitation outcomes.

5. **Precision and Personalized Medicine and Digital Transformation:** Delve into the digital transformation of healthcare through precision and personalized medicine and IoMT-based interventions. Explore the concept of SMART rehab hospitals, gamification of rehabilitation, and the future of at-home rehabilitation solutions.

6. **Research and Innovation**: Explore the latest research and innovations in functional neurosciences, including data analytics, artificial intelligence, and predictive modeling for improved patient outcomes. Discover how these advancements are shaping the future of neurology and rehabilitation.

Through engaging narratives, case studies, and expert insights, we aim to inform, inspire, and empower readers to advocate for neuro-justice and embrace the transformative potential of functional neurosciences in improving the lives of individuals with neurological disabilities.

As we come to a halt here, I want to remind you that we will always be here for you. You may close this book, but the chapters of your life will keep writing themselves. The challenges and struggles don't stop here, nor does my contribution to our society.

Our journey has shown us that the brain is fantastic but also tricky to understand. By working together and keeping an open mind, we can make significant strides in helping people with brain, spine, and nerve injuries lead better lives.

Even though we've made progress, there's still a lot to learn and do. We need to keep researching, learning, and supporting each other. As we move forward, let's remember to be kind, compassionate, and understanding to everyone facing challenges, especially neurological ones.

Signing off...until we meet again.

Till then, remember to wear your helmets, put on your seat belts, and take your hypertension and diabetic medications on time!!! And enjoy life...

QR Codes

Prologue

Chapter 1

Chapter 2

Chapter 3

Chapter 4

Chapter 5

Chapter 6

Chapter 7

Chapter 8

Chapter 9

Chapter 10

Chapter 11

Chapter 12

Chapter 13

Chapter 14

Chapter 15

Web Series

Documentary

Bheja Unfry: Dive into a delectable web series where laughter meets drama, promising a feast for your senses and a craving for more. What more? It's the world's first-ever web series on functional neurosciences.

Rebooting the Brain®: Embark on a riveting documentary journey into the depths of neuroscience, ready to spark wonder and ignite your intellect.

Scan the QR codes for instant access on YouTube, and indulge in an immersive experience of entertainment and enlightenment.

EDITORS & CONTRIBUTORS

Editor-in-Chief:

Prof. Dr. Sharan Srinivasan
Stereotactic & Functional Neurosurgeon
Chairman, Managing Director & Founder
PRS Neurosciences and Mechatronics Research Institute (PNMRI)
HOD of Neurosciences, Bhagwan Mahaveer Jain Hospital, Bengaluru, India.
special interests: movement disorders, spasticity, pain & Neuro rehabilitation
FELLOWSHIPS: (from TWMU - Tokyo, Japan)
1. Stereotactic & Functional Neurosurgery
2. Stereotactic Radiosurgery

Editorial team:

Mr.V. Siddharth
Masters of Occupational Therapy, Developmental Disabilities, AIIPMR
Sr. Occupational Therapist,
AGM- Research & Development,
Advanced Neuro Rehab Specialist
PRS Neurosciences

Miss. Sneha Hari
Bachelor of Audiology and Speech-Language Pathology (BASLP), Mangalore University
In charge- SLP department
Manager- Content & Digitalization,
Advanced Neuro Rehab Specialist- Under Training
PRS Neurosciences

Prof. Stafford Michahial,
(P.hd) Medical Image Processing, VTU, Karnataka
M.Tech Digital Electronics and Communication, VTU, Karnataka
B.Tech Electronics and Communication, VTU, Karnataka
IEEE(Member),IETE (Member), VRARA(President Bangalore chapter(2017- 2020)).
Group Chief Technology Officer (Group-CTO) & Co-Founder
NEWRO-KAAYA INNOVATIVE SOLUTIONS PRIVATE LIMITED
PRS Neurosciences

Dr. Prathiba Sharan
MBBS, (BMCRI)
PGDPC, Neuropsychology (NIMHANS),
Fellowship in Neuro Rehabilitation (Apollo Hospitals)
CEO and **CMRD,**

Co-Founder of PRS Neurosciences

Contributors from PRS Neurosciences:

Content:

Mr. Nikhil CH
Masters of Physiotherapy (Neurosciences), **Dr.MGR Medical University**
Head Of Department - Physiotherapy,
AGM- Operations
Advanced Neuro Rehab Specialist
PRS Neurosciences

Mr. Ganapathy Arumugham
Master of Occupational Therapy (Paediatrics), **Dr.MGR Medical University**
HOD- Occupational Therapy
AGM- Academics & Training
Advanced Neuro Rehab Specialist PRS Neurosciences

Mr.V.Siddharth
Masters of Occupational Therapy, Developmental Disabilities, AIIPMR
Sr. Occupational Therapist,
AGM- Research & Development,
Advanced Neuro Rehab Specialist
PRS Neurosciences

Miss. Sneha Hari
Bachelors of Audiology and Speech-Language Pathology (BASLP),
In charge- SLP department
Manager- Digitalization,
Advanced Neuro Rehab Specialist- Under Training
PRS Neurosciences

Miss. Yashaswini D.S
Bachelor of Commerce (B.Com), Mount Carmel College, Bengaluru
Social Media Coordinator
PRS Neurosciences

Prof. Stafford Michahial,
(P.hd) Medical Image Processing, VTU, Karnataka
M.Tech Digital Electronics and Communication, VTU, Karnataka
B.Tech Electronics and Communication, VTU, Karnataka
IEEE(Member),IETE (Member), VRARA(President Bangalore chapter(2017- 2020)).
Co-Founder
NEWRO-KAAYA INNOVATIVE SOLUTIONS PRIVATE LIMITED
Group Chief Technology Officer (Group CTO)
PRS Neurosciences

Illustrations:

Mr. Rishab Gupta
Bachelors of Product Design (B.Des), MIT, Pune
Co-founder,
NEWRO-KAAYA INNOVATIVE SOLUTIONS PRIVATE LIMITED

Mr. Prathitah Sharan
Data Scientist & Co-founder,
NEWRO-KAAYA INNOVATIVE SOLUTIONS PRIVATE LIMITED

INTELLECTUAL PROPERTIES (IP)

Owned by PRS Neurosciences

Trademarks

SI No	Brand Name	Class
1	Rebooting The Brain	44
2	Newrologix	9
3	Newrologix	35
4	Newrologix	44
5	SEFA	44
6	CarePa-Re	44
7	Vost	44
8	Newro	9
9	Newro	44
10	Rehab Redefined	44
11	ayur newro	5
12	ayur newro	35
13	PRS Exploring New Frontiers	44
14	Newrologix	9
15	Energizing Rehab	44
16	CVC4H	44
17	CVC4S	44
18	MAASS	44
19	SMART REHAB	44
20	SAREEES	44
21	Brain(M)apps	44

Patents (Indian & Global – PCT)

	Description
1	Complete Patent application filed. Application number 201941038618 for your proposed patent titled **"A NOVEL AND ROBUST CURRICULUM FOR ADVANCED NEURO REHABILITATION"**
2	Complete Patent application filed. Application number 202241067553 for your proposed patent titled **"A System And Methodology For Assessment, Prognostication And Tracking Recovery Of Damaged 'Functional' Brain Circuits For Predicting Functional Independence."**
3	**CAREPa-Re Framework: A 360° Evidence-Based Matrix for Precision and Personalized Medicine in Functional Neurosciences, to achieve '8W-4W: X-Y' using data analytics & AI.**

Copyrights

SI No	Logo Name
1	Rebooting The Brain - 142678
2	NewRo - 94555
3	Newrologix - 94068
4	C2C - Literary Copyright - 20609
5	Ayur Newro - 114385
6	NewRo Rebooting The Brain - 14008

Madrid

Sl No	Description
1	Rebooting the Brain
2	Rebooting the Brain USA designation
3	Rebooting the Brain UK designation

ABOUT THE AUTHORS

Dr. Sharan Srinivasan

Prof. Dr. Sharan Srinivasan is a distinguished figure in neurosurgery, renowned for his stereotactic and functional neurosurgery expertise. With a comprehensive educational background, including an MBBS and DNB in neurosurgery, alongside fellowships from prestigious institutions in Tokyo, Japan, Dr. Sharan has honed his skills to become a leading authority in his field.

Currently serving as the Head of Neurosciences at Bhagwan Mahaveer Jain Hospital in Bengaluru, India, Dr. Sharan is deeply committed to advancing the understanding and treatment of neurological disorders. His affiliation as a Visiting Professor at Zubeita University in La Paz, Bolivia, further demonstrates his global impact and recognition.

Dr. Sharan's contributions extend beyond clinical practice. As the founder and Chief Managing Director of PRS Neurosciences & Mechatronics Research Institute (PNMRI), he pioneers innovative approaches to neuro modulation and rehabilitation, aiming to enhance the lives of individuals with neurological disabilities.

Recognized for his outstanding achievements, Dr. Sharan has received numerous accolades, including winning the grand finale of India's prestigious Bio Entrepreneurship competition, #NBEC2022. His groundbreaking surgeries, such as the celebrated 'guitar surgery' for focal hand dystonia, have garnered international attention and acclaim.

In addition to his clinical and entrepreneurial endeavors, Dr. Sharan is a prolific author and researcher. His essential publication, documenting the first unilateral pallid-thalamic tractotomy for Parkinson's Disease in India, highlights his commitment to advancing the frontiers of neurosurgery.

Dr. Sharan's expertise is unparalleled, and he has over 8,000 major brain and spine surgeries to his credit. His dedication to improving functional independence and quality of life for patients with neurological disorders is evident in his trademarked concept of "Rebooting The Brain®."

Driven by a passion for innovation and compassionate patient care, Dr. Sharan Srinivasan continues to inspire and lead in the field of neurosurgery, shaping the future of neurological treatment and rehabilitation worldwide.

Dr. Prathiba Sharan

Dr. Prathiba Sharan is a distinguished figure in the fields of neuro rehabilitation and neuropsychology, renowned for her holistic approach to patient care and rehabilitation. As the Co-Founder & CEO of PRS Neurosciences & Mechatronics Research Institute and the Medical and Rehab Director of newro, she has been instrumental in shaping innovative approaches to neurological rehabilitation.

Dr. Prathiba Sharan's medical journey began with her graduation from Bangalore Medical College and Research Institute. After that, she pursued specialized training in psychological counseling and neuropsychology, culminating in a Fellowship in Neurological Rehabilitation from Apollo Hospitals, Hyderabad, India. Her diverse skill set, encompassing psychological counseling, neuropsychology, and Ashtanga yoga practice, reflects her commitment to holistic patient care.

With a career spanning over two decades, Dr. Prathiba Sharan has emerged as a leading authority in neuro rehabilitation. She has helped thousands of neurologically disabled patients achieve their maximum functional potential. Her approach emphasizes individualized care, empowering patients and caregivers to navigate the challenges of neurological disorders effectively.

A former Junior National Champion in swimming, yoga, and roller skating, Dr. Prathiba brings a resilient "Never Give Up" attitude to her practice. She draws inspiration from adversity to fuel innovation and customization in therapy. Her expertise in customizing therapies to suit each patient's, and their family's unique needs has led to consistently superior outcomes and inspired her colleagues to follow suit.

Beyond her clinical practice, Dr. Prathiba Sharan is a dedicated educator and advocate for wellness. She has conducted numerous workshops in stress management, soft skills training, and lifestyle modification programs, contributing to the overall well-being of her community.

Complementing her professional endeavors, Dr. Prathiba is deeply committed to philanthropy. She runs the Swaasthya Aarogya Foundation (SAF), which provides essential healthcare services to underserved populations.

In her leisure time, Dr. Prathiba Sharan indulges in various artistic pursuits, including painting, drawing, artwork, and stitching, finding solace and inspiration in creativity and spirituality.

With her unwavering empathy, passion, and multidisciplinary expertise, Dr. Prathiba Sharan continues redefining care standards in neuro rehabilitation, embodying the essence of compassionate and holistic medicine.

NOTE FROM THE AUTHORS

Getting started on the awesome neuroscience journey!
Your instructions for this flight

Dear reader,
Greetings!

This book is huge, isn't it? Don't worry. We love solving problems!

If you are a caregiver for a loved one, a therapist trying to help a patient, or simply a medical professional, this book can lend you a helping hand in that journey.

Each chapter is a small book itself. It provides the context for various neurologic ailments, some intriguing stories, and neuroscience specially curated to give you a wholesome experience of the topic.

Do not rush through the book. Take your time. Start with the chapters that are most important to you and move to those you find interesting. Finally, reach the chapter that will fulfill your 'readers' curiosity'! Remember to share this knowledge about what you read with your family, friends, and others! **Rehearsals are essential to improve retention of learning.**

Remember**, there is no rush. Read each line and visualize! Believe me, you will thank me for reading this book. This will definitely transform your life! Walk as you read; it's good for your cardiac health and builds endurance. Listen to some soothing music as you read to reduce anxiety.** It will help you read longer!

This book will guide you as we share our journey, which includes triumphs, peculiarities, and success story anecdotes. Pick up this book to understand what goes on upstairs. Learn the intricacies of the most vital organ to start caring for it better. It's high time to shift focus from leg and arm days to brain days. We are always available for you!

Reach out to us using any of the following:

1. Follow and message us on Instagram @ PRS Neurosciences or search on Facebook for PRS Neurosciences.
2. Call or WhatsApp +91-8884022088
3. Send an email to reach out to us at info@newrorehab.com or info@prsneurosciences.com

You can scan the QR code and visit our YouTube channel! Use the QR code on the right - Proceeds from the book's sales will contribute to the Poor Patients Fund at Swaasthya Aarogya Foundation, our NGO committed to supporting those in need and making top-tier neuromodulation and neuro rehabilitation care accessible to everyone, no matter their social or financial status.

Yours truly,

Dr. Sharan Srinivasan and Dr. Prathiba Sharan

National Bio Enterpreneurship Competition #NBEC2022
Winner of #NBEC2022 Grand Finale
Dr. Sharan Srinivasan, PRS Neurosciences & Mechatronics Research Institute

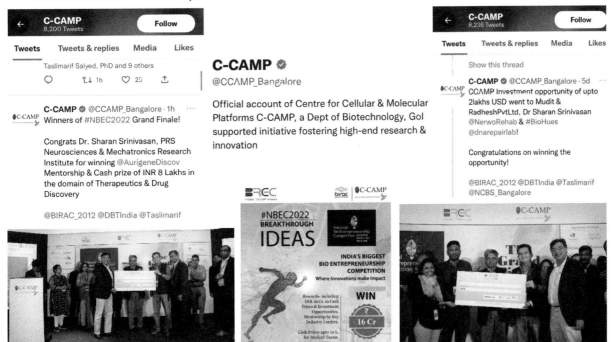

C-CAMP
8,200 Tweets
Follow

Tweets   Tweets & replies   Media   Likes

Taslimarif Saiyed, PhD and 9 others

💬   🔁 16   ♡ 25   ⬆️

C-CAMP ✔ @CCAMP_Bangalore · 1h
Winners of #NBEC2022 Grand Finale!

Congrats Dr. Sharan Srinivasan, PRS
Neurosciences & Mechatronics Research
Institute for winning @AurigeneDiscov
Mentorship & Cash prize of INR 8 Lakhs in
the domain of Therapeutics & Drug
Discovery

@BIRAC_2012 @DBTIndia @Taslimarif

C-CAMP ✔
@CCAMP_Bangalore

Official account of Centre for Cellular & Molecular
Platforms C-CAMP, a Dept of Biotechnology, GoI
supported initiative fostering high-end research &
innovation

C-CAMP
8,236 Tweets
Follow

Tweets   Tweets & replies   Media   Likes

Show this thread

C-CAMP ✔ @CCAMP_Bangalore · 5d
CCAMP Investment opportunity of upto
2lakhs USD went to Mudit &
RadheshPvtLtd, Dr Sharan Srinivasan
@NerwoRehab & #BioHues
@dnarepairlab!

Congratulations on winning the
opportunity!

@BIRAC_2012 @DBTIndia @Taslimarif
@NCBS_Bangalore

#NBEC2022
BREAKTHROUGH
IDEAS

INDIA'S BIGGEST
BIO ENTREPRENEURSHIP
COMPETITION
Where Innovations make impact

Rewards- including
INR 16 Cr. in Cash
Prizes & Investment
Opportunities.
Mentorship by Key
Industry Leaders.

WIN
₹
16 Cr

Cash Prizes upto 10 L.
for Student Teams.